"No longer the province of party hacks and budding politicians, social movements are today joyful and erotic eruptions. While Americans may be aware of explosive convulsions abroad, domestic histories of self-directed opposition are often hidden suppressed. Benjamin Shepard gives flesh to the zeitgeist of joyful opposition in the US, recounting playful episodes of autonomously organized resistance to the forces of seriousness

—George N. Katsiaficas, activist and author of *The subversion of politics: European autonomous social movements and the decolonization of everyday life*

"A historically and theoretically sophisticated study of play and humor in the service of political goals . . . Believing that politics is too funny to be left to the politicians and comedy too serious to be left to the professional funny-men, Benjamin Shepard takes us on a hilarious tour of the streets and parks of America to show us what a little imagination and a outsized sense of fun, mixed in with just enough courage, can do in the struggle for a more human world. Highly recommended!"

—Bertell Ollman, Dept. of Politics, NYU, and author of *Dance of the Dialectic*

"At a time of social and ecological crisis, the idea of playful protest might seem somewhat irrelevant, yet Shepard's brilliant overview of the ludic spirit of social movements shows us clearly that play is exactly what is needed at times like this. From Dada to Reclaim the Streets, via Act Up and community gardening, every page of this book brings another story of acts of play that enable social movement actors to imagine other worlds through liberating their minds and bodies. Best of all, *Play, Creativity, and Social Movements: If I Can't Dance, It's Not My Revolution* shows us that when academics leave the safety of their desks for the playground of the streets, the result is not only intelligent, powerful new forms of action, but critique that is alive and kicking."

—John Jordan, art activist and co-author of *Paths Through Utopias* and *We Are Everywhere: The Irresistible Rise of Global Anticapitalism*

"This is the book I'd have found as a 23 year old and flipped out to—like George McKay's *Party and Protest in 90's Britain*, discovering the MC5 or my first RTS protest. His project, exploring the ludic within movements for social change, comes to our contemporary moment. It is a book of theory, criticism, tactics, documentation and most significantly an insiders perspective on some of the most interesting plays for social change engaged with in the United States over the last 40 years. I love this book. Herein contains the voices of those who have most inspired and challenged me to scheme then act wildly for a more just world."

—Robby Herbst, Llano Del Rio
Collective, Co-founder *Journal of
Aesthetics & Protest*

"Benjamin Shepard theorizes on play and protest--and he lives it. His real experience with the playful struggle in the streets, whether wearing a red nose or a feather boa, comes through in every chapter of this compelling and provocative book."

—L. M. Bogad, UC Davis, *Electoral
Guerilla Theatre: Radical Ridicule and
Social Movements*

Play, Creativity, and
Social Movements

Routledge Advances in Sociology

Play, Creativity, and Social Movements

If I Can't Dance, It's Not My Revolution

Benjamin Shepard

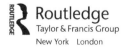

Routledge
Taylor & Francis Group
New York London

First published 2011
by Routledge
711 Third Avenue, New York, NY 10017

Simultaneously published in the UK
by Routledge
2 Park Square, Milton Park, Abingdon, Oxon OX14 4RN

Routledge is an imprint of the Taylor & Francis Group, an informa business

Typeset in Sabon by IBT Global.

First issued in paperback 2013

Library of Congress Cataloging-in-Publication Data
Shepard, Benjamin Heim.
   Play, creativity, and social movements : if I can't dance, it's not my revolution / by
Benjamin Shepard.
   p. cm. — (Routledge advances in sociology ; 57)
   Includes bibliographical references and index.
   1. Social movements.   2. Play—Social aspects.   3. Play—Psychological aspects.
I. Title.
   HM881.S532 2011
   303.48'409—dc22
                           2010034680

ISBN13: 978-0-415-84919-7 (pbk)
ISBN13: 978-0-415-96324-4 (hbk)
ISBN13: 978-0-203-83148-9 (ebk)

*For my comrades from the Lower East Side Collective,
Reclaim the Streets New York, ACT UP, Time's Up!
and its Bike Lane Liberation Clowns and every other
activist who ever had the courage to smile, shake, dance,
wink, nudge, crack a joke, cruise or otherwise create
some pleasure on their way to the revolution!*

Contents

Figures

Foreword

As the police turn fire hoses on teenagers at a civil rights protest in Birmingham, Alabama, in 1963, a young man, perhaps thirteen or fourteen years old, does an impromptu jig, smiling broadly, as he playfully moves out from behind a tree whose bark the fire hoses are shredding.

In October 2005, thousands of New York City cyclists defy a ban on group bicycling without a permit and pedal the streets of Manhattan to the beat of boom boxes carried on bicycles ridden by chanting, singing, and wildly costumed riders, many giddy with the excitement of defying the increasingly repressive rule of public order imposed in the city.

Members of the civil liberties group Sex Panic!, dressed in G-strings and wearing makeup, cheerfully perform a kick-line in front of a New York City police station in response to laws targeting gay men's cruising activities.

As the United States invades Iraq in 2003, a grandmother of sixty-four attends an antiwar demonstration. She watches several queer marching bands, anarcho-punk people, and Radical Faeries prepare for the march with a feeling of "excitement and liberation, of joy and possibility," in part because she "doesn't know what will happen" as she commits civil disobedience with thousands of others during the Direct Action to Stop the War.

AIDS activists, angered and frustrated by the inattention to the AIDS epidemic, debate and discuss how to force Wall Street to reduce drug costs, unsure of what will work, and with a short time frame. They decide to carry out a "die-in" on Wall Street in May of 1987.

What are we to make of these snippets of politics? "Activism" and "social movements" typically conjure up images of serious encounters and debates, dour meetings, and endless strategy sessions, or what often appear to be sophomoric attempts to unsettle the status quo with no particular strategy behind them. But the images here are something else: they are moments of play that are endemic to social movements. Play is the experimental and sometimes joyful quality of activism in which participants imagine and enact new selves, social relationships, and means of politics. It can include self-conscious forms of playing—laughter and humor, theater and music— the spontaneous moments of resistance and liberation in the face of danger or victory, and the "making up" of new selves and forms of politics. Largely ignored by both the "rationalist" approaches that have dominated the study of American social movements, and the post-liberal "identity" frameworks that have characterized much European social movement theorizing, play is an essential part of all social movements.

Activists have always had to find ways to make their views known and to formulate new social relationships. Contemporary activists draw on existing repertoires of action, but they often adapt them in new ways. As Benjamin Shepard shows in this richly theorized book, Brechtian theater, traditions of humor and mockery in American and other politics, and groups such as the Situationists form an important basis of contemporary play in social movements. Bodies, streets, organizations, and buildings, among others, are sites of play in which past repertoires are elaborated and challenged, discarded and reinvented. Because the cultural and political milieu in which the actions and ideals of opponents, supporters, and members are endlessly shifting and competition for attention is fierce, in both conscious and unconscious ways, even activists in the most dire of circumstances— the midst of the AIDS epidemic—use play as a way to draw attention to their claims and to engage in fuller expressions of human possibility.

This book demonstrates the importance of play for understanding the trajectories and significance of contemporary social movements. Highly theorized but written in an accessible fashion, Play, Creativity and Social Movements illustrates the inventive and experimental qualities of activism. Readers familiar with contemporary urban, antiglobalization, sexual politics, and civil rights movements will see them in new ways, and those to whom they are new will see them through the lens of an important new framework for understanding how and why social movements matter.

—Kelly Moore
Chicago, Illinois

Acknowledgments

A qualitative project on social movements is as much a result of a collective zeitgeist as the hand of any one writer. In the time that this project was in gestation during my years at the City University of New York, a handful of writers, sages, and unsung heroes shuffled off this mortal coil. This project is very much a response and a channeling of their experience. Only weeks after starting my PhD program to formally begin this research, thousands of New Yorkers perished in the third Monday of our fall semester on September 11; in the years which followed, uncounted hundreds of thousands of people around the world were decimated in the post-attack vengeance; throughout these years countless untold souls who lived in the Manhattan and Bronx SRO hotel rooms were lost to drug overdoses, HIV, Hepatitis C, physical attack, and the structural violence which characterize life in our ever-dwindling welfare state; homeless advocate Sylvia 'Ray' Rivera passed in the spring of 2002; and garden advocate Francoise Cachelin, who understood what was truly radical about a community garden and why they were threats to the established order, passed in October 2003; housing, harm reduction, pleasure activist, and personal friend Keith Cylar, of Housing Works, passed in April of 2004; Yippie Stew Albert, whose February 2006 obituary read "Used Laughter to Protest a War," and Jane Jacobs, one of the few to fight big real estate and win, both made the big proverbial transition in the spring of 2006. Albert's death was announced the day I was finished with the Yippie chapter. Between summer 2006 and fall 2010, four activists whose voices so informed this project—Eric Rofes, Bob Kohler, Brad Will, and Michael Shenker—all passed. I spent hours and hours talking about and practicing activism with each of these heroes. Kohler, Rofes, and Shenker sat down for formal interviews for this project, and this study is very much a response to their lives and struggles, experiences and legacies. I only wish our culture could learn a little more from their experiences.

I am grateful to Caroline, our playful daughters Dodi, who was born only weeks before the bombings in Iraq, and Scarlett, who was born three years later, for putting up with Dad in and out of jail, protests, arrests, bike rides and the like. You have all taught me more than I can ever imagine about the subversive nature of play. "To have fun, you have to get in a little trouble Dad," Dodi explained just the other day.

At Hunter College, Harold Weissman helped me begin this research on play and organizational innovation. Mike Smith and Mike Fabricant were consistently supportive of my writing and activism, even when it meant missing their classes because of my arrest for protesting war profiteering at the Carlyle group. Mimi Abramovitz offered constant encouragement of my writing and activism. Steve Burghardt offered supportive counsel throughout the dissertation committee process. And Irwin Epstein offered everything a great mentor, supporter, and intellectual counselor could offer in a very messy, open-ended journey from proposal drafts to a completed dissertation.

Outside of Hunter, of course, there are the many mentors and scholar activists who helped me bridge the line between practice and praxis. Stephen Duncombe, who I had known from the streets, first agreed to serve on my committee while we sat around waiting for legal counsel at the Center for Constitutional Rights. If there is one person who made the idea of playful engagement with difficult politics a living, breathing expression it was Professor Duncombe, who first suggested I study play after one of our clown rehearsals before the RNC actions. That same week, David Graeber suggested I read *Homo Ludens* during one of the RNC spokes councils. Another scholar activist at the clown rehearsals was L.M. Bogad, who served as an intellectual catalyst for my introduction to the field of performance studies where the play element is considered serious business. A different scholar/activist who served as an informal committee member and intellectual mentor was Professor Kelly Moore, who I first encountered during the garden auction period in NYC and who helped shape the way I think about politics, embodied experience, and social movements. Countless others, including Ron Hayduk, L.A. Kauffman, and Peter Nardi offered guidance counsel, support, fun, and inspiration. And when arrests took place while trying to complete this material, the Center for Constitutional Rights was there to speak up for those who still believe in quaint notions of democracy and First Amendment expression. Bill DiPaola, of Time's Up!, has remained a constant fixture of support in the world of activism. His Time's Up! archives proved tremendously helpful for this project.

Three other activists who helped catapult this project from rough edges into polished prose were Ian Landau, Kate Crane, Spencer Sunshine, Liz Highleyman, and Carmen McClish. Highleyman and Sunshine provided a critical reading of the manuscript which helped pull it together.

Thank you to the team at Routledge—Benjamin Holtzman, Max Novic, Jennifer Morrow, Rachel Markowitz, and Eleanor Chan—for their interest and ongoing support in making this project happen.

My mom and dad provided ongoing insight into what the process would be like, what it would take, and what would be fun about it, all while offering a helping hand. Al and Penelope and the rest of the Smiths helped make life in New York a wonderful klezmer smorgasbord. And Regine dropped off diapers and helped Caroline and me with becoming new parents until her passing in fall 2005.

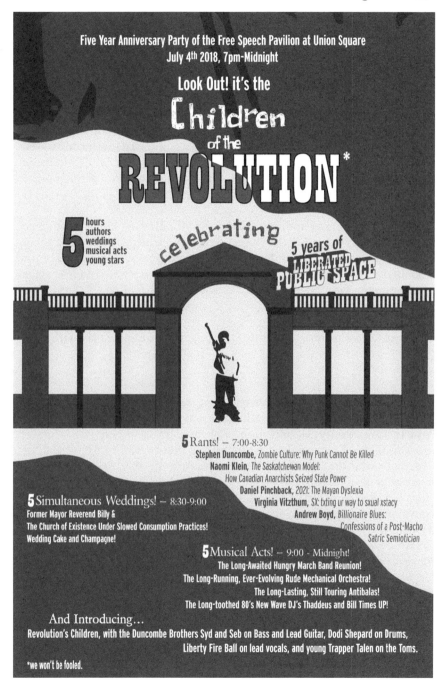

Figure A.1 The Children of the Revolution by Mark Read and Gregg Osofsky highlights much of the warmth of a cohort of activists who have grown over the last decade, had children, and contributed to this project as well as the movement it represents.

Of course, no qualitative study can happen without those who help make the news and the stories. Ben Holtzman, my faaabulous editor at Routledge, took immediate interest in the project, supporting its progress. Max Novick helped move it from production into a final finished project. Chuck and Christine from RTS and all the other activists who shared of themselves. Sixty-plus activists took time out of their lives to tell their stories over repeated occasions. Those such as Elizabeth Meixell, Karan Ramspacher, James Wagner, Steve Quester, and Aresh Javadi even opened up their files of photos, images, and activist paraphernalia for me to use. Thanks to the Schulman and Jim Hubbard, with the ACT UP Oral History Project, Aresh, with More Gardens!, and Bill DiPaulo, for permissions to quote and reprint material from their activist archives.

Throughout this period, another group of citizens—Dorothy Imogene Shepard and her sister, Scarlett Renee Shepard, Sydney Slingsby and Sebastion Yves Raila-Duncombe, Rita Kalet Hayduk-Jones, Corinne Alice and Desmond Clyde Kauffman-O'Hehir, Wiley Casmer and Maveric Jacey Mouchowski—were born while the war raged. The hope is this baby block will live to grow up in a world with less war and more playdates as they come of age.

Thanks to all of you, especially Caroline, for letting me play with you!

*   *   *

I would like to thank four journals for granting me permission to republish material which first saw light in their journals. "Four Narratives of Anti Poverty Community Mobilization" appeared in *Humanity and Society: Journal of the Association of Humanist Sociology* 33 (4): 317–40. "Play, Creativity, and the New Community Organizing" originally appeared in *Journal of Progressive Human Services* 16 (2): 47–69 (Copyright 2005, Haworth Press, Binghamton, NY). Article copies available from The Haworth Document Delivery Service: 1–800-HAWORTH. E-mail address: docdelivery@haworthpress.com. "Toward a Ludic Counter-Public: Play, Creativity, and the New Street Activism" originally appeared in *Drain—A Journal of Contemporary Art and Culture*. And, finally, Mark and Robby Herbst first suggested I write about ludic politics in their journal. Some of the first drafts of the writing which inspired this project first found the light of day in *Journal of Aesthetics and Protest*. They deserve acknowledgment and thanks for friendship and encouragement.

Notes toward an Introduction
From Play to Eternity

There is no clear dividing line between this play and life.

Mikhail Bakhtin (1984, p. 265)

Life does not cease to be funny when people die, any more than it ceases to be serious when people laugh.

George Bernard Shaw (quoted in Shepard, 2005, p. 50).

All play means something.

Johanna Huizinga (1950/2004, p. 117)

It is a Saturday morning in New York in 2008. As drivers pass through the intersection of the Hudson Valley, New York P.O.W.-M.I.A. Highway on Route 9, they are greeted with an antiwar chorus. Standing in front of signs with the words "PEACE" spray-painted in bright orange letters, a banjo player and a group of musicians lead the music. The man on banjo, of course, is none other than the iconic ninety-year-old folk singer Pete Seeger. Most do not even recognize him among the half-dozen activists at the weekly vigil. And that is fine with him. If Seeger wanted more publicity, he could hold a press conference. In between songs, Seeger walks to the other side of the six-lane freeway to make common cause with pro-war protesters holding a counterdemonstration. "They always have more flags," Seeger notes. "But our signs are more fun" (Gaffney, 2008). Of course, this is the point. This lighthearted dimension of the antiwar vigil is not lost on the participants, nor should it be for observers of social movements. The mix of play and protest, songs and colorful signs only help such movements gain vitality. "One plays only if and when one wishes to," argues play theorist Roger Caillois (1961/1979, p. 6), "In this sense, play is free activity." It certainly is for Seeger and those involved in the ongoing vigil.

In many ways, this spirit has kept Seeger going through decades on the front lines of social struggle. In the years since his refusal to invoke the Fifth Amendment during questioning at the House Un-American Activities Committee, Seeger's highly participatory chorus has engaged and enticed generations of audiences, often directly into social action. "Participation!

It's what all my work has been about," muses Seeger (Denning, 1997; Eyerman and Jamison, 1998; Isserman 1993). The "fun" part of the participating Seeger describes can be a transformative part of the process of social change. "To play together is to commit to one another, to affirm that these moments spent together . . . are valuable," notes sociologist Thomas Henricks (2006, 14).

During his June 1963 concert at Carnegie Hall just weeks before the March on Washington, Seeger talked about this ethos. "Nobody who's never actually faced one of those policemen can know exactly how much bravery it takes to be just this gay and cheerful in the face of all this." He was referring to the civil rights protesters who stared down police dogs and riot cops just weeks before in Birmingham, Alabama. "They have a little dance called the wobble a dance," Seeger (1963) explained. "I ain't afraid of no jail 'cause I want my freedom, I want my freedom now." Seeger, a supporter of the movement, recounted that King was adamant that participants must be solemn before an action, especially if they were leaving church to get there. "'No songs, no slogans until you are arrested,'" he noted King would warn. But once the arrests started, activists sang and danced: "I ain't afraid of no jail 'cause I want my freedom, I want my freedom now." The crowd at Carnegie Hall erupted in laughter and applause as Seeger finished the story. Seeger would reflect on the image of children dancing in streets as they fought for justice for the next five decades. "Humans have especially developed capacities to play, that is, to hold the world lightly and creatively," notes play theorist Thomas Henricks (2006, p. 11). "Our species, it seems can step back from grim necessities of life. In our minds, we can see new possibilities and together plot a common future" (p. 11). And quite often there is a pleasure and satisfaction to be gained in doing so. The lure of joy and justice is hard to contain. This impulse to play is the subject of this book.

Toward the end of her 2007 work, *Dancing in the Streets: A History of Collective Joy*, Barbara Ehrenreich offers a telling observation about this sentiment. "[W]hatever its shortcomings as a means to social change, protest movements keep reinventing carnival . . . Almost every demonstration I have been to—has featured some element of the carnivalesque: costumes, music, impromptu dancing, the sharing of food and drink" (p. 259). For Ehrenreich, such forms of 'collective joy' are essential components of social movement practice. "People must find, in their movement, the immediate joy of solidarity, if only because, in the face of overwhelming state or corporate power, solidarity is their sole source of strength" (ibid.). Most organizers recognize that such activities offer a useful compliment to an ongoing organizing campaign. They add a little flavor to an all-too-common mix of movement tactics. Without a little seasoning, the stew of social protest becomes bland.

Still critics remain (Loew, 2005; Taibbi, 2004; Weissberg, 2005). "The media often deride the carnival spirit of such protests, as if it were a self-indulgent distraction from the serious political point," Ehrenreich explains (2007b, p. 259). This line of logic has deep roots in a Protestant ethic which favors work over play and a general rejection of the Bacchanalian carnival. "Devotion to work was a Christian virtue; and play, the enemy of work, was reluctantly and only charily permitted to children," writes anthropologist Victor Turner (1982, p. 39). "Even now, these values are far from extinct in our nation, and the old admonition that play is the devil's handiwork continued to live in secular thought" (ibid.). Only recently, have critics come to acknowledge this form of expression as a vital part of human experience. "[I]t is still something in which we 'indulge' (as in sexual acts), a form of moral laxness" (ibid.).

Yet, increasingly activists and scholars take issue with this line of logic. "[I]t is somewhat short-sighted to equivocally dismiss playful protest as insignificant," argues Carmen McClish (2009, pp. 1–2) in highlighting the tactical uses of play in an anti-corporate campaign. For McClish, such "felt anger" can find its expression in any number of ways. "[T]his tactic when employed in interrupting the 'flow' of business not only disrupts but ultimately can influence corporate practices" (ibid.). Such play is important not only strategically, but also in terms of affect and emotional need. "[S]easoned organizers know that gratification cannot be deferred until after the 'revolution,'" Ehrenreich elaborates (2007b, p. 259). Despite the contention that such activities are counterproductive, movements continue to put the right to party on the table as a part of a larger process of social change; the logic being that humor and pleasure disrupt monotony while disarming systems of power. When we play we challenge a series of social mores (Turner, 1982). For a social movement to create a place to play is to challenge core workings of capitalist social arrangements. Yet, there is more to it than that. It is also a lot of fun.

Examples of such practices abound. The Dutch Provos illegally distributed blank leaflets as they declared, "Write Your Own Manifestos" in 1966 (Bogad, 2005a). Queer youth formed a Rockette kick-line and sang, "We are the Stonewall Girls" as they thwarted riot cops during the Stonewall Riots of June 1969 (Carter, 2004). Members of ACT UP taunted white-gloved police officers with the jeer, "Your gloves don't match your shoes, we'll see you in the news!" as they were arrested at the Food and Drug Administration in 1988 (Crimp and Rolston, 1990). Anarchists catapulted teddy bears over a fence mocking tear gas–wielding police during the Free Trade of the Americas actions of April 2001 in Quebec. And antiwar protesters performed the hokeypokey amidst riots and red alerts in New York City during the largest day of antiwar protest in world history on February 15, 2003. These are just a few of an endless list of examples from the streets of cities around the world.

Elements of fun, improvisation, and humor are cornerstones of such moments. As for a simple working definition, *play* is a term for drag, ACT UP zaps, pranks, the use of food and mariachi bands in the Latino community, dance dramaturgy, culture jamming, the carnival, and other creative community-building activities. It is the exhilarating feeling of pleasure, the joy of building a more emancipatory, caring world. This is a fundamentally free activity.

In the pages to follow I explore notions of play as a social movement activity. With this introduction, I attempt to situate the study, considering some of the meanings, applications, and history of the concept in relation to social organizing and movement activities. *Play, Creativity and Social Movements: If I Can't Dance* is the second of a two-part study on the topic. The first, *Queer Political Performance and Protest: Play, Pleasure, and Social Movement*, concerned queer uses of play (Shepard, 2009). For this reason, this book is limited to an overview of queer direct action groups the Cockettes, OutRage, and ACT UP in Chapters 2 and 3. They serve as a bridge between activist cohorts and movements from 1968 to the global justice years and subsequent movements which make up the bulk of the study. Yet much of the spirit and philosophy of ludic movement practices dates back to Dada, Surrealism, and Situationism, briefly explored in the first chapter of this work. They ground a practice which is anything but new. Yet, rather than insist "they all do play! it's all carnivalesque!" *Play, Creativity, and Social Movements* considers the ways in which groups and movements have explored the relation between play to fantasy, arts, activism, and social change, tying a sense of the practice in the *particularity* of different social, cultural, and historic contexts.

This study follows a brief overview of Dada, Surrealism, and Situationism with a review of the ludic campaigns of the Yippies, who made use of the prank as a means of political protest, in contrast with the street actions of the Young Lords. Each builds on the legacies of civil rights activists who danced in the face of Jim Crowe era social controls Pete Seeger describes (Reed, 2005; Zinn, 2002). From here, it traces the work of AIDS/ queer direct-action groups which made arts, design, and a defense of pleasure cornerstones of their struggle against oblivion (Crimp, 2002). It considers the ways do-it-yourself (DIY) agitational groups sought to break down the lines between art and life while connecting play and pleasure, creativity and fantasy into activism (Duncombe, 2007; Jordan, 1998). With events such as Critical Mass, festive bicyclists created protests as amoeba-like bike cavalcades. In New York City, community garden activists created their own Central Park within the rubble of neighborhood vacant lots, and DJs transformed bland streets into spaces for dance, protest, and community building (Duncombe, 2002b; Ferguson, 1999). The work begins and ends with campaigns which conceptualize play as an appropriate response to the lunacy of wars stretching from WWI to Viet Nam to Iraq.

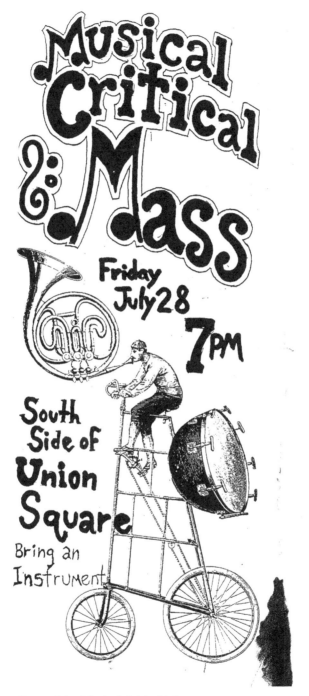

Figure I.1   Musical Critical Mass.

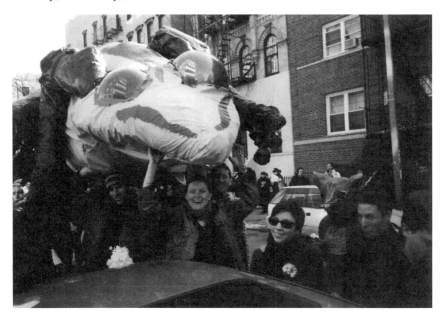

Figure I.2 Garden activists carry coqui. With garden activists carrying giant frogs and bike riders carrying musical instruments, activism took on an increasingly fun, theatrical quality. Bike rides and community garden activism embody a ludic turn in movement activism. Courtesy www.times-up.org.

Some of these campaigns make use of play as a prefigurative model of the world which activists hope to create actualized through the process of organizing. Here, play helps sustain and nourish campaigns. Others utilize creativity to achieve policy victories. Yet, can play and the social organizing which accompanies it bridge these two streams of social change practice? This is the core question of this study. To answer this one must grapple with additional questions. To what extent does play really contribute to or undermine such social change activism? What is the play of social protest? Has the practice changed and why? What are best practices which have actually shown results in movements? And finally, how does play fit into an organizing campaign, if at all?

CONCEPTUALLY SPEAKING

There is a slipperiness to any one conception of the term. Like a rabbit in a briar patch, just as one closes in, the concept eludes categorization (Huizinga, 1950; Hyde, 1998). Nonetheless, in the remaining pages of this introduction, I will consider some of the ways play has been conceived over time, provide a few examples, offer a short overview of the methods used, and briefly frame the cases to follow. While I consider the ways the term is defined, emphasis is placed on process rather than out-come; here play is seen less in terms of one definition or another as much as a process involving an impulse toward unfettered freedom.

Play takes shape in a number of different contexts, with widely diverg-ing cultural understandings and definitions. What links the questions and gestures described in this introduction is a recognition of the multiple possibilities of the free activity understood as play. For historian Johan Huizinga (1950, p. 3), play is anything but serious. It is a space for joy, experimentation, make believe, cultural interaction, and exchange of ideas. "In Huizinga's judgment, history is not only the accounting of tech-nological process or economic movements but also the analysis of cultural interchange and development," notes Henricks (2006, p. 10). For Richard Schechner (2002), play involves doing something that is not exactly "real." It is looser; it is "double edged, ambiguous, moving in several directions simultaneously" (p. 79).

The *Oxford English Dictionary* lists of definitions for play as both a noun and a verb. As a verb, it is used to describe the state of being "busily engaged," to "leap for joy, rejoice." It involves "living being[s]" that "move about swiftly with a lively, irregular, or capricious motion, spring, sly, or dart to and fro, gambol, frisk, or flutter." The third defi-nition suggests that to play is to "cause to bubble or roll about as in boiling liquid." The fourth defines it as: "to carry out or perform (an action), perform or execute (a movement), perform or practice (a trick, a joke, etc.) in the way or sport, deceit, etc." As a noun, *play* is under-stood as an "active bodily exercise, brisk and vigorous action of the body or limbs in fencing, dancing, or leaping." It can be thought of as "an action, activity, operation, working, esp. with rapid movement or change, or variety."

In terms of this project, the ever-slippery concept is conceived of as a practice, theatrical activity, or street action. This performative spirit supports social movements in countless ways. While some forms of political performance and guerilla theater may not feel inherently light, silly, or playful, the struggle to create a space for such activity has every-thing to do with creating a space for the most democratic of pursuits of happiness. Any number of struggles—such as the chance to surf on a nonpolluted beach or go to a public space where gay men cruise and connect—involve an ambition to play in the public arena. In this sense, notions of serious play function as cornerstones of a struggle for a pub-lic commons for ideas, debate, pleasure and experimentation (Addams, 1910/1998, 1914; Bogad, 2005a, 2005b; Ornstein, 1998).

The verb "to play" is the operative function for expressions related to games, such as "ball" or "Russian Roulette." "The layers of meaning of 'play' also are part of the intricacies behind ideas of truth and illusion, between appearances and reality, what is play and what is for real," argues sociologist Peter Nardi (2006, p. 286). "Let's avoid thinking about 'play' as something not serious. Playing requires an active agency and the creative use of our sociological imagination" (ibid., pp. 287). This work contends with the term's panorama of uses, sometimes as dramatic gestures, street theatrics, subversive forms of humor, and other times as various modes of communication and meaning creation. Play is best understood along a continuum from its meanings as a noun—a performance/means of communication—towards those as verb—as a liberatory, sometimes subversive form of action, as well as a resource for group support. Here, play is considered in the context of social movement activity encompassing a range of affects and outcomes, including experimentation, social eros, liberation, and healthy exchange—all a part of the ins and outs of everyday living. It can be both affective and instructive.

For the purposes of this study, a few core assumptions are useful. The first is that play is near impossible to completely define. Instead it is useful to think of it as a spirit, which encompasses theatrical presentation as improvisation, motion, and an ethos of action. "It is a mood, an activity, an eruption, of liberty" Schechner (2002, p. 79) explains. But it is also paradoxical (Bateson, 1972). Sometimes play takes the shape of a formal commercial or competitive activity one participates in or enjoys; examples include a tennis match at the US Open or an off-Broadway show. These socially sanctioned, well choreographed forms of play are palatable with a Puritanical culture which condemns looser, less regimented forms of play as "time wasted" (Turner, 1982, p. 39). In its less formal incarnations, play can involve a pick-up soccer game in Prospect Park, or occur at social gatherings, in playgrounds, sidewalks, or streets. Yet, from time to time, it departs from the mundane, expanding into a status quo threatening endeavor (see Turner, 1969, 1982).

This, of course, is Johan Huizinga's (1950) thesis. As far as he was concerned, play served as a central ingredient in the development and transformation of societies and cultures. "Thus, tennis courts, courts of law, debating and scientific societies, song duels, parliaments, potlatch festivals, and philosophic bantering find their places as crucibles of social change," explains Henricks (2006, p. 10). In South Africa, for example, the game of soccer has become a public means with which to challenge social mores around public discussion of HIV prevention. "It's a way to address something that nobody wants to talk about through a game that everybody loves," explained one of the organizers of the campaign (Longman, 2010). Amazing things happen when people commit to such endeavors together. The play element makes it easier. "[P]lay is not to be sought within some separate institution of a society. Rather, it is a distinctive relationship that stands at the center of public imagination and contact" (Henricks, 2006, p. 10).

Because of its capacities to ignite the unexpected, those who favor law and order remain wary of its unsanctioned manifestations. "Play may involve an erosion or inversion of social status," such as with the Trinidad

Carnival, Boxing Day, or other role-reversal holidays (Bial, 2004, p. 115). For this reason, authorities often seek to close spaces where improvised play takes place. Recent crackdowns include: Critical Mass bike rides and immigrant rights marches (Karmazin, 2005; Shepard, 2007). Even spontaneous gatherings, such as New Orleans funeral marches, drum circles, and dance parties are increasingly hyper-regulated, controlled, and even prohibited (Blumenfeld, 2007; Williams, 2008). "Dance clubs all over the country have faced the threat of shut downs," writes Barbara Ehrenreich (2007a, p. 14). To the extent that such play spaces invert social hierarchies, they take on a subversive dimension which draws the attention of authorities.

A few words about these conflicts inform an understanding of the interplay between ludic and social movement activities at the center of this study. Struggles for control over public space and expression extend into countless spaces for social gatherings, including protests. For example, when the Pope visited New York in April of 2008, I joined a group of New York activists who formed a clown bike block to "Welcome the Big German Clown to Town!" While we were not able to get anywhere near where the Pope was holding mass, we did encounter the Popemobile traveling East on 42nd Street as we rode past Grand Central Station. As we moved closer to the Popemobile, a group of police swept in to push us away. We were surrounded and questioned. When we finally got to the designated protest areas, we were far beyond sight and sound of the Pope's appearance. Queer activist Bill Dobbs, who took part in the clown action, noted: "Mayor Bloomberg and [Police Commissioner] Ray Kelly used police state tactics on Saturday to push protest so far away from the Pope that it was Siberia" (Humm, 2008). This was anything but an isolated example.

Over and over the state, "projects phantasms of Dionysian disorder and pantomimes of insurrection at the site of the smallest examples of protest activity," writes Alecia Simmonds from Australia (2007, p. 13). "Protestors are greeted with water cannons, spies, mounted police and dog handlers. The streets are locked down. Police powers reach vertiginous heights." If democracy thrives as "a dialogue between the nation and its leaders, then, [the state] has succeeded in killing the conversation. There are no jokes, public criticism or robust celebration, only private terrors, isolation and insanity" (ibid.). In the face of such encroachments, activists have come to recognize ludic activity as a practical response to political repression. Here play serves as a device for group solidarity, as well as a tool used to both disrupt what is wrong with the world and generate images of what a better one might look like (Bogad, 2005a, 2005b; Huizinga, 1950; McClish, 2009; Schechter, 2002).

Conceptually, play can be seen as part of a continuum from work to leisure, pleasure and games, as Stanley Aronowitz (1972/1992), Herbert Marcuse (1955), the Situationists (1958), Victor Turner (1982), and even

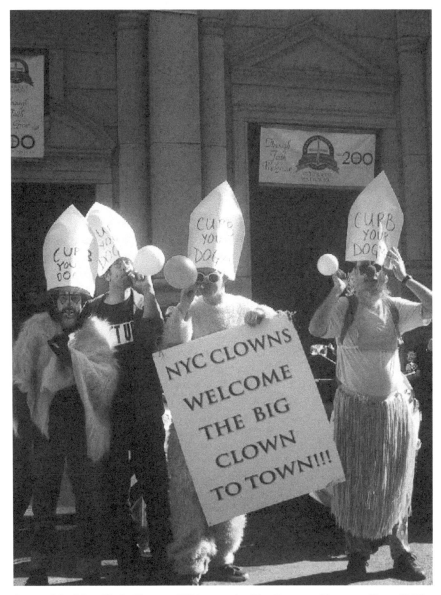

Figure I.3 New York Clowns "Welcome the Big German Clown to Town!" The police were not so interested in a group of clowns accompanying the big clown's Popemobile to the service. Photos by Andy Humm.

Max Weber (1946/1968) discuss. Roger Caillois (1961, p. 9) suggests that play is essentially separate from commerce, it is about freedom: "playing is not obligatory; if it were, it would at once lose its attractive and joyous quality." Play is utterly engaging. For this reason, thinkers from Weber (1946/1968) to Herodotus (1942) have considered its appeal as a diversion

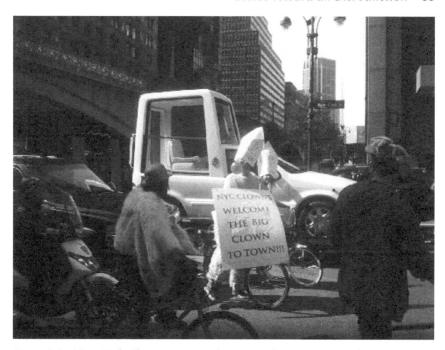

Figure I.4　New York Clowns attempted to escort the Big German Clown, the Pope, to Yankee Stadium.

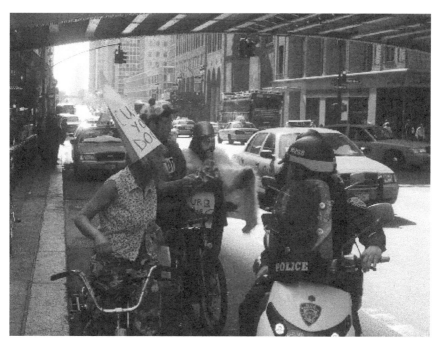

Figure I.5　Yet, the NYPD apprehended the clowns before they could begin their escort.

from life's pain, misery, and tedium. This liberatory quality is part of what links play to movement activity and thought. "Once free of wage-slavery, humankind will immediately redesign its labor so that it will not be work at all, but play. Today's society, unfortunately, has all but forgotten to play," writes Chicago Surrealist Penelope Rosemont (2002, p. 396). "What workers need most is to rediscover play—collective, imaginative, liberating, non-competitive, and full of fun" (ibid.).

For the Situationists, the contestation of play extends into the questions about the very nature of modern life. "The ethos of need, labor, and sacrifice, is unnecessarily perpetuated, serving only to maintain the capitalist system," writes sociologist Sadie Plant in a work on the Situationists; "the idea that we must continue to struggle to survive hinders human development and precludes a life of playful opportunity," she continues (1992, p. 2). Here, the practice offers a counterbalance to forces of alienation.

Such sentiment is increasingly echoed in the clinical realm. "Free, imaginative play is crucial for normal social, emotional, and cognitive development," Melinda Wenner (2009) writes in *Scientific American*. "Play has to be reframed and not seen as an opposite to work, but rather as a compliment . . . Curiosity, imagination, and creativity are like muscles. If you don't use them, you lose them." Here play is recognized as a mechanism to cultivate creativity, solve problems, and generate ideas (Brown, 2009; Linn, 2008; Weissman, 1990).

HOMO LUDENS—HUIZINGA AND CAILLOIS

While there are countless ways to consider the concept, it is useful to ground such discussion with Johan Huizinga's 1938 work *Homo Ludens: A Study of the Play Element in Culture*. His definition encompasses many of the threads already discussed:

> Summing up the formal characteristics of play we might call it a free activity standing quite consciously outside the ordinary life as being "not serious," but at the same time absorbing the player intensely and utterly. It is an activity connected with no material interest, and no profit can be gained by it. It proceeds within its own proper boundaries of time and space according to fixed rules and in an orderly manner. It promises the formation of social groupings which tend to surround themselves with secrecy and to stress their difference from the common world by disguise or other means. (1950, p. 13)

Huizinga goes on to suggest it is accompanied by a "feeling of tension, joy and consciousness that it is different from ordinary life" (p. 28). In the chapters which follow, organizers reflect on their experiences with these vexing combinations of feelings.

Huizinga was a German medievalist and cultural historian in the tradition of Jacob Burckhardt. Many of his works address the theme of play in culture, but it was not until the Nazi ascent to power that he collected his thoughts on the subject with *Homo Ludens*. For Huizinga, play was a central element of human life, one that provides the foundation for music, poetry, dancing, and even philosophy. Five years after *Homo Ludens* was published, Huizinga was caught by the Nazis. He spent his final days in a prison camp, before his death in 1945 (Henricks, 2006). Throughout this work, play is considered part of a framework for meaning creation, struggle, and adaptation. In this respect, play serves as a coping mechanism and resource for those struggling against oppression. In the years after his passing, countless theorists and activists would look to his work (Debord, 1967; Duncombe, 2007; Jordan, 1998; Turner, 1982).

Roger Caillois (1961/1979), a colleague of Andre Breton and George Bataille, wrote *Man, Play, and Games* as a response to Huizinga's *Homo Ludens*. Caillois saw play activity as unproductive and free, spontaneous and make-believe. He suggested it took place within an evolving continuum from highly energetic, active, tumultuous, spontaneous, and exuberant realms of activity, toward ludic endeavors involving calculating, contrived subversion of rules (Barash, 1961/1979). It was also a part of everyday life.

Caillois was acutely aware that play functioned as an inherently subversive endeavor. Caillois began his study of play as he fought the rise of fascism in the 1930's in Europe. Throughout these years, he came to see play as intricately involved with questions about power and world-making. It could also be recognized as a cultural resource (Barash, 1961). He joined the Surrealists in 1932 and in 1938 he helped found the College of Sociology. Yet, unlike his colleagues in the Surrealists, Caillois suggested play required engagement with the here and now rather than the world of fantasy. Caillois (2003) was quick to argue that the Dionysian impulse offered ample satisfactions within the realm of the everyday . "Indeed, the essential value of Dionysianism was precisely that it brought people together . . . participating in ecstasy," he wrote (2003, p. 158). Yet not everyone saw this capacity to bring people together as a good thing.

This perspective provides insight into some of the long-standing hostilities toward the liberatory activities involved with Bacchanalia. Such activities, including drink, dancing, and sexual transgression, tend to be viewed as with suspicion, particularly by those in charge. In Rome, they were specifically forbidden (Caillois, 2003). Today, ludic activities such as unpermitted street parties, even pillow fights, merit close scrutiny by police intelligence (Parascandola, 2010). Such disputes "are at least as old as civilization," notes Barbara Ehrenreich (2007a, p. 14). They stem from a "long standing conflict between the forces of order and hierarchy . . . and the deep human craving for free-spirited joy" (ibid.). For Callois, the play of social life represented an entirely relevant context in which to consider social change. He was not alone in thinking so.

ON PLAYING—THEORY AND METHOD OF STUDY

Social welfare scholar Harold Weissman (1990, p. xxi) argues that the mere act of imagining alternative visions of the world brings an element of creativity into organizational life. By connecting bodies and actions, ideas and experiences, creative play helps inject a dose of vitality into often routinized organizational practices. Building on this sentiment, this project examines some of the ways in which practices associated with "play" do and do not inform a wide range of contemporary movements. The primary data sources are stories of key informants; data was collected from a purposeful sample of sixty-nine interviews with activists reflecting on their lived experiences, actions, and groups (Patton, 2002). Each completed a forty-five to ninety minute semi-structured interview (McCracken,1988), which I transcribed, coded, and conceptualized as a distinct narrative of action (Holland et al., 1998; Patton, 2002). In order to account for discrepancies and contradictions among accounts, I compared archival resources with other sources, including complimentary histories, newspaper accounts, e-mails, blogs, and participant observation data. From here, data was categorized, organized, grouped according to theme, and formed into distinct case histories (Snow and Trom, 2002; Strauss and Corbin, 1990; Yin, 1994). The case studies which follow are organized from these bundles of stories.

In *The Interpretation of Cultures*, Clifford Geertz (1973) suggests that much of ethnography involves a degree of confession. Full disclosure: I have worked closely with a number of the groups considered in the case studies, some for well over a decade. In doing so, I have engaged in activities ranging from outreach to organizing affinity group meetings, to being arrested and put through the system—even being targeted by police when repressive structures set in (Shepard, 2005). Building on these experiences, my perspective as an observing participant informs the work (see Butters, 1983; Hume and Mulcock, 2004; Juris, 2007; Myerhoff and Ruby, 1982/1992; Kohut, 1959/1978; Lichterman, 2002; Tedlock, 1991). In this respect, the reader is invited to observe elements of the study of play interact between personal narrative and case study, as a reflexive process and coherent whole (Myerhoff and Ruby, 1982/1992; Snow and Trom, 2002). (For a closer review of the process, see "Methodological Notes on the Study of Play in Social Movements" in the appendix of Part I of this study—Shepard, 2009.)

The work's qualitative nature is also a direct nod to Johan Huizinga (1950, p. 2). He worried that critics failed to grasp the visceral, lived experience of play. They "attack play direct with the quantitative methods of experimental science" and "only deal incidentally with what play is *in itself* and what it means for the player" (ibid.). In contrast, this work is constructed of narrative reflections on the messy means and motivations, failures, historically grounded observations, conversations, and insights of regular people, 'organic intellectuals' who share their stories (Gramsci, 1971/1992). Through the qualitative method, I attempt to grapple with the meaning of such experiences (Patton, 2002).

After all, "meaning construction is a social movement's primary function" movement scholar Sidney Tarrow reminds us (1998, p. 17). Through such stories people come to grips with their lives and struggles, connecting personal challenges with larger contests over meaning (Fine, 1995; Holland et al., 1998; McAdams, 1985; Nepstad, 2002; Somers, 1994). "[P]eople do things with stories," writes sociologist Francesca Polletta (2006, p. 14). "They entertain and persuade, build social bonds and break them, make sense of their worlds and, in the process, create those worlds."

This work is constructed of stories detailing efforts to organize, play, succeed, resist social controls, and inject alternative perspectives into public discourse. Here, social actors utilize multiple means—some earnest, others quite nonsensical, "expressive," and "sometimes downright silly" (Polletta, 2002, p. ix). The context in which this "expressive" protest takes place is a joyous tradition of actors using every tool possible—to make one's arguments heard to create change. "Play activities may be structured into the conduct of public institutions or they may simply erupt there by stopping or transforming ordinary affairs" (Henricks 2006, p. 14). Such "[p]lay is often connected to everyday life." Over the years, this experience has been a source of profound social change (Lefebvre, 1947/1991).

In an interview toward the end of his life, French philosopher Michel Foucault commented on this spirit as he ruminated about the changes he had seen in his life. "There has been political innovation, political creation and political experimentation outside of the great political parties, and outside of the normal ordinary program" (quoted in Gallagher and Wilson, 1987/2005, p. 35). This "innovation" included changes in the way people gather, organize, socialize, and interact. "It's a fact that people's everyday lives have changed from the early 1960s to now, and certainly within my own life," Foucault elaborated, "And surely, that is not due to political parties but is the result of many movements" (ibid.).

Much of this innovation took shape within social movements themselves. "In the most recent upheaval," Foucault explained in a different interview, referring to the events of May 1968, "the intellectual discovered that the masses no longer need him to gain knowledge: they know perfectly well, without illusion; they know far better than he, and they are certainly capable of expressing themselves" (Foucault and Deleuze, 1977, pp. 207–8). Grounded within the stories of just this sort of activist experience, this work strives to honor Foucault's call for intellectuals to value the ways nonlinear social knowledge and practice contributes to social innovation and change. For many, ludic activism functions as a lived theory and practice (Duncombe, 2007; Jordan, 1998). "In this sense," Foucault noted, "theory does not express, translate, or serve to apply practice: it is practice" (Foucault and Deleuze, 1977, pp. 207–8).

Certainly movement practices have shifted and evolved. Yet, there has been no consensus about their meanings or function, especially those more ludic endeavors such as pranks, sexual play, display, or street theatrics. While Johan Huizinga (1950/2004, p. 120) notes that in Shakespeare's day "[i]t was the fashion to liken the world to a stage" with the rise of capitalism the meaning of such activity has been obscured (see Tawney, 1937; Turner, 1982). "[P]lay has normally been under esteemed as a human activity (devalued by the doubtful antithesis between it and seriousness and the narrow assumption that it is, at best, 'merely' play)," notes literary critic R. Rawdon Wilson (1990, p. 8). There are any number of reasons for this. Huizinga (1950) postulated that as the world has become more and more automated, space for play has been devalued. The Industrial Revolution, with factories and mass production, squeezed away room for such spaces or activity (Henricks, 2006). The frenzy of quantification, of management, evaluation of education, and performance measures of even the very young merely extend the process. And today young children spend their days preparing for standardized tests in time once used for recess (Flaxman, 2000; Linn, 2008).

Throughout their writings, both Marx and Huizinga pine for a bygone, less regimented life. A more authentic and satisfying experience in living could be reclaimed if social mores shifted or were transformed (Henricks, 2006). Such a vantage point helps explain the appeal of play for anticapitalist movements of recent years (Duncombe, 2007; Jordan, 1998; Yuen, 2004). Here, the practice serves as an alternative to the systems of work, mind-numbing drudgery, and capitalist exploitation (Harvey, 2005; Kauffman, 2004). The later chapters of this book consider the work and play of some of these anticapitalist movements. By opening up less regimented forms of social interaction, a wide range of often neglected voices find expression.

The challenge remains how to situate such practices critically. Complicating this picture, social movement scholarship has long been dominated by a rationalist perspective on social behavior (McAdam et al., 1988; McCarthy and Zald, 1973). The limitations of such a view are many. In the first place, humans do not always behave or make decisions in a rational fashion (Simon, 1957). The rationalist view fails to acknowledge any number of the motivations and pleasures in the chase to create a better world (Jasper, 1997). "[W]orkers often want to go on strike, even when economists doing their calculations later say their wage concessions don't make up for their wage losses," notes movement scholar Frances Fox Piven (quoted in Sheaprd, 2008, p. 14).

Given this, it is not surprising that questions about political efficacy tend to accompany discussion about the occasional frivolity of movement practices (Chvasta, 2006; Ebert, 2006; McClish, 2009; Weissberg, 2005). Such a view is not a surprise. While meaning could be found in the expressive behavior seen at protests (Ehrenreich, 2007a), well into the 1960s, many argued such action betrayed rational thought (Jasper, 1997). The dynamics of crowds were seen as forms of deviance (Le Bon, 1896). And critical consideration of the meanings of desire and creativity, expression and destruction were left to psychoanalysis and the writings of those in the Frankfurt School, German heterodox Marxists who combined Marxism with insights from Weber, Freud, Nietzsche, and others to create a new kind of social theory (Martin, 1973). Some of Frankfurt theorist Herbert Marcuse's (1955) first writings on play were born of this milieu. Other movement scholars took the dim view of crowd behavior and its association with postwar memories of fascism (Goodwin et al., 2001). Still Huizinga, who witnessed the rise of Nazism and perished in a German prison camp, was quick to question the benefits of cold, calculated rationality (Henricks, 2006).

Others, such as Max Weber, suggested that organizational life was best based on logical thought. Emotions would be minimized within view. The problem with the "rational turn" in social movement scholarship, of course, was that it failed to explain why people got involved, what excited or motivated them to join movements (Goodwin et al., 2001). It wasn't until Gramsci (1971/1992) that movement scholars started asking why people did or did not get involved in efforts aimed at social change. And this attitude began to shift. Saul Alinsky (1989) would argue that there was always a place for emotions as a complement to larger, more coherent organizing strategies (Goodwin et al., 2001). And newer approaches to social movement scholarship came to stand in stark contrast to dominant linear approaches (Jasper, 1997).

Gradually theorists came to recognize that less rational behaviors, including play, offered a far different route toward social knowledge and investigation. "Rather than only looking at the social world as a construction of institutions and roles, consider instead using illusions and play in the search for meaning and truths," Pacific Sociological Association president Peter Nardi (2006, pp. 288) counseled at the group's 2006 meetings. Instead of engaging in positivist-style prediction, Nardi argued the study of play compels practitioners and scholars to consider different forms of efficacy and outcomes which extend beyond positivism.

Others would come to agree with this sentiment. "There is another aspect to it that I think we should talk and act on more," suggested movement scholar Frances Fox Piven (quoted in Shepard, 2008, p. 14). "There is a lot of joy in it . . . We should have purple umbrellas. We should have good songs." After all, "any game has its thrills," noted movement scholar James Jasper (1997, p. 26). The game was often the draw, even if some still did not see it. "Those who would reduce social movements to instrumental actors engaged in power struggles on a battlefield called 'political opportunity structure' have made an ontological choice," put movement theorists Eyerman and Jamison (2003, p. 368). They choose "to see the world in terms of structures and processes which exist outside the meanings actors attach to them" (ibid.).

Perhaps the most consistent criticism of play in movement building is that ludic activity is a class-bound form of engagement, which only those with leisure time can enjoy. Andrew Boyd (the founder of the Billionaires for Bush), Steve Duncombe (one of the founders of New York's chapter of

Reclaim the Streets), and I had to confront this line of questioning after we all presented on activist performance, play, and fantasy during a conference on the legacies of 1968. On the train on the way back from the talk, we reflected on this recurring line of criticism. Boyd recounted a famous story. "All power to the imagination"—that was the graffiti painted on the streets of Paris in 1968, Boyd noted. Yet, some argued this sentiment betrayed the class struggle. "All power to the workers," a labor activist insisted in a debate with Paul Virilio. "Comrade, are you denying the workers have an imagination?" Virilio responded, dismissing this myopic charge. Boyd smiled recalling Virilio's pithy retort to the reductionist line of criticism. While play has long been a part of class-based labor movements (Fuoss, 1997), its role in such movements is often undervalued or not even recognized.

Even a cursory glimpse of movement history indicates play is anything but a class-bound activity. Letters from civil rights workers who participated in the Freedom Summer of 1964 suggest social eros, dancing, beer drinking, singing, hooking up, and an unbridled sense of social connection were an ongoing component of the experience. The struggle to break down racial, social, cultural, and sexual barriers included a great deal of play and social experimentation. Those in the movement described these feelings and practices as part of the "freedom high" (McAdam, 1988, p. 72).

"When you are locked arm in arm with your friends and you are running into a line of police and you tell them to screw off, why wouldn't that be play?" Frances Fox Piven (2008) commented at a recent conference. The point is fighting authority can be a joyous endeavor (Shepard, 2008).

Yet, there is more to it than that. Play serves as a powerful coping mechanism, even in the most difficult of circumstances, including war. According to classical historian Herodotus, when one of the armies faced a famine during the Persian Wars, they devised a play-based strategy to divert the troops. "The plan adopted during the famine was to engage in games one day so entirely as not to feel any craving for food," Herodotus wrote, "and the next day to eat and abstain from games" (Csikszentmihalyi, 1975, p. ix). They followed this pattern for nearly two decades. "[P]eople get immersed in games so deeply as to forget hunger and other problems," explained Mihaly Csikszentmihalyi (ibid.). "What power does play have that men relinquish basic needs for its sake?" Perhaps it is that people continually strive to find ways to cope.

Faced with a different kind of crisis—the AIDS pandemic—those on the front lines looked to a different kind of play. In Chapter 3 of this study, AIDS activists discuss ACT UP's ludic organizational culture, which included an abiding faith in the political possibilities of pleasure, camp, and the liberatory potential of direct action. Here play served as a powerful draw and release value for activists contending with the AIDS carnage (Takemoto, 2003). These antiheroic aesthetics were tremendously appealing for those who had grown weary of the overused rhetoric of the often dour Left

(Critchley, 2007; Crimp, 2002). In so doing, play supports creative community building, which fosters engaged citizenship. And gradually such forms of low-threshold fun build social solidarity among participants and their movements.

A TRAGICOMIC TURN

In any number of circumstances, this play element connects participants in a lusty encounter with a world outside rationality. Here, play extends into areas of pleasure and experimentation, manifesting itself in ecstatic, risky, often creative, sometimes destructive, carnivalesque experiments in living (Bakhtin, 1981, 1984). Some involve sex; others different forms of play (Mains, 1984/2002). The shadow of Dionysus takes countless often paradoxical forms—some comic and others tragic (Aeschylus, 1984; Maffesoli, 1993; Neitzche, 1967). "'Tragic' denotes a sense that one has to come to terms with inherently flawed and painful realities; 'comic' captures the more pragmatic, problem solving view that changes can be made to bring about a happy ending," psychoanalyst Nancy McWilliams (2004, p. 28) concurs. An awareness of this tragicomic quality of experience opens room for agency and a capacity to act, even amidst the ruins. The specter of tragedy, for example, allowed audiences of the Greek stage to reconcile their lives with the "fact that they had to make their decisions in a world that was not entirely rational, in which rationality was sometimes violently disrupted, in which rationality itself could be used for irrational ends," writes philosopher Johnathan Lear (1998, p. 29). For Lear, the lessons of Greek tragedy are simple: those who ignore the meanings of the irrational engage in a form of hubris which puts them at risk of reliving Oedipus's fate. From this perspective, the irrational is not thought to imply something opposed to rationality. Rather, it invites us into a world not governed by reason alone; this is a world outside the parameters of the rational (Jung, 1923).

Max Weber recognized that the rational turn in modern life had its downsides. Weber's writings are filled with musings about unyielding prison-like work conditions. He worried about the lack of meaning, a despair of life in bureaucratized society (Weber 1930/1992). In response to such pressures, he acknowledged the appeal of play, frivolity, and even game activity (1946/1968). For Weber, such activities served any number of purposes, including helping the individual to create space, adapt, cope, divert oneself, and find pleasure in a cold world. "The game also occupies a most serious and important position," Weber (1946/1968) explained. "It constitutes a counterpole to all economically rational action" (p. 1106). He lamented that the time for such activity had been eclipsed, "eliminated by every rationalization of life" (p. 1105). Still, the impulse to dress up, dance, and play remained. Through such activity, he argued regular people reveled in "rejecting purposeful-rational control"; more than a "superfluous" endeavor; such activity served as a "means of self assertion" (p. 1106). In the years to follow, efforts to assert a sense of self outside of work would galvanize a range of movements—from labor to anarchism, Situationism to today's movement of movements (Aronowitz 1972/1992; Bogad, 2005a, 2005b; Sunshine, 2003; Vaneigem, 1967/2003). After all, "In play, there is something 'at play' which transcends the immediate needs of life and imparts meaning to the action," Huizinga explains (1950/2004, p. 117). Yet, the question remains: what is this play of social movements?

CONTEXTS AND CASES

For the purposes of this book, play is a shorthand way of describing free activities, often finding expression as a gesture, performance, or ritual. The result is quite often a form of social eros—a connection among minds and bodies, tribes and movements (Katsiaficas, 2002; Maffesoli, 1996). Gay men in the AIDS Coalition to Unleash Power (ACT UP) were known to use most every occasion which presented itself to take off their T-shirts and start making out. Here, defiant gestures of pleasure found their way into street actions whenever possible (Gould, 2009; Chapter 3, this volume). Dressed as garden vegetables and butterflies, community garden activists framed their garden defense actions as a struggle between towers, flowers, and swarming butterflies (Martinez, 2009, Chapters 4 and 5, this volume). Before moving on to Chapter 1, the following is a brief overview of the case studies which comprise the rest of this study (Snow and Trom, 2002; Yin, 1994).

Theorists from Marx to Huizinga argued that the frenzy of capitalism steamrollered the quieter spaces of life and leisure, replacing them with a drive to accumulate goods, trade, fight, control, and wage war. The first two chapters of this book consider the work of antiwar activists who hoped to create a different kind of experience in living. Challenging the ruthless logic of conflicts from the First World War to Vietnam, antiwar activists responded to the drive to war with an impulse to recreate space for play and affect, performance and poetry. The first chapter considers the impulse from the vantage point of WWI and the artistic movements from Dada to Surrealism. The realization of the use of play as political prank found rich expression with the Situationists and the Yippies in the 1960s. The second chapter explores the dadaesque, ludic impulse which propelled the 1960s era Youth International Party (the Yippies) in contrast with the highly creative, yet earnest Young Lords Party of the same period.

Throughout the 1970s, the politics of play continued via the DIY practices of Gay Liberation, the anarchist queer theatrics of the Cockettes, and the later punk movements which very much built on the legacies of Dada, Surrealism, and Situationism (Marcus, 1989). For Gay Liberationists, pleasure and play were intimately connected with their work. The play only continued over the next decade. With Gay Liberation and AIDS activism, play functioned as both subversive tools and means of pleasure. An understanding of the political possibilities of play as a vehicle for pleasure and personal freedom became a cornerstone of movements for sexual freedom. With ACT UP, notions of play as both a theatrical device and coping mechanism became a cornerstone of the group's work (Crimp, 2002; Gould, 2009; Reed, 2005). Chapter 3 highlights the clownish pranks of ACT UP's Operation Ridiculous as well as OutRage, and harm reduction housing group Stand Up Harlem. This chapter situates play as a means of DIY cultural resistance in a struggle against oblivion.

By the 1990s, the streets of Seattle offered a telling example of a generation finding a way to engage and joke, work and create change within a distinct form of engagement (Boyd, 2002). Rather than repeat exhausted models, many embraced the Groucho-Marxist approach of the Situationists and other pranksters using culture, music, joking, and performance to involve people in community organizing (see Chrysler, 2003; Duncombe, 2002A,B). Here, play evolved into an understanding of a wide range of movement strategies—including social and cultural activity, creative and disruptive engagement, "hard" fun and game playing, as well as carnival, community building, and storytelling. And pranks the Situationists imagined found expression within the culture-jamming ethos of the movement's antic, anti-corporate disruptions (Duncombe, 2007; Lasn, 1999; McClish, 2009).

In New York, this movement took shape within the stories of activists involved in struggles for public space. A central theme of this activism involved campaigns against restrictions and removal of open public spaces, in particular community gardens. And gradually this struggle overlapped with the rise of the Global Justice Movement. Here, activists helped demonstrate the ways humor and theater could work as surprisingly effective tools, especially in communicating a message. Jesters carry no weapons; thus they apparently offer less of a threat to the powers-that-be. These light-handed approaches get the audience's attention in ways that "dangerous" political agitators rarely accomplish. By serving as comics instead of lobbyists, jesters maintain face time after others have been shooed away. When gardeners converged on New York City Hall in their campaign to save community gardens from 1998 to 2002, the media delighted in the idea of lobbyists dressed as giant sunflowers and tomatoes. The stories and public pressure mounted, and an usually obstinate mayor became willing to cut a deal. The result was a compromise. When asked why he imposed a temporary restraining order against bulldozing community gardens in 2000, New York Attorney General Elliot Spitzer responded, "because a giant tomato asked me to do it." Chapters 4 and 5 consider the links between a struggle for local spaces as they overlapped with a burgeoning movement.

The sixth and seventh chapters consider the stories of activists involved in organizing as the Global Justice Movement became a global peace and justice movement after 9/11. Their story addresses the struggles of these urban actors to grapple with the limitations of the carnival model of protest so popularized during the years before 9/11. The study follows the struggles of a movement once propelled by play, which found the tactic less appropriate for the times. As activists were tagged terrorists, the struggle for a place to play become increasingly complicated within a politics of terror and war. Groups involved included the Reclaim the Streets spin-off group, an Absurd Response to an Absurd War.

The eighth chapter considers the use of the new tools to challenge the politics of neoliberalism in contrast to more conventional politics. Questioning the accustomed lesser evil electoral politics, the boring rallies, the bursts of direct action, and frustrated tears of routine cycles of protest, a new cohort of political actors emerged with a new series of tactically silly approaches to organizing for social change. This chapter traces the upsurge and limitations of political clowning as the image of clowns rummaging through the streets found its way into the public consciousness. Building on the previous chapters, the conclusion outlines some of the limitations and possibilities of the ludic approaches to social change practice.

A burning ambition to include more people in the performance of political change churns throughout the chapters to follow. "The play is a problem," declared the Zapatista public spokesman, Subcomandante Insurgente Marcos (2001, p. 154). Following the passage of the North American Free Trade Agreement (NAFTA) in 1994, the Zapatistas started an uprising. Their highly creative approach marked the upsurge of a global movement (Mertes, 2003). This movement actually envisioned their struggle as a theatrical performance: "Those directing it are making a huge effort to convince the audience that it's already over. Not only is the public not leaving the premises, they're also insisting on getting up onto the stage," wrote movement spokesperson Subcommandante Marcos (2001, p. 154). Yet, more and more people are getting up on stage. "It is no longer possible to know where the stage is and where the seats are," Marcos continued, echoing the Surrealists and Situationists (ibid.). The play is the thing after all.

Through an appreciation of the play of social change, movement actors come to recognize the narrative contours, which construct of social reality. As sociologist Peter Nardi (2006, p. 288) counsels: "The institutions of society . . . while they do in fact coerce us, appear at the same time as dramatic conventions, even fictions." Through play with these conventions, we come to see these stories of our world as increasingly mutable. If reality is but a series of fictions, then the task of social movements is to create more compelling intersections of movement narratives within the struggles of people's lives. Here, social actors use play to communicate truth through illusion, prank, and street performance (Marcos, 2001; Nardi, 2006). The stage becomes a site for social engagement as actors and activists, citizens and noncitizens cultivate a theatrical pageant of everyday life. Each actor faces a choice: either to remain on the sidewalk or to step onto the street, into an open-ended, participatory experience in democratic living. Action takes place when social actors start improvising with their roles and their lives, rather than follow the stage directions. And gradually, everyday life becomes an arena of performance and struggle. While the Zapatista narratives assert there are different ways of thinking about political power, this study asserts that different kinds of social relations are produced when people play with politics and power.

Much of the new organizing aims to create a truly direct democratic political globalization project that honors countless points of view—not just those of the richest corporations. Building on a wide range of influences, this movement of movements values creativity, anger, defiant politics, culture jamming, sexual nonconformity, the rejection of shame, and protest pranks which include expressions of affection, care, and connection rather than social isolation (Gould, 2009; Lasn, 1999). Here, Zapatismo theatrics combine with queer aesthetics to merge creative protest and radical play into a new philosophy of political engagement. Instead of taking power, a new cohort has come to favor a richer form of engagement with power (Solnit, 2004). Yet, the process remains in constant flux. *Play, Creativity and Social Movements* considers some of the ways play does and does not find its way into these stories.

1 Surrealists, Situations, and Street Parties
History, Play, and Social Movements

The study of play in social movements opens up any number of questions about social and cultural change. Did the Commedia dell' Arte improvisational performances as clowns, the Zannis, prefigure the French Revolution (Grantham, 2001)? It is difficult to say. Yet surely enough, when Richard Schechner conceptualizes play as an "eruption of liberty" (2002, p. 79), it is not a stretch to imagine Liberty with her breast bared, waving a tricolor banner. But this does not answer the question, what is the relationship between play and social movement activity? Is storming the Bastille play? It depends on whom you ask. "I've no idea," one of Gustave Flaubert's (1869/2008, p. 27) characters explained when asked what provoked a disturbance during the French Revolution, "and neither have they . . . It's a habit of theirs these days. What an excellent joke." Everyone broke out in laughter. Individual motives are rarely pure. While revolution has traditionally been viewed as a response to desperation, the compulsion to act is rarely simple or heroic. The motivations of those involved in social movements are often a combination of dissatisfaction, affect, anger, love, and maybe a bit of a desire to be a part of the action. A protest over sex-segregated university housing is said to have set off the uprising of 1968 in Paris. During pro-democracy struggles in China in 1989 one of the students was asked what he wanted in Tiananmen Square. "I'm not sure, but I want more of it," he answered. The public theater of the streets takes any number of manifestations from an embrace of the 'grotesque' to a 'theatre of the ridiculous' (Kaufman, 2002; Mitchell, 1999). There is something telling about being moved to take the streets, even if one cannot put words around why. Yet, sometimes we know exactly what it means to do so. I will never forget the righteous, yet cathartic plea of a fellow student, who was African American, during the post-verdict street actions during the riots in Los Angeles in 1992. "It's been four hundred years, baby! Four hundred years!!!" he exclaimed as he sang, skipped, and chanted with the others as riots erupted. "It's a lot of fun to confront authority," Frances Fox Piven noted in a recent oral history on her life's work (Shepard, 2008, p. 14).

If anything, such activity is born out of the motivation to live in a more caring, just world. The subtitle of this study, "If I Can't Dance," refers to the famous adage attributed to US anarchist Emma Goldman, "If I can't dance, it's not my revolution" (although she did not actually say it). As the story goes, she was taken aside at a dance by a young comrade who told her that revolutionaries should not be seen dancing. Goldman is said to have responded:

> I did not believe that a cause which stood for a beautiful ideal, for anarchism, for release and freedom from conventions and prejudice, should demand the denial of life and joy. I insisted that our cause could not expect me to become a nun and that the movement should not be turned into a cloister. If it meant that, I did not want it. (quoted in Highleyman, 2004, p. 501)

Much of Goldman's philosophy was based on a broad belief in personal freedom. For her, joy and justice intermingled, neither able to exist without the other. Today, Goldman's adage on dance and revolution provides the underpinnings for the street party–style protest of Reclaim the Streets and the global justice "movement of movements" to create a far more colorful public sphere (see Chapters 4 and 5).

This spirit can be found in the call for a "Pink Silver March—Tactical Frivolity" during the G8 meetings and convergence actions of 2001 in Genoa, Italy. "Dance Down the G8!!" the communiqué declared.

> We are a colorful party in the street, a carnival with theatre, pink fairies and radical cheerleaders, clowns and music, a creative, magical and confrontational dance that takes decisions in a horizontal manner through affinity groups. We want to reduce aggressively to the minimum with imagination, samba, art, playing with space (and with the police), to create a relaxed atmosphere with good vibes. While we dance we denounce the brutality of capitalism, patriarchy, racism and all the forms of oppression and domination. (Archives of Global Protests, 2001)

A lineage of such activism leads directly back to the topsy-turvy experimentation of Marcel Duchamp, Dada, the Surrealists, Bertholt Brecht's theater, and the liberatory gender play witnessed in the Berlin cabarets of Weimar Era Germany (Kaes et al., 1994; Buhle and Schulman, 2005; Ferrell, 2001, Marcus, 1989). The Situationists specifically located their project within this milieu. The group recognized the liberatory potential of the intersection between art and play found in the Dada spectacle. "It was in fact from art that play broke free. The eruption was called Dada," argued Situationist Raoul Vaneigem (1967/2003, p. 257). "The Dadaist events awoke the primitive-irrational play instinct which had been held down (ibid.) This lineage represents a vital chapter in the history of play in social movements. It is the subject of the following chapter.

DADA AND SURREALISM

Formed in 1916, the Dadaists juxtaposed their delight in paradox with the ridiculous, up is down, down is up world of the years after the First World War (Hopkins, 2004). With mass carnage and the stench of the trenches in mind, Dada yearned "for a changed world" (Plant, 1992, p. 39). Tristan Tzara (1918) opens the Dada Manifesto with these words, which hint at the anarchistic impulse of the new movement:

> DADA EXCITES EVERYTHING.
> DADA knows everything. DADA spits everything out.

A sense of silliness and "wordplay" characterizes much of the movement (Marcus, 1989, p. 4). Its absurdity stood in stark contast to the rationalizations used to justify overwork, nationalism, stress, and ultimately war. Tzara (1918) begs the question:

> HAS DADA EVER SPOKEN TO YOU:
> about the fatherland
> about sardines
> about Art (you exaggerate my friend)
> about heroism
> about mustaches
> about lewdness
> about genius, about genius, about genius
> about the eight-hour day
> about heroism.

Instead of asking about "work" or "heroism" or the "fatherland," Dada was a movement for which those things no longer mattered. "NEVER NEVER NEVER" has Dada asked these things, Tzara (1918) conceded. "DADA doesn't speak. DADA has no fixed idea." Tzara addressed those reading along:

> If you have serious ideas about life,
> If you make artistic discoveries
> and if all of a sudden your head begins to crackle with laughter,
> If you find all your ideas useless and ridiculous, know that
> IT IS DADA BEGINNING TO SPEAK TO YOU.

The absurdity of Dada served as a provocation and homage to a topsy-turvy world. The movement's targets: work, war, capital—all of which seemed to be making everyone crazy. Even Freud (1961) conceeded that only a few of us could actually sublimate our desires into our work. There had to be more to life than this.

Dada would help the world ask questions about what that could be. One of the movement's foremost practitioners was artist Marcel Duchamp, whose readymades put into question the very ways we understand art and culture. It all started in 1917 when he responded to a call from the New York Society for Independent Artists. Anyone willing to pay six dollars could display two works. Duchamp submitted a urinal and said it was ready to be presented, "readymade." This readymade "art" object conjured up images of men urinating, among other provocations (Mink, 2006). Yet, mostly it was a joke on the world of art and bourgeois social mores. "In Duchamp's slapstick-infused readymades, the idea and the actuality of play offer possibilities for examining the tangled knot of work and leisure in everyday life," suggests Helen Molesworth (1998). In another work, Duchamp penciled a postcard of the Mona Lisa with a moustache, adding "L.H.O.O.Q." French shorthand for "she's got a hot ass" (Mink, 2006, p. 63). Through such juvenile humor and silliness, the realm of play, jokes, and humor found their way into social critique (Molesworth, 1998).

Sexuality was also part of the art, activism, and cultural experimentation of the era. Throughout the decade, movements in radical ecology, aesthetics, and gender play contributed to the pulsing public sphere of the Berlin Cabaret (Kaes et al., 1994). Here, an ethos of pleasure and generativity marked a stark contrast to the authoritarian, nationalist impulses that had driven Germany into WWI in the first place. Sex as a relational activity, as play and pleasure rather than procreation (and production of children with material needs), represented a new way of living (Foote, 1954; Turner, 1982).

By 1924, Surrealism established itself as Dada's heir. For the Surrealists human nature was best understood as an irrational social force (Hopkins, 2004). If it was modern civilization which set forth to divide up, take sides, and conduct four years of slow suicide, then these movements wanted nothing to do with its morality. The group rejected work "in favor of play" while experimenting "with forms of expression disallowed in capitalist society," explains Sadie Plant (1992, p. 40). Rather than dedicating life to producing and consuming, the Surrealists "argued and played with the system of values which entrapped them," disordering the senses through "antibourgeois free play" (Hopkins, 2004, p. 16; Plant, 1992, pp. 40, 42). Much of this took shape via new kinds of relatedness, supported within the active interplay between the conscious mind and an inner world of ideas of daydreams. Here, a movement pulsed within a space between a cacophony of ideas, free association, word soup, and fantasy (Breton, 1924/1972; Plant, 1992; Molesworth, 1998).

For the Surrealists, play offered a space to excavate, imagine, and meander through the recesses of the unconscious mind. The movement was profoundly influenced by psychoanalysis, where thinkers also grappled with the meanings of play and dreams (Freud, 1961; Piaget, 1962). Within play "the child or adult is free to be creative," argued psychoanalyst D.W. Winnicott (1971, p. 53). In child's play, the child is free to traverse the edges between pleasure and reality, dream and material worlds, and even self and external object (Freud, 1961). Here "real" objects are incorporated into a world of "make-believe" where the child maintains a sense of agency. And, the playground functions as a psychic space for creative exploration of "complete freedom" (Freud, 1914, pp. 147–56).

"Surrealism is not a new means or expression, or an easier one, nor even a metaphysic of poetry," wrote Surrealist Andre Breton (1924/1972). "It is a means of total liberation of the mind and of all that resembles it." For Breton and company, this was a movement in support of complete "freedom of thought." For only here could humans approximate the possibility of happiness. "Imagination alone offers me some intimation of what can be," mused Breton (1924/1972, pp. 4–5).

In his essay "Surrealism," German social critical Walter Benjamin (1978, p. 189) confessed that he found the group's "energies of intoxication for the revolution" tantalizing. For Benjamin, this revolutionary project came as close as anything he knew to realizing the humanist promise of Marx. "[O]nly the Surrealists have understood its present commands. They exchange, to a man, the play of human features for the face of an alarm clock" (p. 192).

Much of this revolution was buttressed within an ethos which favored eros over repression, the free expression of "desires, pleasures, and imaginations" (Plant, 1992, p. 49). Yet, it seemed as soon as it began, the life-affirming possibility of the Surrealists and the Weimar cabaret was forced to contend with oblivion. The Nazis specifically targeted the cabarets and Magnus Hirshfeld's Institute for Sexual Research for destruction in their first weeks in power (Gordan, 2000). Yet, the era's legacy persevered. Throughout the postwar period, Dada and Surrealist thought influenced any number of movements (Crimp and Rolston, 1990; Jordan, 1998; Rosemont and Radcliffe, 2005; Sakolsky, 2002). Surrealist calls "to make a Revolution" of the imagination were largely echoed by graffiti from Paris in 1968: "All Power to the Imagination" (Breton, 1924/1972; Marcus, 1989). Here, eruptions of play, festivity, and spontaneity burst into the political consciousness of a generation.

THE SITUATIONISTS

By the late 1950s and 1960s, the Situationists recognized that the impulse to play and create had not been—and could not be—rendered extinct by capital, war, fascism, rationality, or more overt efforts to contain their anarchistic contours (Debord, 1967). "The desire to play has returned to destroy the hierarchical society which banished it," declared Situationist theorist Raoul Vaneigem (1967/2003, p. 257). Still, much of the edgy, volatile character of play had been marginalized, exiled to a periphery of peoples' lives (Marcuse, 1955, 1964). All reification is forgetting, Herbert Marcuse (1978) would explain (though he was neither a member of nor influence for members of the group). In response to this pattern of flattening out, activists looked to art, culture, and play to animate social life. In order for these elements to break free, lines demarcating work and play would have to be dissolved. Escape valves would have to be shut off before pressure built for the system explode. Here, art and play would move out of the galleries and playgrounds and into the streets. "[W]ith the crisis of the spectacle, playfulness, distorted in every imaginable way, is being reborn everywhere," Raoul Vaneigem elaborated (1967/2003, p. 256). The group saw play as means to escape an all-encompassing "spectacle" that colonizes countless aspects of our lives (Debord, 1967).

The Situationists combined Hegelian Marxist social theory with radical impulses of the avant-garde. Influences ranged from Rimbaud to Marx, Lukacs to Lefebvre. For the Situationists, there had to be something outside of work and necessity. "Economic necessity and play don't mix," Raoul Vaneigem explained (1967/2003, p. 256). The group recognized that mechanisms of alienation existed not just in labor, but the ins and outs of everyday life (Aufheben, n.d.). The time had come to eclipse this "iron cage of despair." In one of its earliest papers, the *Situationist International* (1958) looked to practices including pranks, jokes, and game playing aimed at provoking and cultivating authentic experience. Play would serve as a site of resistance (Vaneigem, 1967/2003), infusing desire and vitality into everyday living (Sunshine, 2003). Here, play was thought to be the vehicle for a new type of society.

"All true play involves rules and playing with rules," Vaneigem asserted, invoking the image of the playground: "Watch children at play. They know the rules of the game, they can remember them perfectly well, but they are always breaking them, always dreaming up new ways of getting around them" (1967/2003, p. 258). Play with new rules could shift the experience of the everyday into a game without losers. "Play, pleasure, and participation were to be hallmarks of a new form of social organization appropriate to a world in which the imperatives of survival no longer legitimate relations of domination, alienation, and separation" (Plant, 1992, p. 71).

To achieve this end, the Situationists talked, thought, and strove to create a theory of practice around the struggles of the everyday. A primary intellectual supporter for this disposition was French Marxist philosopher Henri Lefebvre. Lefebvre suggested that thinkers make sense of the difference between "fulfilling" authentic engagements of the lived moment, and "alienating" "negative elements" (Harvey, 1991, p. 42).

In 1958, he was suspended from the French Communist Party, having spoken out about the events in Hungary two years prior. Yet, it was his forgery of Marx—"Art is the highest joy that man can give himself"—that was listed as an official reason (Lefebvre, 1947/1991, pp. 255, 69–70). In the years to follow, Lefebvre developed an increasingly festive, exuberant, even playful Marxist urbanism. Asked if he had become an anarchist, he is known to have replied, "I'm a Marxist, of course . . . so that one day we can all become anarchists" (quoted in Merrifield, 2002, p. 72). The decidedly playful answer was reflective of both the author's sense of humor and his increasing emphasis on a flexible, open-ended practice over a heavy-handed fixation on ideology. Lefebvre suggested a new praxis could be developed within the enactment of differential space (p. 72). He called for urbanists to demand a new "right to the city," achieved through a new jouissance, of sensual pleasure, free conscious movement, protest, carnival, theater, rent strikes, and recognition of the radical possibility of a lived moment (p. 84). He loved Paris and hoped it could remain a space for art and ideas, the sexy, creative space it had always been. "Are we entering a city of joy or the world of unredeemable boredom?" he wondered, contemplating its fate (p. 81). Faced with high rents and imagination-crushing imperatives of labor, he called for an urban experience of spontaneity and vitality, laughter and even mockery. "[R]evolutions of the past," including 1789 or even the Paris Commune of 1871, "were festivals," he noted (p. 83). Without space for such activities, urban spaces lose their connection with the imagination. He called for citizens to carve out spaces where "use" was prioritized over "exchange"; and improvisation and conversation were considered part of the "right to urban life" (p. 85). "Power . . . regards spontaneity as the enemy" (p. 87). The streets were the rightful space for such a politics, street parties a rightful heir to such thinking.

In 1957, Lefebvre taught in Strasbourg, where he met a group of young radicals who had been involved in occupations and demonstrations. Through these students, he came in contact with the burgeoning Situationist movement and inadvertently became a mentor to one of its leaders: Guy Debord. Both shared a fascination with the workings of everyday life, the limitations of docile urbanism, and a disdain for Baron Georges Haussman's Paris. "Today's urbanism's main problem is ensuring the smooth circulation of a rapidly increasing quantity of motor vehicles," Debord quipped (1967, p. 94). Both worried that the modern metropolis of drab order was gradually suffocating the life-affirming creativity of the city (p. 95).

Like the Dadaists and Surrealists before them, Lefebvre and Debord recognized the potential for a new kind of ludic experience. "[T]he Situationists defended the urban mix, wanted to get beyond the rational city, strove to reassert daring, imagination and play in social life and urban culture," notes geographer Andy Merrifield (2002, p. 96). The crux of such a politics was the construction of heightened lived moments. "Play, as well as politics, was fundamental to any Situationist situation," Merrifield continues. "In fact, play was fundamental to any politics, too. Play nourished politics and political man was very much *Homo Ludens*" (ibid.). Debord spent much of the 1950s not only studying Huizinga's (1950) work, but integrating this thinking into a Situationist brand of activism, emphasizing freedom of the mind, body, and urban space (Merrifield, 2002).

To achieve these ends, the Situationists cooked up spontaneous disruptions, injecting the "realm for play" into the everyday (Vaneigem, 1967/2003, p. 131). To do so, the group deployed a series of guerilla activist interventions termed "détournement" and "derive." "Détournement" referred to the rearrangement of popular signs to create new meanings, while disrupting expectations of such spaces (Lefebvre, 1974/1991; Merrifield, 2002; Thompson and Sholette, 2004). "Derive," on the other hand, referred to short meandering walks designed to resist the work- and control-oriented patterns of Georges Haussmann's redesign of Paris and remapping a city as a reflection of one's own imagination (Thompson and Sholette, 2004). The point was to trigger up new thoughts, daydreams, and associations which might inspire viewers to second-guess or rethink a few of the givens of modern living (Aufheben, n.d.). "The derive acted as something of a model for the 'playful creation'" (Plant, 1992, p. 59). Through such tactics, ludic activist practice was thought to highlight a sense of individual agency, that one could actually control the way he or she participates within the world (Plant, 1992).

"The revolutionary project," argued Debord, "a generalized historical life, is also the project of a withering away of the social measure of time in favor of an individual and collective irreversible time which is playful in character" (1967). Such a revolution was thought to find its expression within the rejection of story-crushing, everyday monotony in favor of authentic engagement with the everyday. The Situationists reached their apex with the days of May 1968 when the Metro shut down, the shops closed, and play really did supersede work. Yet, as soon as the temporary autonomous zone was born, it ended (as these things tend to do, see Bey, 1991). And everyone returned to work. Lefebvre and Debord had already split over a paper on the Commune. The relationship would not survive Debord's disappointment in his sixty-eight-year-old mentor's failure to take to the streets. Lefebvre was less moved with the chaos of 1968; his life had meant a great many things before it and would continue to do so afterward. Debord's life, on the other hand, would become increasingly dark. He killed himself in 1994 (Merrifield, 2002, pp. 86–111). In the years after 1968, Lefebvre continued with his investigations of the mechanisms of power in everyday life (Lefebvre, 1947/1991, 1974/1991).

PARADOX AND PREFIGURATIVE ORGANIZING

Countless thinkers would build on Lefebvre's study of the constant flux of space, place, and culture, and their impacts on everyday life. Play seemed to straddle any number of the endless dualisms— inhibition and expression, pleasure and pain, repression and transgression—of the modern epoch (Gardiner, 1997; Mains, Mains, 1984/2002).. Under capitalism, "everything is pregnant with its contrary," Karl Marx would contend; good things are intimately linked with the bad (Merrifield, 2002, p. 5). Keenly aware of these contradictions, Walter Benjamin remained fixated with the high and low culture of his Paris. He is said to have wanted to leave the decadence of the city, just not today (Berman, 1982, p. 146). The pulse of the city thrives in just such a jazz-like urban dialectic, a contrast between the dark and light, the cruelty as well as the unsuspected random acts of kindness and even humor. Much of the politics of play takes place within just such a tragicomic stage. Herein, play offers a useful intermediating space between what is real and what is fantasy, between liberation and repression, possibility and pain (Aronowitz, 1972/1992; Bateson, 1972; Marcuse, 1955, Wilson, 1990).

If there is one thinker who truly grappled with the inherent tensions between work and play, politics and pleasure, it was Frankfurt School social theorist Herbert Marcuse. In *Eros and Civilization*, Marcuse suggests, "The play impulse does not aim at playing 'with' something; rather it is the play of life itself, beyond want and external compulsion—the manifestation of an existence without fear and anxiety, and thus the manifestation of freedom itself" (1955, p. 187). Borrowing from Marx, he viewed this schism as a differentiation between a "realm of necessity" and "the realm of freedom" in which imagination, freedom, and play thrive (1969). Friedrich Schiller's letter *On the Aesthetic Education of Man* and Immanuel Kant's *Critique of Judgment* influenced Marcuse's study of the "play influence" on culture and the transformative possibilities of art. They would influence countless theorists of play (Wilson, 1990).

Yet, for each of play's possibilities, limitations would soon follow. "[T]here can be alienation in leisure just as in work," Lefebvre would suggest (1947/1991, p. 42). "Play is *unproductive* and *useless* because it cancels the repressive and exploitive traits of labor and leisure; it 'just plays' with reality," Marcuse (1955, p. 195) continues.

While "just playing" with reality may have had its limits for movements aimed at changing the world, the idea would influence social movements for decades to come. Yet so would the idea of violence in the name of social change. For many in the antiwar movement of the 1960s, the response to the lack of direct results from years of antiwar activism was despair. In 1969, a faction of the Students for a Democratic Society (SDS) known as the Weather Underground (WU) turned to an audacious—perhaps crazed—response. Instead of creating an ethical form of refusal, the WU and the Red Army Faction turned to violence as a form of transcendent action (Varon, 2004). Marcuse, who by this point had become a guru of sorts for the New Left, counseled that activism had to include an affirmative component, which included a vision of something better than what one opposes. "The goal, free human beings, must already be evident in the means," argued Marcuse (Varon, 2004, pp. 237–39).

In the following decades, a number of movement scholars and activists (Burghardt, 1982; Duncombe, 2002b; Epstein, 1991; McKay, 1998) built on this sentiment to identify an approach understood as prefigurative community organizing (although its practice dates back decades to at least as far as the writings of Gandhi). Quite simply, prefigurative community building assumes that the means of organizing are as important as the ends. Here those involved must actually create the world they want to live in as part of their actions and organizing (Hudema, 2004).

Another way to describe such practices is "immediatism." The practice was a central theme of the Situationist emphasis on everyday life (Plant, 1992). Hakim Bey, whose concept of the "temporary autonomous zone" (1991) was an inspiration for many in these movements, describes the practice, "[W]e nevertheless demand of ourselves an extreme awareness of *immediacy*. A direct means of implementing this consciousness is through an appreciation of the possibilities of play, immediately (at once) & immediately (without mediation)" (2003). For Bey, "immediatism" is not so much of a movement as an awareness. "It may take the form of any kind of creative play which can be performed by two or more people, by and for themselves, face-to-face and together. In this sense it is like a game." Such creativity is difficult to limit to mere aesthetic or even political purposes: "Real art is play, and play is one of the most immediate of all experiences." Here, the everyday is seen as a source of contestation, daily interactions a means of resistance. "[I]mmediatism" becomes a way to break down the lines between art and life, while introducing "creativity, imagination," and "play" into struggles for a better world in the here and now (Jordan, 1998, p. 129). While not everyone was enamored with such thinking, the appeal of the practice found its way into cohort after cohort of direct action projects.

Over the years, much of movement organizing seemed to divide between play infused prefigurative and conventional organizational models. Both approaches aimed to address similar issues. Yet, the question was which model best addressed a given movement's needs? Organizers with a "play emphasis" placed a premium on creativity; those who approached organizing with little or "no play" tended to approach their work with a linear, functionalist view of the task at hand. Prefigurative organizers viewed the way one plays the game as imperative, while those in the traditional left suggested the ends justify the means and left little room for play or cultural work (Isserman, 1993). Proponents of "play" based strategies noted cultural work makes organizing enjoyable and entry easy. The underlying logic remained that there is joy in changing the world (Burghardt, 1982).

Even Martin Luther King Jr. was caught between these tensions and influences. King was profoundly effective at using street theatrics and direct action to demonstrate what was wrong with apartheid in the United States (McAdam, 1996; Payne, 1995). He was also aware that activists in the movement loved to sing and dance. Opponents constantly sought to stop such cultural activities. After a group was arrested in Albany, Georgia, in 1961, one sheriff informed those arrested, "We don't have no singin', no prayin', and no clappin' here" (Zinn, 2002, p. 51). Such tools helped activists resist social controls, maintain esprit de corps, and challenge seemingly insurmountable targets. They were also a lot of fun.

By the late 1960s, many such ambitions found their expressions in the milieu of the Youth International Party (better known as the Yippies), who were heavily influenced by pop culture as well as the civil rights movement. Pranks, play, and pleasure seeking were a central part of their practice. Many suggested they lacked sufficient seriousness. Despite this, the disruption of everyday life would become a storied practice of the era. So would tensions over the role of play within the movement. The second chapter of this study considers the contrasting activist practices and story lines of two late 1960s New York City direct action groups—the Yippies and Young Lords—whose contrasting styles embodied this conflict.

2 Play as Prank
From the Yippies to the Young Lords

Never doubt that a small and dedicated group of people with pies can change the world. Indeed, it is the only thing that ever has.

—Communiqué from the Biotic Baking Brigade (BBB)
—Ecotopia Cell, 2000

"All roads lead to Rome," classical historians used to repeat. Yet, for scholars of twentieth-century US social movements, these roads often lead back to 1968. I have never been as enamored of this era. Yet, interviewee after interviewee connects their own activist narrative to the Yippies and Chicago 1968. "I trace it all to the Democratic Convention in 1968," explained AIDS activist Jeanne Bergman. "I wasn't there but I watched it on TV and I understood which side I was on." "The Yippies, in 1968 in Chicago, were doing all sorts of wild stuff," noted longtime AIDS Coalition to Unleash Power (ACT UP) facilitator Ann Northrop, in our interview. Andrew Boyd, the founder of the Billionaires for Bush, began his interview this way. "When we talk about the uses of play, the way I talk about it is using artistic strategies, thinking like an artist about doing political action. Abbie Hoffman says that all protest, and you can extend that to political action, is theater." During the G8 protests in Scotland during the summer of 2005, the Clandestine Insurgent Rebel Clown Army (CIRCA) referred to the Yippies in much of their propaganda. "One of the worst mistakes any revolution can make is to become boring," the group website quotes Abbie Hoffman.

This chapter assesses the competing forms of play and protest advanced by the silly yet subversive Situationist-influenced Yippie style street performance, in contrast with the highly creative, occasionally violent forms of direct action of the Young Lords, a South Bronx organizing group. Throughout the chapter, two of the last few remaining members of the New York Yippies, Dana Beal and Aaron Kay, speak about their life and work, slapstick and pranks. Vicente "Panama" Alba, a close associate of Richie Perez, recalls his work with the Young Lords. This chapter considers the way two of these groups—the Yippies and Young Lords—did and did not make use of play within their organizing and approaches to political performance. While the Young Lords hoped to change the rules of urban life, which grinds people down within a concrete jungle, they rarely conceptualized their action as play. The Yippies, on the other hand, looked to practical jokes and drugs to cultivate a politics of disorder and pleasure. The verb for engaging in a prank is, after all, "to play." "It's a game—revolution is a game that's just more fun," Yippie founder Abbie Hoffman explained in an interview in 1986. "I met philosophers in France . . . and they said, 'You came up with the idea that revolution could be fun. No one in history had thought of that, and only an American could have been so goddamned silly.'" That was Abbie Hoffman's line and he was sticking to it. It would keep him involved in organizing for the better part of two decades. "It was a lot of fun," he explained (Pranksters, 1987, pp. 65–66). Generations of activists followed his rambunctious lead.

Much of Yippie legend begins in 1968. By 1968, the rules of the game felt like they had to change. Activists had worked, agitated, marched, written statements, yet the war continued. "It is difficult to communicate at a distance the sense of helplessness and suppressed rage we all felt by the end of 1967," historian David Schalk recalled (2000, p. 501). Still, protest felt like a dull Kabuki ritual. People arrived, marched, and screamed; they knew the end destination before they began. There was little room for play. "[I]t is the game that must be changed, not the pieces," surrealist Andre Breton observed after a similarly absurd war from 1914 to 1918 (Sakolsky, 2002, p. 201). By 1968, they were about to.

The Yippies converged on the "Festival of Life" during the 1968 Democratic National Convention with ambitions to change US politics and culture. There, they held their own mock convention, nominating a pig to become president in Lincoln Park. While the week began with this silly "charade," within days, a darker form of play would find expression in the streets of Chicago (Mailer, 1986). There, gestures that began as forms of simple bravado would descend into theater of violent confrontations between protesters and police (Schechner, 2002, p. 107). And protest would not be the same (Ayers, 2001; Varon, 2004). Throughout the era, play functioned as a transgressive performance in freedom and direct action, a part of the drama and poetry of the movement (Bail, 2004).

ABBIE HOFFMAN: THE POLITICS OF 'PROP'AGANDA AND THE STRUGGLE AGAINST BOREDOM

The Youth International Party, the Yippies, were first and foremost proponents of "a politics of ecstasy and joy" (Jasper, 1997, p. 212). Yippie founder Abbie Hoffman specifically noted that if he had to choose, his ideal revolution would create a space for "free play" (Hoffman, 1989, p. 245). For the Yippies, activism was best organized around affect and pleasure. The group aspired to create rambunctious mischief—dropping LSD in the NYC water supply or having public 'fuck-ins.' In the same way the Dadaists and Surrealists questioned the logic of a culture hell-bent on sending youth to war, the Yippies contrasted the 1968 Democratic Convention of Death with their Festival of Light (Guttman, 2007). Hoffman's political approach has been described as a nonlinear "assault on rational sensibilities" (Simon,

1989, p. xii). "I really did it because it was fun. That's what I tell my friends," explained Abbie Hoffman, who after all had been a student of one of the primary theorists of play, Herbert Marcuse. "To my brothers I tell the real truth, which is that I don't know why I did it . . . any explanation I give is made up" (Hoffman, 1989, p. 13).

Unlike other direct action groups, "who were always in battle mode, both Abbie Hoffman and Jerry Rubin played the revolutionaries for laughs," noted Osha Neumann (2008), who was a part of Up Against the Wall Motherfucker, an anarchist-inspired Lower East Side direct action group of the same era. "Prancing in front of television cameras they acted the part of revolutionaries having fun playing at being revolutionaries" (Neumann, 2008, p. 96).

Hoffman recognized that most of the United States is anti-pleasure; people are taught to deprioritize fun, except when pleasure is associated with consumption and shopping. In order to disrupt this line of logic, the Yippies created situations aimed at forcing people to rethink these associations, to upend such social mores while opening up alternate perspectives. Simultaneously, they reinforced the point that one could have fun while organizing to change the world (Guttman, 2007, p. 507).

"The key to the puzzle lies in theater," explained Hoffman (1989, p. 17). "We are theatre on the streets: total and committed. We aim to involve people and use (unlike other movements locked in ideology) any weapon (prop) we can find." "The play's the thing," Hoffman (ibid.) argued in a nod to English Queen Elizabeth's day when Shakespeare's plays and popular dramas were a central feature of public life (Bevington, 1962). Here, the aim was to create a highly participatory theater in which audience members could take part. "Theatre will capture the attention of the country" (Hoffman, 1989, p. 18). "Give them a new, positive, authentic frame of reference," he argued. "Just do your thing; the press eats it up. Make News!" (1989, pp. 24–25). Use cultural resources. "Do it all fast. Like slapstick movies. Make sure everyone has a good time" (p. 17).

Play and paradox permeate Hoffman's Dada-like line of thought. "Accept contradictions, that's what life is all about . . . Have a good time . . . laugh—it's a riot." (pp. 20, 17).

Rather than lecture or give didactic speeches, he recognized that public debate was increasingly influenced by signs, symbols, and media filters. "MEDIA is the message," Hoffman (p. 19) declared, echoing Marshall McLuhan.

"Don't rely on words . . . Rely on doing." Here, regular people are invited to become active partners, not passive spectators in the spectacle. And once everyone is involved in the performance, shake it up, keep it fresh, he urged, echoing Saul Alinsky (1989). The worst thing an activist can do is lose the sympathies of the crowd: "When they get bored, they are turned off. They are not receiving information. Get their attention, leave a few clues and vanish" (Hoffman, 1989, p. 19).

For Hoffman and the Yippies, the problem was too many movements were "locked in ideology" which discouraged creativity and engaged participation (1989, pp. 17–19). Supporting a 'New Left' politics which rejected racism, sexism, and homophobia in favor of a new democracy of pleasure and social change, the Yippies tried to distinguish themselves from the orthodoxies of the 'Old Left,' which viewed pleasure as antithetical to class struggle (Guttman, 2007; Isserman, 1993). "The thing about the old left was they were not very funny," Yippie Dana Beal explained. Bob Kohler, a member of the civil rights group Congress on Racial Equality and the Gay Liberation Front, concurred, noting there was "no humor in the old leftist movement." The Situationists referred to hair shirt, dour political activists as the 'militants.' Their gripe was that the 'Militants' delineated "politics" from personal desires; they charged the 'militants' allowed social change work to become a tedious chore in which ends were separated from the means. Recognizing such practices turned activism into a form of "alienated labor," the Situationists declared: "Boredom is always counter-revolutionary" (Aufheben, n.d.).

The politics of play offered far more flexibility. Aaron Kay, who joined the Yippies in 1972, explains how this worked. "When it comes to issues, there's an old Abbie Hoffman line that I use. 'Isms are wasms.' We deal with issues, not dogma."[1] The Situationists described such thinking as "critique of isms" (Vaneigem, 1967/2003, p. 24). Theory is when you have ideas. Ideology is when ideas have you. For the Yippies, pop culture was more important than adherence to ideology. "When we were thinking of dogma, we used to think of Groucho Marx and the Three Stooges," Kay explains. "Nobody wants to hear about Karl or Lenin, unless it's John Lennon. You have to use entertainment. You have to use what cultural tools are there." Hoffman revered his former teacher, Frankfurt School philosopher Herbert Marcuse, because, among other things, the noted social critic was willing to smoke pot with him instead of debating social theory. Politics was better served with a light touch (Hoffman, 1989).

ENTER DANA BEAL

Beyond his silliness, Abbie Hoffman was a thoughtful, experienced organizer. He understood that effective organizers must make an effort to understand what people need and then help them find a way to achieve that. "Dropouts dig flowers, don't give them I.F. Stone weeklies. Bowery bums dig wine, don't give them Bibles," cautioned Hoffman (1989, p. 20). "Become aware of the most effective props . . . On the Lower East Side pot is an effective prop, it is the least common denominator. It makes us all outlaws, brothers" (ibid.). This is where Beal came in, as he explained in our interview. "He (Hoffman) was twenty-seven and I was around twenty. There was about a ten-year

---

1. This expression predates the Yippies, dating back to the 1940s or 1950s.

difference. I was a younger guy who could get the kids to do a lot of stuff. I was able to bring people in," noted Beal as he described his entrance into the Yippies. "I was at a party at Abbie's. I was part of the scene that preceded the Yippies." It was this scene which witnessed the New York Stock Exchange and Pentagon pranks. "They were proto-Yippie," explained Beal. "Technically the Yippies did not exist until New Year's Eve of 1968. They came up with the name around Christmastime, and by New Year's Eve they were having a party at Abbie's and they asked people to join."

Today, Beal still lives in the Yippie headquarters at 9 Bleecker Street, where he has resided since 1973. Also known as "the Yippie Museum," the old three-story brick building at Bleecker and Bowery, just adjacent to the now closed CBGB's, has served as the central meeting space for the quirky group for some thirty-plus years (Moynihan, 2001). As I walked in for my interview with Beal, my senses were jolted with the scent of cat urine. Psychedelic posters, with pulsing colors, filled the walls. Walking upstairs, the cat smell gave way to the smell of pot. I noted an iconic sticker from recent activist lore, with the words "NYC—AIDS Disaster Area" from ACT UP's second anniversary action in 1989. Relics of literally decades of street activism crowded the wall-to-wall bookshelves.

Beal greeted me wearing his trademark blue jeans half unzipped, no shirt, and cowboy boots. With white hair and a drooping Mark

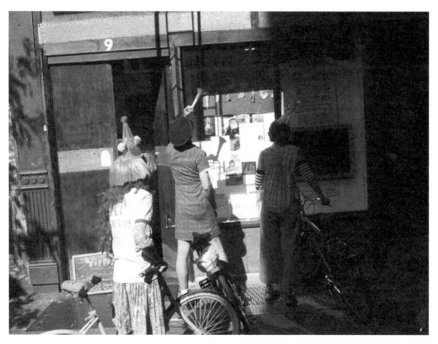

Figure 2.1 New York's bike clowns paying homage to the Yippie's longtime home at 9 Bleecker Street. Photo by James Nova.

Twain–like handlebar moustache, Beal is a striking sight. For much of the interview, Beal answered other phone calls and e-mails and smoked a joint. His office was cluttered with decades of old issues of the *Yipster Times*, posters, boxes of literature on ibogaine, and other relics and paraphernalia from the underground. At one point after returning from a phone call, he settled back down into his chair and realized he had lost his joint. So we both walked around the second floor to look for it. When we finally found it we returned to the interview. Beal answered questions and we chatted. I asked what first got him involved in political organizing. Like many, he was drawn into organizing with the civil rights movement in 1963. "I was a precocious protester. I tried to organize a protest when I was sixteen. The first real action was when the Klan blew up a church, which blew up four little girls. I just loved demonstrations. I always have."

"The interesting thing is Abbie came out of the civil rights movement," Beal elaborated. "His roots are not in antiwar, but in the civil rights movement. Abbie was working with Freedom Summer and something called, I think, Freedom House." Here, both Beal and Hoffman witnessed the use of songs and cultural resistance in support of social struggle. Social eros, dancing, drinking beer, singing, and sexual experimentation were all part of the "Freedom High" of those years (McAdam., 1988, p. 72).

For activists of this generation, music and song served as vital resources for communicating messages, maintaining group cohesion, and promoting strength in the face of very hostile opposition. Bob Kohler, who took part in any number of sit-ins and blockades with CORE, explains, "It was the best way to break that awful tension, turning it around." Many civil rights activists were well aware of this. "Jesus Loves Me, This I Know," civil rights activists sang, highlighting the hypocrisy of white apartheid with updated verses of the old Sunday school song. "Jesus loves me 'cause I'm white / Lynch a nigger every night (Payne, 1995, pp. 263, 242–43). The humor of the songs also helped alleviate fear. After all, something had to lighten things up; without a little levity the liberatory "Freedom High" would be lost (Burdell, 2003). The white apartheid system depended on this fear. In the face of this, freedom songs tapped into a spirit of defiant humor which helped movement players stay the course (Reed, 2005).

Coming out of this experience, Hoffman and the Yippies recognized that laughter created spaces for social actors to engage otherwise insurmountable problems. It also helped support organizing efforts. If spectators saw others having fun while fighting for social change, they might be compelled to jump off the fence and join the struggle (Guttman, 2007; Pranksters, 1987). It also helped the movement renew itself and stay vital. "That was really important," Dana Beal explained. "[If] you have a really good vibe and you are playful and joyful, you are going to be more attractive to people than if you are kind of somber and bummed out. I've always said that."

LOVE-INS, SMOKE-INS, AND PLAY IN PUBLIC SPACE

By 1967, Beal and Hoffman "transitioned from civil rights to antiwar movement." During this period, Beal learned another important lesson: police always want to be in charge, especially if a movement is gaining support. So the police seek to control public space. In the face of an ongoing clash between protesters and police, Beal came up with an innovative solution. "We had gigantic smoke-ins" explained Beal.

> There had been a riot over in the park where the police beat up peace people. They manhandled people, even a pregnant lady . . . It was a big overreaction. But that somehow set off nights of rioting. And so the smoke-ins arose to pacify things. Actually, it worked quite well. You could see people calming down. If it had been alcohol, there would be fights.

The same dynamic was taking place across the country. In Los Angeles, future Yippie Aaron Kay was busy organizing "love-ins" aimed at bringing people together in the fragmented metropolis of Los Angeles. "The cops did not like the communities coming together," Kay speculated.

> It was a weekend hippie get-together. People would gather every Sunday in the park. And we'd have free music. Just party hardy. People came in from all over Southern California for that. The scene in Los Angeles was very fragmented. People are all in their own orbit. With the love-ins, the scene kind of came together. Everybody would know about it. The cops did not like everybody in LA coming together. They used all sorts of excuses. But what it was, was an all-class sort of situation. Upper-middle-class kids hanging out with kids who came from 'the other side of the tracks,' the ghetto kids from the barrio and "white trailer trash," all hangin' together and partyin'. They did not like that at all.

Kay, in turn, organized against the crackdowns on public gatherings. I asked Kay if he made use of any pranks as part of the campaign. "We were being conventional with this one," Kay explained, acknowledging the need to be aware of the tactical strengths and weaknesses of a given organizing strategy. "We were trying to draw a broader element," Kay noted, acknowledging that as much as anything, a prank's utility depends on its circumstances. This theme ran throughout our conversation. "Some things are more tailored for the prank type of situation," Kay explained. When, for example, a politician has been particularly hypocritical, it can be useful to deliver a pie in their face. "That's like committing a nonviolent assassination without a bullet. You are dissolving their ego with a pie," notes Kay, also known as "Pieman." Over the years, Kay has hurled pies at the likes of former California Governor Jerry Brown, former New York Senator James L. Buckley, Nixon aide G. Gordon Liddy, and even Phyllis Schlafley (Moynihan, 2001). "A pie in the face . . . has no equal in slapstick comedy. It can reduce dignity to nothing in seconds," explains Mack Sennett in *Pie Any Means Necessary* (quoted in Crane, 2004).

For Kay, the most appropriate targets for pieing are the super-powerful. "Like Pat Buchanan, for example. He spoke on Cesar Chavez's birthday. He deserved a Cesar salad pie in honor of Cesar Chavez and the farmworkers." Others are pied because they are "turncoats" or just plain "obnoxious and pompous," Kay added. "Someone like that you want to take down all the way. Buchanan, I have my own ax to grind with him 'cause of the anti-Semitism, he says the Holocaust didn't happen. It's totally obnoxious."

Yet, when the BBB pied former San Francisco Mayor Willie Brown, Kay did not think it felt right. "I personally had a criticism of the Willie Brown action," he said. While Kay understood why Brown had been pied, he worried about the symbolism of three white activists attacking an African American man, albeit with a pie. For Kay, it was not effective political theater. "Someone told me it was like the South," mused Kay. The Cherry Pie 3, as they were dubbed, would spend the next four months behind bars. Yet they retained a sense of humor. As Agent Cherry Rhubarb Tart explained, "Sticks and stones may break your bones, but a pie is just flour, sugar, water and fruit for fuck's sake. Get over it!" (Crane, 2004).

Cherry Rhubarb Tart's response is part of a long tradition among the Yippies and neo-Yippie humor. The Yippies found their muse in the slapstick shtick of Lenny Bruce and the Marx Brothers (Crane, 2004). "It goes back to the 1940s," noted Kay. "Charlie Chaplin, there was lots of pieing in Three Stooges movies . . . who would go in there and make fools of these guys." The point was to take opponents down a notch.

THE POLITICS OF ENTERTAINMENT AND DISRUPTION

"You are hippies and you are here to have a demonstration and we cannot allow that in the Stock Exchange," a security guard is said to have told Abbie Hoffman on his way to conduct one of the most famous Yippie actions, the August 24, 1967, Yippie invasion of the New York Stock Exchange. "Who's a hippie? I'm Jewish and besides, we don't do demonstrations, see we have no picket signs," Hoffman replied, doing his best stand-up. Hoffman was not at the Stock Exchange to conduct a simple demonstration. He was there for a prank which combined slapstick humor with cultural resistance. Such pranks have long taken shape through such "mischievous" gestures or "practical jokes" (Pranksters, 1987). Hoffman was eventually admitted into the exchange because, he reasoned, "the guards decided it was not a good idea to keep a Jew out of the Stock Exchange" (1989, p. 21).

"I think probably my all-time favorite Yippie action is the Stock Exchange," Beal ruminated. "A few people went down. They had an open balcony at the time where you could look down on the exchange floor and they started throwing dollar bills. And it completely shut down the biggest financial trading thing in the world 'cause everybody stopped what they were doing and started chasing dollar bills, which of course were worth almost nothing. It created a frenzy." News of the anticapitalist zap at the Stock Exchange was covered by the media and told around the world (Moynihan, 2001).

"When we got out, I carried on in front of the press," mused Hoffman. "How much money did you throw out?" one reporter asked. "A thousand dollars in small bills," retorted Hoffman. "We danced in front of the Stock Exchange, celebrating the end of money. I burned a fiver. Some guy said it was disgusting and I agree with him, calling my comrades 'Filthy Commies'" (1989, p. 21).

Similar disruptions would only continue in the decades to follow. In 1972, Yippies released white rats at a dinner for Pat Nixon. Another favorite activity for the Yippies was to streak through public places in Nixon masks. For Kay, all the pranks involved a basic philosophic understanding. "They are the buffoons. Listen, everyone knows someone who should get pied. People would like to pie their boss, their landlord. It humanizes things, gets people to laugh. It breaks the barriers down." So Yippies set their aim on the everyday lives of any number of policymakers. "These fucks disrupted our lives with the Vietnam War; they disrupted our lives with depression; they disrupted our lives with their stinking economic policy," Kay explained.

While other groups, including SDS, wanted to march on Washington, the Yippies converged in Washington in 1967 to levitate the Pentagon. "Humor breaks barriers," Kay explained. "Sometimes you gotta use silliness to open people's eyes, because these people are dangerous but they are also silly. These people are very silly." Sounding every bit like Andre Breton and the Surrealists, Hoffman reasoned: "Our alternative fantasy will match in zaniness the war in Vietnam. Fantasy is freedom . . . The Pentagon will rise 300 feet in the air" (1989, p. 29). The call for the Pentagon action framed it as a carnival. "Anybody can do anything." Here, the line between audience and leader blurred. "No rules, speeches won't do, leaders are full of shit. Pull your clothes off. . . . jump a wall, do a dance, sing a song, paint the building, charge, and get inside" (ibid.).

"The people who did the action knew that if you surrounded the Pentagon, the government, the police would freak out," recalled Dana Beal. "They had a regulation saying that you could not surround the Pentagon." The mere announcement of an action at the Pentagon created a stir. "We applied for permits to raise the Pentagon one hundred feet; we measured it—me and a friend got busted measuring the Pentagon," Abbie Hoffman explained. "The Pentagon cannot be surrounded by peaceful civilians at, like, a distance closer than one hundred yards or something like that," Beal noted. So this is exactly what the Yippies did: "I think they had an inkling . . . there would be a big confrontation."

"We knew the blue meanies were not going to let us defy the law of gravity because they were not letting us defy any of the other seven million laws of the country," mused Hoffman (Pranksters, 1987, pp. 65–66).

ALIENATION, VIOLENCE, AND THE LIMITATIONS OF A MODEL

"I tried to do something that was funny" Beal reflected on a lifetime of pranks, "not just like the Left with a lot of slogans." Yet, not everyone was enamored with the Yippie mode of action. "We weren't interested in floating Monroe High School," quipped Panama Vincente Alba, a member of the Young Lords Party. While many found the Yippies entertaining, the Yippies were profoundly alienating to working classes, who harbored animosities toward the movement (Freeman, 1990; Graeber, 2009). "People always resented us," Beal acknowledged. Still, the Yippies gravitated to the more subversive voices in the culture. Explained Beal: "The sensibility was they were not from the old—the kind of people who were running the country in the 1950s."

Along the way, the Yippie carnival brought a whole new cohort into the antiwar movement. "There were a lot of positive responses from much of the Left and the people they were trying to incorporate," explained Beal. "They were trying to get kids who were antiestablishment. How do you get to the hippies?" For the Yippies, the answer was to reach out to their disaffection. The Yippie hook was a combination of pot and playful political engagement, others turned to more extreme methods (see Ayers, 2001; Varon, 2004). "There were some groups who had some success, like the Weathermen, but even they were not that funny," noted Beal. "The only problem was that then people started to get serious. And there was this kind of split in the Left." The conflict was reflective of an aesthetic conflict over models of protest which continues to this day. The ludic Yippie approach was certainly not for everyone. Others took a different track.

FROM THE LOWER EAST SIDE TO THE SOUTH BRONX

New York City's Lexington Avenue subway line stops on Bleecker Street just down the street from 9 Bleecker, where the Yippies have met since the early 1970s. From there, it is a thirty-minute subway ride north through Manhattan to the South Bronx, where the Young Lords Party got their start in 1969 (Melendez et al., 2003; Young Lords and Abramson, (1971). Though geographically close, the cultural gap between 9 Bleecker Street and 149th Street is beyond measure; it is reflected in the differing approaches to organizing taken by the Yippies and the Young Lords. While the Yippies sought to make activism spontaneous and infused with pop culture, the Young Lords used every trick they could imagine to deal with issues of poverty, police brutality, and social inequality. The Yippies were primarily white, middle-class hippies and anarchists, while the Young Lords consisted of a cross-section of Puerto Ricans and Nuyoricans (New York Puerto Ricans). While the Yippies had no dress code, the Young Lords adopted the "revolutionary dress code of US Amy–issued field jackets, combat boots, and purple berets with a 'YLO' button" (Melendez et al., 2003, p. 94).

Despite these differences, the groups actually shared a number of similarities. Both had a knack for attention-grabbing gestures which highlighted social inequalities. While the Yippies threw cash at the New York Stock Exchange, the Young Lords piled garbage on Third Avenue and set it on fire when the city refused to pick it up (Lee, 2009). Both groups were heavily influenced by the Black Panther Party model of engaged praxis, linking tactics, including direct action, with community based direct services (Melendez et al., 2003). The Young Lords went as far as taking control of city medical equipment in order to make sure those who needed it got access. Echoing the Black Panthers, the Young Lords occupied a church and turned it into a children's breakfast program for its community (Lee, 2009).

For some in the group, the model of the Black Panthers was enough to inspire them to act. In the spring of 1967, the Black Panthers staged one of their most audacious actions—the choreographed entrance of armed Panthers into the California State Capitol building in Sacramento (Reed, 2005). A coast away a nineteen-year-old Bronx resident named Vicente "Panama" Alba watched the event on TV (Alba, 2004). For students of social movements, the Panthers' action is recognized as perhaps the most thrilling act of guerilla theater in history (Reed, 2005). "The guerilla theatre siege of Sacramento was one of many dramatic moments in what was a very dramatic time," Panama explained in our interview. Panama was mesmerized. Someone was actually fighting back, he thought to himself. Not long after, Alba quit heroin and joined the Young Lords. "I wanted to be a revolutionary, not understanding what it took. I started off wanting to fight; I was motivated by anger," noted Panama. "I started developing a love of people. And I realized that if you wanted to move people from where they were from to where they were going, you needed to have organizing." A conflict between love and anger characterizes much of Alba's story. Born in Panama City before immigrating to the Bronx in 1961, Alba began his political activism protesting against the Vietnam War. In 1970, he joined the Young Lords and supported their ambition to disrupt the oppressive mechanisms of everyday.

THE YOUNG LORDS: A DIFFERENT KIND OF DRAMA

Throughout most of our lives, there is something at play—sometimes it is a wave we hope to surf. When something important is taking place, we understand something is in play. During such moments, regular people find some element of agency. Here we imagine new ways of seeing things, new relations to the streets and our lives. As we play, we step away from stark reality and means or necessity to conjure up new possibilities for both the present and our common future. Much of the Young Lords story was about using any means necessary, from direct action to poetry, to put a more affirming future into play (see Chang, 2005).

The overlapping themes of culture and play, drama and street theatrics run throughout my interview with Panama Alba. When we talked about the Black Panther trip to the California statehouse bearing weapons, I referred to the action as a form of theater as Reed (2005) had. Alba respectfully disagreed with this interpretation. "Again, this is where you talk about the cultural difference underlying this. That was not theater. That shit was dramatic. There is a difference." Still, he acknowledged, "It was a dramatic moment so people interpret it as theater." As Alba's narrative suggests, understandings of play are culturally and contextually determined. Such differences highlight long-standing conflicts between theater and drama, play and political performance. After all, Johan Huizinga (1950, p. 17) reminds us "dramatization is played." While, *theater* implies more structure and an audience, *drama* involves individual action in a given social context. Drama is synonymous with creative play, which does not have to be structured or involve an audience. As Alba argued, the Black Panthers went in the statehouse in Sacramento with guns, but the action was not "structured" like a play such as Hamlet. The Black Panthers did not know how their performance was going to end. Yet, as it turns out, there was an audience. The whole media loved the stunt (Bogad, 2005b).

Such tensions have everything to do with the play of social movements. After all, "[t]he function of play can largely be derived from the two basic aspects in which we meet it: as a contest for something or a representation of something" (Huizinga, 1950, p. 13). Both elements were present in the Black Panther and later Young Lords confrontations with the police. Through such actions, the challenge or "game becomes a context for the best representation of something" (ibid.). Much of the play of movement messaging involves similar contests over meaning and representation.

I asked Panama about the line between work and play within the movements in which he worked. "The ones that used play were the Yippies, who had their parties in the Lower East Side," he explained:

> That appealed to the white youth. We were into the long hair, too. The most serious aspect of that was the antiwar piece. There was a lot of self-indulgence, a lot of theater, a lot of partying, free love, drugs, sex, and rock and roll. But as far as our communities were concerned, that was happening in conjunction with the rise of the civil rights movement and the Black Panthers, national liberation movements around the world, and empowerment struggles in our communities. That's very serious. That's life and death. You are talking about drug epidemics that were killing thousands; you're talking about poverty; you're talking about hunger; you're talking about racial discrimination, racial prostitution.

Still, an element of play was part of the scene: "The Young Lords," Alba paused before acknowledging, "had a bit of both. We came out of that time period. I remember many a time going to the office and we had the Stones and Santana blaring on the radio." Yet, the play was not a driving dynamic.

Unlike the ludic Yippies, the Young Lords practiced a starkly dramatic form of direct action-based street activism. On one occasion the group took over Lincoln Hospital to force the facility to become more responsive; on another, the group commandeered a medical truck so they could perform TB tests in their neighborhood (see Nelson, 2001; Perez, 2000). "We were action-oriented," explained Panama. "If a hospital was not working, we would make it work; if a janitor was refusing to make a repair in a building, we would organize a rent strike; if the trash men were not picking up the trash, we would burn the trash in the street until they picked it up." As Richie Perez (2000) wrote, "if confrontation or breaking the law was necessary to move an issue or campaign forward," the Young Lords were willing to do it. And tangible successes followed. Many of their proposals were later incorporated into city policy (Lee, 2009; Melendez et al., 2003). "In our community, what was effective was the dramatic," Panama recalled. "The garbage action was dramatic—and people could see the impact." For Alba, "all of those things had drama in them. But they were not theater pieces." The media gravitated to those actions and the community supported the group's efforts.

DAYS OF RAGE: VIOLENCE, COMMUNITY INVOLVEMENT, AND PREFIGURATIVE POLITICS

The Surrealists were quick to argue that lived fantasy should be part of social activism (Breton, 1924/1972). Dreams and schemes for building a better world often begin with fantasies (Duncombe, 2007). In 1971, the Young Lords planned for an action at the Puerto Rican Day Parade, which extended this line of thought. "We in the Young Lords were very clear on the role of the police" noted Panama. "We, as we say today, recognized them as an occupational force in our community and a source of brutality and death against people in our community." So, the group sent in "suicide squads" to push back the police who were leading the parade. "We were going to take the police head-on on Fifth Avenue to prevent them from taking part in the Puerto Rican Parade," Alba recalled. While the group felt the police had no right to lead the parade; this was not a consensus in the community. The action fell apart as soon as it began, as the police responded violently. "When they retaliated, they did not count who was carrying the purple beret. They started stomping over women with baby carriages, it was nasty," Alba explained. "And I guess in a sense correctly, the community held us responsible for that. And our relationship changed dramatically and forever after that Puerto Rican Day Parade," he lamented. "If we would have done the groundwork ahead of the time and made an effort to hear the needs and concerns of the people, things might have been different. We didn't have the right to risk the safety of everyone." After all, "That was not the understanding of the people."

Panama reflected on the emotions which inspired the action.

> By and large what happens is that people get to that point of consciousness very quickly when a loved one is victimized that way. We went and we planned this. I was invited to participate in a suicide squad in 1971. It wasn't killing, it was Weatherman-style direct confrontations with cops, with helmets ready to fight. We certainly had the right to attack the police, who treated us as colonial subjects. Yet I think again when you have clichés that say that 'true revolutionaries are guided by true feelings of love,' those clichés are way more than clichés. At least the way I think about that action is, there are a lot of levels of questions to think about. I think that a lot of us, myself included, who went into the Young Lords and went into the Black Panther Party, we were motivated by feelings of rage and anger.

Most certainly, there is a place for the kind of anger which inspires direct action (Neumann, 2000). But Alba is quick to differentiate: "You know, there is righteous anger and righteous rage. However, that should not be the driving force behind what you should do." Direct action involves any number of questions about strategy and tactics, as well as motivation.

While some view the practice in terms of its tactical application toward movement goals, others view it as a gesture of desire and freedom. Each approach has impacts and consequences. Each action creates a reaction and sometimes a backlash, as Alba conceded. "I think that the agents within the organization understood that that rage was there. That there was a propensity among us and some adventurism, and maybe some romanticism on some people's part," Alba confessed. "And we had just lived a year, two years [since] the Days of Rage in Chicago, and we should have learned."

In many ways, the 1969 Days of Rage, in which the WU confronted police in Chicago, and the 1971 Puerto Rican Parade actions helped activists confront the limits of a politics of rage. Such action was part of a lived dream. "Part of it was my own fantasy to fight back against the cops, who we viewed as our oppressors, by actually organizing a confrontation," noted Panama. He was not alone in feeling this way. "Fighting cops was romantic." "I tingled with freedom, it danced around and through me," mused Bill Ayers (2001, p. 71), who helped organize the Days of Rage. Many reveled in the 'freedom high' of the era (McAdam, 1988). Yet as Ayers (2001) started losing friends to this pursuit, the high turned to a jittery buzz of peaks and crashes. Fantasy inevitably recedes into stark reality. At least, this was the case for the Young Lords.

For Alba, the Puerto Rican Parade action was a tactical failure. "It violates every tenet of guerilla warfare that you are going to take on a better equipped and trained enemy than us. But we did all that." Yet, most importantly, "I think that revolutionaries who truly love their people judge their actions by how is it going to benefit the people you live with and you are fighting for." Alba conceded:

> The reason for the revolution is not so you can have an outlet for your rage. And I think that that coupled with ignorance, coupled with immaturity, coupled with police infiltration. And so we wound up in a place where we started battling with the police. Those of us that made it to the middle of the street got our asses whooped. We made a gallant effort at winning. But there was no fucking way we were going to do that.

The action had a wide range of impacts. "We brought on the wrath of the police department, not [just] on the Young Lords, but on the Puerto Rican community," Alba noted, acknowledging the unintended consequences. "The police fought back against everyone."

"Our goals, our values, our morality, must be visible already in our actions," philosopher Herbert Marcuse wrote after watching the social movements of the late 1960s (quoted in Neumann, 2000, p. 89). The Young Lords aspired to a similar sensibility. "The new man was not just against the state," Alba explained, echoing Marcuse's admonition: "The new human beings we want to create—we must already be these human beings right here and now" (quoted in Neumann, 2000, p. 89). "The struggle was also within," Alba reflected. "It was against the biases he had within the individual. The Young Lords was the first place I ever found open acceptance of gay people." For the Young Lords, "The question was, are you challenging the internal 'isms'—the racism, the homophobia, the sexism? We challenged internal forms of oppression and concepts of beauty—'ballo mallo, ballo bueno,' bad hair, good hair." Yet, the question was how to integrate such thinking into organizational practices so as to create a healthy movement culture. "It was about teaching people to use meetings in ways which were useful, without personal attacks."

All the while, the group, "refused to be limited to tactics that were defined as 'legal' as they intervened in the social issues of the day" (Perez, 2000). This approach presented a double-edged sword, producing some beneficial results as well as heat from agent provocateurs and other police. "I dare say that was quintessentially how the Young Lords were destroyed," Alba conceded.

Probably the most difficult outcome of the 1971 Puerto Rican Parade action was that it diminished much of the goodwill the group had garnered with earlier direct actions that served the practical needs of people in the neighborhood (Melendez et al., 2003). "People loved us," Panama lamented. "Before the Puerto Rican Day Parade, our community fed us, kept us warm, hid us when we had to run from the police. After that day, our relationship was very different."

For much of their short history, the group's actions helped fuse a love between community and group. In the years after their demise, this social eros continued in the movement's poetry and direct actions. Throughout the 1970s, Alba worked on multiple actions with a similar focus—to push his Young Lord counternarrative into the public sphere. In 1977, a group of former Young Lords hung a banner on the Statue of Liberty: "Everybody says that it was a Young Lords–type action—taking over the Statue of Liberty—but it was post–Young Lords. But the people who planned it and executed it were all Young Lords—Richie Perez, Mickey Melendez, and I." All three worried the action would not make the news. "We did not have a full sense of how dramatic something would be," mused Panama. They were not even sure *El Dario*, New York's Spanish-language paper, would cover it. As it turned out, "We were way off target. Photos of the Puerto Rican flag on the Statue of Liberty went around the world. People sent us front-page pictures from the Netherlands, everywhere. . . . In our imagination, we never dreamed it would go out like that."

The action helped build on an ever-expanding story, around which regular people could build meaning and connect with their own experience. Stories are reality-creating machines. "You gotta imagine it" Alba mused, acknowledging the storied dimension of his activism. "Eddy Tiguero used to say, 'we are writing a script.'" The elaborate banner drop was part of a larger solidarity-building effort, part and parcel of a culture of resistance, which included art, direct action, politics, poetry, music, storytelling, and mythmaking. Miguel Melendez's uncle, the legendary Puerto Rican jazz musician Tito Puente, even offered his band's services to play a free show to help those involved with the banner drop pay off their fines to the city (Melendez et al., 2003). Play supports movement action in any number of ways. Between the music at the meetings and the dancing and performances at fundraisers, play was part of what sustained the activism.

Throughout the mid-2000s, I worked in a syringe exchange program across the street from Lincoln Hospital. Panama served on our board of directors. Three decades after the Lincoln Hospital takeover, the neighborhood included the highest rates of homeless people coping with HIV and chemical dependency in the city. We used to circle, play drums and read poetry during our advisory meetings or memorials after one of the program members had passed. Some of these deaths involved HIV, Hepatitis C, or overdose. On one occasion, a transgender client was thrown out the window of a single-room-occupancy hotel. The despair was unending. Yet, group members knew they could make it through the grief when a chuckle or smile crept onto their faces during one of the memorials. And members knew they had faced the negative, moved through it, and come out the other side. The tenacity of those in the circle made the scene one of the most pulsing spaces I have seen. In their daily transforming of the negative into a new way of living, those in the program achieved a kind of magical power (Berman, 2007). Play and resiliency meander in any number of directions throughout social movements.

THE USE OF CULTURE

While the Young Lords had little interest in the ludic antics of the Yippies, elements of direct action, drama, and performance were integral parts of their activism. A great deal was in play. "What you had was the first generation on the mainland of a group of Nuyoricans (New York Puerto Ricans)," Alba explained. "There were some people who were very artistic. We had Pietri's poetry. What we didn't have was a cultural ministry. Yet we had cultural players." Poetry was part of propelling a worldmaking counternarrative of Puerto Rican identity.

In the summer of 1969, Pedro Pietri (1974) stood up at one of the first Young Lords rallies and read from "Puerto Rican Obituary," a poem about the complex relationship between New York and Puerto Rican identity. Like the banner drop eight years later, the poem would find an audience the world over. Today, the Nuyorican poetry remains a testament to a tragicomic panorama (Algarin and Pinero, 1975). Some have suggested that Pietri's poem helped launch this movement. Like Situationists and Surrealists before them, Pietri's poetry functions as an homage to the liberatory possibilities of the radical imagination. And the legacy of this writing, activism, and storytelling extended well beyond the life of the group itself (Chang, 2005).

IN THE END

The Young Lords did not last much past the early 1970s. Like many activist groups from that era, they were hounded by government provocateurs until they ground to a halt. Yet Alba continued his activism. In 1977, he was arrested and spent six months in jail for alleged ties to Fuerzas Armadas de Liberación Nacional. Five years later, he was acquitted. Alba was involved in two takeovers of the Statue of Liberty as part of campaigns supporting Puerto Rican nationalist prisoners and in support of the people of the island of Vieques. In 2003, the US Navy ended its training exercises in Puerto Rico. And Panama celebrated the culmination of years of activism. He remains active to this day.

In the years after 1968, the Yippies would welcome delegates with pranks and direct confrontations, or zaps, at most every major party convention over the next forty years. Highlights would include the RNCs in Kansas City in 1976, Dallas in 1984, one in their own backyard in New York in 2004 (Anderson, 2004), and St. Paul in 2008. Controversy never eluded the group. "We had a smoke-in at the DNC in 1972 and they said that the only issue was the war," Dana sighed. "The war, in case you didn't notice, is winding down and there were certain [other] issues, which we had put aside in 1968, but we never really dropped them." Many held a grudge over the Yippie frivolousness. "That wing of the movement sort of stayed in a snit over that. And we started organizing [marijuana] smoke-ins in 1972. . . . they didn't consider them to be socially conscious." Yet, they were mobilizing people. "We were getting thousands of people out for the 'wrong reasons.' But when you have ten thousand kids marching to Central Park, that's a hell of a community." The tension between ludic and more conventional forms of protest would continue. Still, the Yippies persevered, even when facing the blue meanies.

For Beal, the high point of the Yippies' playful zaps came at the 1976 RNC in Kansas City:

> The apogee, the highest point of the ludicrous protests, was the incident of the clowns. In 1976, Wavy Gravy ran a "Nobody for President" campaign. That was big that year. A lot of jokes about—Who's gonna solve all your problems?—nobody. And we were going around in clown noses. So it got to the point where the Kansas City police were going around arresting people for no reason and they kind of cornered people and they were down an alley, and real quick, Wavy Gravy handed out all these clown noses, and they got away. They didn't get beaten up. They didn't get arrested.

Such ludic approaches have often been recognized as useful tactics with which to play with power and elude social controls. Over the next three decades, similar ludic theatrics were employed by groups ranging from ACT UP to Reclaim the Streets and the Clandestine Insurgent Rebel Clown Army (highlighted in the later chapters of this book). Over and over, the tactic helped disarm political opponents and alter mechanisms of power. "It punctured the tension, particularly in that situation," Beal mused.

Yet, there were always those who opposed the liberatory politics of play. And even with the rise of a Temperance era Comstockery taking hold of New York's public commons, Dana continued his pot parades. By the late 1990s, the yearly parades resulted in hundreds of arrests. And the city sought to stop the rallies. "We have survived it," Beal reflected. "If there is one thing they cannot handle, it's a sustained campaign of civil disobedience." This was also the case in Vieques, Puerto Rico, when years of civil disobedience compelled the US Navy to stop its trainings there.

AFTERWARD

The Yippie and Young Lords stories offer countless insights about play in community organizing. One group rejected the lighter elements of the politics of play; the other advanced a framework for a politics of madcap antics. Both made use of drama and extreme situations, direct action and pranks, to plant ideas and stories into the public consciousness. In the years after the Yippies hit their peak, others built on Abbie Hoffman's prank-infused model and helped reinvent it. Hoffman passed in 1989 (Carr, 1993). Richie Perez, of the Young Lords, died in 2004. One of the first to speak about Perez was his longtime friend and fellow activist, Vincente "Panama" Alba.

After I finished the first draft of this chapter, I went over to the Yippie Museum to meet Dana Beal for dinner. At one point in the evening, Dana informed everyone that Stew Albert, one of the Yippies who had helped nominate Pigasus outside the Democratic National Convention, had died. "There are only a few of us left," Dana noted. "Stew Albert, 66, Dies; Used Laughter to Protest a War" was the headline for the *New York Times* obituary for the passing of the former prankster (Martin, 2006). The obit featured a gentleman smiling, surrounded by a multicultural crowd, as he burnt his draft card in front of a municipal building. It recounted Albert's absurdist lecture to the 82nd Airborne on the inherent lessons of the Lone Ranger during the march on the Pentagon in 1967. Ever the clown, Albert inspired laughter from onlookers even after he was arrested during the Pigasus stunt during the Democratic National Convention in 1968. Once out, he talked about the banter with the police while he was locked up. "I have bad news for you boys," he recalled a cop telling the arrestees. "The pig [which they ran for president] squealed on you" (quoted in Martin, 2006). While significant portions of the Left found them off-putting or insufficiently serious, at its core, the group articulated a philosophy which favored action and laughter rather than fear or guilt. Countless movements found this message inspiring. And these ideas moved through the tributaries of movements over the decades to come.

FROM RIOTS TO RHINESTONES

One evening while visiting Dana at 9 Bleecker, I sat chatting with a gentleman about Yippie politics, pot, Gay Liberation, and Harvey Milk. Shortly after finishing a joint, the man started to say good-bye. I asked his name again. Gilbert Baker, he told me, the designer of the Rainbow Flag now seen around the world.

After he left Dana posited that much of the ludic spirit of the Yippies continueed with Gay Liberation. Throughout the 1970s, play found its way into countless social and political expressions (Ginsberg, 1969/2001; Kantrowitz, 1977/1996; Takemoto, 2003). This spirit influenced both organizing and cultural production, including the participatory theatrics of San Francisco's Cockettes' shows and punk performances, which thrived within a similar DIY ethos (Marcus, 1989; Shepard, 2010; Cockettes, The, 2009).

In 1972, the Cockettes made a short film, *Elevator Girls in Bondage*. It embodied the era's campy endeavor to insert the right to fun into social struggle. "We carry the bags. We serve the meals. So why is it that we do not have the diamond rings, fur coats?" one of the gender-bending elevator operators pontificated in a dry soliloquy, delivered to a roomful of fellow elevator operators.

> It's because the bosses have ripped us off. We are but a few of the mighty new that is demanding the right to a decent salary, the right to medical care in case we get our teeth knocked out. And some fringe benefits like maybe a two day vacation once a year. Yea! (Cockettes 2009)

The room full of drag queens roared. She concluded: "All those rights, and above all, the right to have some fun every once in a while." The right to create something bigger and richer of lives and struggles accompanied much of the boundary-transgressing politics of the era (Shepard, 2009).

By the early 1980s, the dance of these movements increasingly found its way onto a tragicomic stage. And many of the most creative minds from the 1970s cultural activism were lost. The former leader of the Cockettes, Hibiscus himself, succumbed to the AIDS virus in 1983. "The article reporting his death in *The Village Voice* was the first time in print I saw the acronym 'AIDS,' followed by its then-obligatory parenthetical expansion '(Acquired Immune Deficiency Syndrome),'" wrote Samuel Delany (1998/2005). The endpoint of such politics tends to represent liberation from pain and alienation, liberation from isolation through innovation, connection, and community building. But play comes with its paradoxes: joyous possibility arrives in tandem with the specter of penalty, harm, even death. But who can resist its siren song? The AIDS years, of course, profoundly shifted our faith in, and understanding of, the politics of pleasure (Crimp, 2002). That is a story for the following chapter.

3 Send in the Clowns
Play, Pleasure, and Struggles against Oblivion

Everyone involved either was personally threatened, or people in their lives were threatened. It was very clear that . . . death was the alternative. It really was. Nothing motivates you like that.

—David Crane

You could not escape the stench of death. It was everywhere. Every meeting of ACT UP on a Monday night would begin with announcements of people who had died the week before. And these are people who just two or three weeks before you had been demonstrating with at the barricades. So, it doesn't get more real; it doesn't slap you in the face harder than that.

—Jay Blotcher

One of the things—among many talents—we, ACT UP, would have— and actually, this is something that was actually really key to the organization, in a funny way, which is that we played a lot together.

—Ron Goldberg, ACT UP Oral History Project, 2003

What I said to the police was, "Look, we're gay. We have tickets tonight for Bette Midler at Radio City Music Hall. We've got to get out of here soon if we're going to make it back to NY in time."

—Andrew Vélez to the police in Meriden, CT, after having chained himself and ACT UP colleagues to the entrance of a biotech company producing bogus medication

Andrew Vélez and company did make it to Bette's show on that evening 1992. Bette had long supported the queer public sphere, performing at the baths. Queers had long reciprocated, showering Midler with their love and support. When Vélez and his colleagues from ACT UP returned for their court date weeks after the concert, "the judge said that rather than being arrested we ought to be applauded for what we're doing as outstanding citizens and he totally threw the case out," Vélez recalled in our interview years later. Getting arrested and going to Bette Midler concerts—for many that was what queer activism was all about. Play, direct action, and performance were essential ingredients of the very serious, but sometimes campy, approach of the AIDS Coalition to Unleash Power (ACT UP) to fighting the AIDS carnage. Susan Sontag (1964/2001, p. 63) reminds us, "There is a seriousness in camp . . . and often a pathos." This was certainly the case with ACT UP.

For the Surrealists play was "a means to contributing to the solutions of the gravest problems of human existence" (Rosemont, 2002, p. 201). For ACT UP, play connected sex, power, and agency. In the face of a crisis which amounted to a struggle at the edge of an abyss, play would live up to its Surrealist promise. Facing oblivion, activists used every tool possible to take on this ever-elusive target. Sometimes, it functioned as a theatrical device, a performance used to communicate movement aims. In other cases, it served as a subversive tool used to support and sustain those in the movement; here it helped activists stay engaged in a highly complicated dance between illness and eros (see Marcuse, 1955; Shepard, 2009). Change the rules of the game, Surrealist Andre Breton admonished (1924/1972, p. 201). And this is what ACT UP tried to do. "After we kick the shit out of this disease, I intend to be able to kick the shit out of this system, so that this never happens again," ACT UP's Vito Russo (1988) declared, summing up the group's queer brand of solidarity. For the last two decades, ACT UP strived to live up to this sentiment.

There are other works which take on the group's tragicomic engagement in much richer fashion (Crimp and Rolston, 1990; Crimp, 2002; Epstein, 1998; Gould, 2009; Reed, 2005; Shepard and Hayduk, 2002; Shepard, 2009). This chapter highlights a small number of approaches used by ACT UP and other queer activist groups as means of resistance and survival. Some included clownish pranks; others squatting buildings. From agitprop to radical ridicule, safer promiscuity to sexual generosity—play found itself into any number of the group's approaches to activism and queer worldmaking. It was a key part and parcel of reversing a highly homophobic cultural script and challenging the insurmountable. This chapter highlights ways that it served as a bridge between the ludic practices of the Yippies and arts groups covered in the first chapters and the DIY Global Justice Movements considered in the remaining chapters. Here, ACT UP and queer direct action groups including OutRage and Stand Up Harlem integrated play into coherent organizing strategies, in which pleasure, possibility, and direct action helped get the goods.

PLAY AS POSSIBILITY, PLEASURE AS A RESOURCE

Social movement scholars often talk about resources to be mobilized (McAdam et al., 1988). For queers, one such resource is eros; pleasure is a resource (Shepard, 2009). It is a way to form relationships and connect distinct groups of people—who build communities that share certain commonalities, including a respect for pleasure, humor, and a recognition of similar forms of oppression. From Jose Sarria's arias informing Black Cat patrons of an imminent raid in postwar San Francisco to drag shows among military service members during the Second World War, play, pleasure, and camp have long served queers in a wide range of contexts (Boyd, 2003; Crimp, 2002; Newton, 1972; Shepard, 2009; Sontag, 1964/2001). "[D]rag performances, wherever they were held, inadvertently opened up a social space in which gay men expanded their own secret culture," wrote historian Allan Bérubé (1990, p. 72). He was referring to clandestine gays who served in the US armed services in WWII. "The joke was always on the unaware members of the audience—a subplot about homosexuality was being created right before their eyes and they didn't even know it" (ibid.). Here, camp was a tool to help those involved cope with an extremely complicated circumstance. "To view camp as, among other things, the communal, historically dense exploration of a variety of reparative practices is to be able to do better justice to many of the defining elements of classic camp performance," explained queer theorist Eve Sedgwick (1997). "[T]he startling juicy displays of excess erudition, for example; the passionate, often hilarious antiquarianism, the prodigal production of alternate historiographies; the 'over'-attachment to fragmentary, marginal, waste" (p. 28). The striking detail of the literary critic's erudite description offers a somewhat over-the-top hint into some of the life-affirming silliness of the performances of the camp genre. When notions of "'over'-attachment to fragmentary, marginal, waste" come to this writer's mind, images of countless performances, former drag icon Divine following a puppy before ingesting her "waste" in John Waters's 1972 film *Pink Flamingos*, or a man pissing on the stage at the Cock, a gay bar in the Lower East Side—these images flash across my mind. It is impossible to recall such moments without a smile (among other visceral responses). Nonetheless the effect is the same. Such performances function in a vexing context, in which laughter helps lighten up an awfully heavy, often very serious, and contradictory experience in living with both pleasure and oppression, an escape from an often hostile outside world. It is a reparative which keeps us moving, acknowledging our messiness and laughing at ourselves. And in this way play is relevant to multiple forms of activism, including the struggle against the AIDS carnage.

These lessons applied to the tragicomic struggle faced by those in ACT UP in any number of ways. "When you're dealing with something like that either you break down and cry and crawl into a hole or you stand up to it defiantly and you blunt the sadness with humor, sarcasm, with black comedy, drag, with defiant street theater," explained Jay Blotcher, the ACT UP media coordinator from some of its peak years.

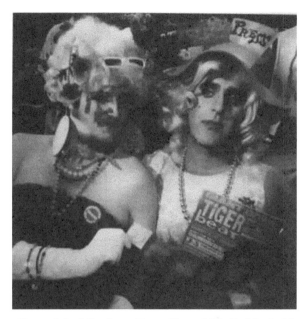

Figure 3.1   Miss Jesse Hems (l), and Media Mavis (r),
Tiger Beat reporter, at Wigstock 1989, New York City:
Ms. Jesse Hems is Leo, longtime activist and theatre
designer. Media Mavis is Blotcher. Used with permission
from the collection of Jay Blotcher.

Douglas Crimp elaborated on the point in his interview with the ACT
UP Oral History Project: "One of the things that I loved about ACT UP was
that it often undercut or punctured or criticized the kind of heroics of activism, even as it also enacted it; the kind of, the macho character of activism." That was absolutely necessary. "But, you also have to be self-reflexive
about that, and to recognize ambivalences" (Crimp, 2007, p. 43). Some
people in the movement were going to die, even those in the room with you
at the meetings. The space became almost unbearable for some and they
could not come back. "[T]he way in which the heroics got punctured by
Rollerena in drag on the floor, or the various jokes that were made, that
sort of punctured the inflated rhetoric, and so on; that's what made those
meetings pleasurable to me," mused Crimp (2007, p. 44). And, like many,
he was able to endure, even revel in that moment as the group embraced a
love of life, sex, camp, queerness, and a culture of resistance as they fought
the unending carnage (Crimp and Rolston, 1990; Crimp, 2002).
    Along the way, ACT UP helped inject queer activism "with a jigger of
play" (Takemeto, 2003). "[M]aybe because we are gay, maybe because we
were staring down death, a tradition of black comedy comes into play here,"

Jay Blotcher elaborated. It just became a way of looking at and living in the world. "And here these people were going about their lives when this epidemic moved in and either you ran away from it or you jumped in and said I'm going to beat the hell out of this thing." It was all part of coping. "A lot of us did this and we became self-educated, self-taught in how we deal with this." Yet, social connection among bodies kept the process going.

For many in the group the play was also about sex and vice versa (Foote, 1954). "[O]ne of the things I treasured in those years that I spent a lot of time around ACT UP was that it was a given that sexual freedom had to be defended in the face of a deadly epidemic and not just that, but the whole atmosphere," explained sexual civil liberties activist Bill Dobbs (2006, p. 18) during his interview for the ACT UP Oral History Project. "ACT UP was a bubbling cauldron of tremendous political energy and ideas and action, and flirting and cruising" (ibid.).

As the alchemy between the streets and the baths, the meetings and cruising congealed, a distinctive cultural politics took shape. This politics cultivated a rich cross-pollination of ideas and forms of social knowledge. "The great thing about ACT UP is it brought people in from all levels of life and disciples and schools of thought," explained Blotcher. He continued:

> There were some people who were very ardent, studied queer studies people, although queer studies hadn't really bloomed then, ardent black studies or political studies people. These people were real serious. They were serious as a crutch. They could recite letter and verse everything of Martin Luther King's "Letter from a Birmingham Jail." They could quote Henry David Thoreau "On Civil Disobedience" or "On Self-Reliance." And then there were some people who were very new age, who come from a love your neighbor, kumbaya. Then there were people who had been longtime activists since the 1960s, like Maxine Wolf. And then there were people who joined ACT UP who had this amazing lineage— Jim Fouratt and Mark Rubin and Arnie Kantrowitz and Bob Kohler. All these people who had either been in Gay Activist Alliance or Gay Liberation Front. You have to be really careful about which is which.

Much of the ACT UP political stew was born of the mix of ideas, practices, hopes, and aspirations. Many, such as Kendall Thomas, Lidell Jackson, and Douglas Crimp argued that the ACT UP meeting continued after the formal meet was over when people went out to dinner, to the bars, or the baths. "We were eating, breathing, sleeping, activism, and then activism went from the demos to the streets to the bedrooms," mused Blotcher.

Throughout these years, ACT UP helped support a distinct sexual politics. "First of all, ACT UP endowed us with a larger-than-life sexual persona," explained Blotcher. "We were not only fearless but we looked good [*laughs*]." Ann Northrop, the group's longtime facilitator, noted that ACT UP was the high school many in the group never had. Here, members of the group built a space to explore alternate social realities, reimagine possibilities, and create spaces for queer living. "We may have been shit under the heels of the jocks and the cheerleaders in high school, but in ACT UP we got to turn that around. We were the cool kids," Blotcher remembered. "When we talk about esprit de corps, we were not only knocking down political sacred cows, but also sexual. It was incumbent upon us to be sexual renegades." For Blotcher and company, there was an obligation to "play out all that talk about sexual liberation and freedom. We had to remind people that the epidemic did not immediately render sex evil." Sex was part of the game. "And so you would go to a demo with somebody, and then you would go to a bar with them, and then you would take them home."

Such play drew legions to the meetings. "It was recruiting. Michelangelo Signorile, I told him about ACT UP and he was all, yea, yea, yea," Blotcher continued. "And then he met a guy named Adam, who was a tall boyishly attractive boy from ACT UP who was out, somewhere in the bars talking it up. And that's what got Michelangelo there. All my beseeching didn't do it." Rather, the draw was "this marvelous aspect of sexuality, these pretty boys who were not only pretty but kick-ass activists." Cruising and organizing, organizing and cruising—the practice dates back to the Gay Liberation years of the 1970s. Some would argue this is part of why the movement has only grown over the decades (Shepard, 1997). It gets people out of the shops into the streets, meetings, and the movement. Certainly, it did with ACT UP. After all, pleasure is a resource.

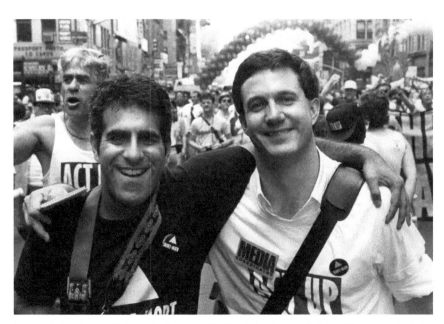

Figure 3.2 ACT UP March, June 1989. Jay Blotcher and ACT UP comrade John Voelcker. Pioneer activist Mark Rubin to the left. Play, camp, and friendship helped fuel ACT UP. Used with permission from the collection of Jay Blotcher.

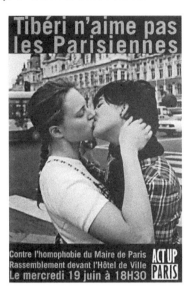

Figure 3.3   ACT UP Paris: "Tiberi does not like Parisian people!" Released when Tiberi was still mayor of Paris. A respect for pleasure (and a willingness to challenge the moralists) helped propel the group's work.

Others had little interest in cruising at the meetings. "I never did anything with anybody in that crowd. I was a real prude that way," David Crane, another early ACT UP member explained. "It was a pretty scary time too. It was difficult to reconcile . . . and all the activism against the disease, and just psychologically it was a really weird scene . . . all of this for me was sublimated into doing the work." Within that sublimation, a great deal of creativity took hold. Yet, even Freud (1961) acknowledged that not everyone could sublimate their desires into work. Instead, many played and experimented with those desires.

Here, boundaries blurred as new social relations took form. "There was John Kelly, one of ACT UP's logistics people, and he was a sweet, bearded, bespectacled Irish boy from Park Slope," Jay explained. "And when he got drunk enough, I got to suck face with John." Although technically John was "straight," Blotcher reveled in the understanding that this was not so important for those in the group. "It was like we're all together."

Politics, play, and pleasure overlapped with activism in any number of ways throughout those years. Take Lidell Jackson, a long-term New York queer activist. The founder of Jacks of Color—New York's longest-running sex party, run by and for men of color and their friends—explained that queers have always known they had to fight for the right to party. Building community through public sexual culture was a given. "And those of us who fought for it remember it very well. It took a lot of work to achieve the rights that we have nowadays," Jackson would note. Yet, to make that happen one needed to understand the politics of pleasure. "It took a lot of work just to have an environment and make it free for us to be able to have a good time. And be able to party with each other." You fight for it. Jackson was always up for that fight.

Play favors a level of freedom and authenticity not found in other experiences (Csikszentmihalyi, 1975). For Jay Blotcher, the joy of so many of the ACT UP moments, being arrested, then lined up in central booking, looking over at a buddy you slept with the night before and giving a wink, this was all part of ACT UP's distinct esprit de corps. "It has such a ferocious aspect to it," he would explain. "And it was so liberating and so enlightening and so exciting. It insinuated itself into every moment."

Through such interactions, the group set the stage for a series of innovations in organizing with alternative forms of power. "We were blacked out, stigmatized by the mainstream media," Jay Blotcher recalled. "So how do you get their attention? You do it with theater. We realized that we had to create great spectacles in the streets in order to get attention." So the group looked to a distinct quasi-Situationist approach to stage street spectacles (Tatchell, 2000). More than entertainment, the aim of the group's camp, stand-up comedy, and agitprop theater was to take down their opponents a notch, as well as communicate a message. Several observers have come to describe such endeavors as "serious play" (Bogad, 2005a; Weissman, 1990). Through such practices, social actors utilize whatever ideas they have to communicate ideas and cultivate new social possibilities (Alinsky, 1989; Schechner, 2002). Along the way, the group's work and play helped shape a collective counter-narrative to a predominantly homophobic cultural script (Gamon, 1991).

"Watching these people become radicalized," mused David Crane. "There were so many people who were writers and in media, as well as lawyers and accountants, people who knew how the system worked and how to make the system work the way they needed it to work." In his twenties at the time, Crane recalled a feeling of awe. "This was like, Wow! This is how the world works."

One of the group's most significant moments would take place in 1989 with the action, Stop the Church. "It was clearly going to be a big event. We were clearly going to be attacking a big controlling interest and it was clearly going to be a defining moment of some sort," David Crane recalled. The plan was to zap St. Patrick's Cathedral during high mass. To do so the group borrowed from a tradition of radical ridicule to undermine the authority of political opponents. "It wasn't going to be about trying to get the president to say the word 'AIDS' like in our initial skirmishes. As a Catholic I was excited by it, but I also really knew what they were up against."

With word of O'Connor's endorsement of the violent tactics of Operation Rescue, members of ACT UP targeted his church. "The fact that the cardinal was so outspoken and really had so much influence made him a target. And a legitimate target," explained Crane. With the mayor and cardinal working in close alliance, discussion of effective HIV/AIDS and reproductive health policies was subsumed within a moralist discourse which had more to do with repressive politics than effective public health. "It was an evil group that explicitly wanted to punish women, that's what it was all about," explained Crane. "All of the rhetoric of punish women, it was men who controlled the organization . . . punish the wayward women who are getting pregnant, make them have their babies. There was nothing about taking care of their children. It was awful, horrible." Like many in ACT UP, Crane had also been involved in reproductive rights advocacy and specifically clinic defense. There he had seen Operation Rescue firsthand. So, when he heard Operation Rescue was going to be at Stop the Church, Crane joined the affinity group organizing to challenge their moral high ground. "You know, the power of ridicule," Crane explained. "I've come to realize how powerful that is. So we dressed up as clowns and we were Operation Ridiculous." The point was to take away their legitimacy, to make fun of them. Such forms of guerilla theater have come to be described as 'radical ridicule' (Bogad, 2005a).

Before the action, the group published its manifesto. "We are Operation Ridiculous. We are comprised of members of ACT UP and WHAM [Women's Health Action Mobilization]. Our mission is to diffuse the energy of the flag-waving, fetus-loving, bible-thumping bigots, we go where no clown has gone before." The manifesto included a clear rationale for the clown action: "It's ridiculous that inert tissue masses are considered more vital than the rights of living women." Further, "It's ridiculous that Operation Rescue—a predominantly white group—preaches carrying all pregnancies to term, while a majority of them are of color." They concluded: "Calling all clowns! Calling all clowns. It's time for Operation Rescue to rescue this demonstration from the hands of the cops" (Diva TV, 1990).

The day of the action, Ray Navarro dressed as Jesus to do color commentary for ACT UP's DIVA TV. Members of Operation Ridiculous arrived dressed as clowns, performed clown skits, and ran around with little doll babies—all highlighting the church's support of social control rather than women's lives. The antics included their own version of the old clown taxi routine, in which Operation Ridiculous members drove a taxi up to St. Patrick's before moving their routine inside the church. With microphone in hand, Navarro interviewed members of Operation Ridiculous. "We're doing this for you, Jesus," one female clown confessed running through the streets to the roars of the crowd before being taken down by a group of five policemen (Diva TV, 1990).

Crane chanted "Save the Babies, Save the Babies" while waving an Ernie doll with a bumper sticker on his chest with the words: "Abortion on Demand Without Apology." He described the scene:

> It didn't get inside the church. It got up front. I was a support person, I had to avoid arrest so I could make sure that they all got out. Had

coffee and donuts when they got out. But since there were no [counter] demonstrators to speak of, and it was impossible to get across Fifth Avenue, because they had barricaded all of Fifth Avenue, they decided to entertain the troops, so they go around the corner, like Sixth Avenue, hop in some taxis, and convince the taxis to go up and down Fifth Avenue, and then they got to like 50th, 51st Street there. So the taxi doors open, and clowns bounded out, and are galloping down the street with the Keystone Cops in hot pursuit, you have three thousand people on the avenue roaring their approval at these antics that the cops had inadvertently participated in.

Of course, this humor did not prevent the police from chasing down and arresting numerous clowns rushing through the streets amid the carnival-like topsy-turvy atmosphere outside the church. "I don't remember who had the idea, but when they said it. I thought, 'Oh my god. Clowns bounding out of taxis pursued by the Keystone Cops. That'll be beautiful circus theater,'" Crane mused. "And the cops played right along with it, and they arrested every damn one of them."

ACT UP was quite useful at using clowning to punch holes in social pretense or to highlight the flaws in a social policy. Operation Ridiculous was not the only occasion when the group made use of radical clowning. Other highlights included the "Send in the Clowns" demo in Washington, DC, when members wore clown masks during a congressional hearing, mirroring what they considered the lunacy of a reactive, moralistic policy approach (see Shepard, 2009).

Countless activists weighed in on the merits of the Stop the Church action. Many, such as Ann Northrop and Charles King, of ACT UP and Housing Works, view it as perhaps the best thing ACT UP did (see Shepard, 2009). Others, such as David Crane, thought the action was a disaster. Crane was critical of the tactics used inside the church to disrupt the service (see Crimp and Rolston, 1990). Coordinating the politics of play and performance is anything but simple.

Others such as Jay Blotcher, who coordinated media for the event, felt it helped propel ACT UP's narrative across the world. "This was beamed all over the planet. They saw angry fags. People had only seen what they thought gay people were, limp-wristed little nellies. And God knows, we are. And [the church action] showed them that we were a formidable adversary," Blotcher explained. On a large scale and small, something changed after that action. Blotcher was told about an exchange that came up at a card game in tony Putnam County shortly after the action. "One of them said, 'You know, my son was part of that.' And the others said, 'You know, I didn't realize gay people could be so angry.'" The image of queer people, as was an understanding of the epidemic, was changing, "because our demonstrations and because of our media." Shortly after Stop the Church, Jason Deparle's (1990) favorable story on the group ran in the *New York*

Times. And the group started receiving more sympathetic treatment in public opinion. "And the perception changed and people started to think, oh well, I guess we have to take these people seriously," Blotcher observed. And ACT UP's perspective helped shape AIDS policy on city, state, federal, and international levels for the next two decades (see Shepard, 2009; Shepard and Hayduk, 2002).

OUTRAGE AND ORGANIZING

Of course, ACT UP was not the only queer direct action group to recognize the utility of play as an organizing tool. "Protests should, wherever possible, be fun as well as serious. That means making them enjoyable for those who take part and witness them," argued Peter Tatchell (2000), of the British direct action group OutRage! "This exultation of 'politics with pleasure' runs against the grain of mainstream political campaigning, which tends to be predicated on duty and sacrifice. Usually involving boring, repetitive methods, conventional politics can also be quite aggressive, with a strong streak of machismo." In order to avoid such pitfalls, organizers with OutRage! turned to play, camp, and pleasure (see Lukas, 1998). They saw them as distinct components of a coherent organizing framework which included the following elements:

> A fusion of art with activism.
> Re-inventing the queer tradition of camp and theatricality.
> Acting out protest as a form of performance.
> The politics of pleasure and the pleasuring of politics.
> Claiming queer space.
> Challenging homophobic institutions and laws. (Tatchell, 2000)

Here, pleasure found its way into much of OutRage's organizing strategy. By extension much of this organizing involved establishing a clear goal, research about the goal, connection with the strengths of the culture and community impacted, mobilization to move the goal, direct action, short- and long-term legal strategies, and an ethos of fun to sustain a campaign. "Why have a march, we ask, when you can have a spectacle?" Tatchell pontificated. "What's the point of boring the pants off passersby if you instead give them political entertainment that makes them stop, listen, and think?"

ACT UP organized in similar fashion. "ACT UP was trying to figure out how to dramatize as many actions as possible," explained Mark Harrington, who briefly worked with one of ACT UP's visual collectives, Gran Fury. For example, ACT UP fused art with activism during the Nine Days of Action in 1988. "They thought if they did nine different days all in a row, focusing on different issues like homophobia, so they had a kiss-in, or syringe exchange, or men use condoms or beat it," explained Harrington. "A lot of the posters came out of that period." The posters accomplished a number of things simultaneously linking ACT UP's queer politics with a politics of pleasure, claiming queer space, and effective movement messaging. At its essence, art was most effective in terms of communicating activist messages, explained Jay Blotcher: "We realized that not only was dissemination of information important but the tone of the information, the tone of the urgency, was important, and then you had to make it colorful. That's where the graffic artists came in," Blotcher said, citing artists artists such as Gran Fury, Ken Woodard, Vincent Gagliostro, and Avram Finkelstein. "These are people who created these really vibrant stickers and posters," Blotcher said (For an overview of art and graphics in ACT UP, see Crimp and Rolston, 1990.)

Harrington, who went on to found the Treatment Action Group, described his work with one of these groups, Gran Fury. "They were temporarily open for new members and I had heard about it. I had a photo with me; it was like a World War II porno photo of two sailors kissing. That was when we made the 'Read my Lips' poster."

Throughout these years, ACT UP and OutRage "had remarkable success in profiling lesbian and gay issues and contributing to changes in public opinion," noted Peter Tatchell. "This must, surely, have something to do with the group's style of campaigning? Whatever its shortcomings, OutRage's 'art of activism' shows that politics doesn't have to be boring, miserablist, or unpopular."

Some of ACT UP's most vital actions built on the Situationist tradition of disruption of everyday life as a form of performance. Patrick Moore, another ACT UP veteran, was a part of the group's Days of Desperation Action, when thousands disrupted rush hour, blocking signs and entrances for trains, creating havoc at Grand Central Station on January 23, 1991. While intended as a nonviolent action, the violence of the commuters was of an intensity few had seen. While being kicked, Patrick Moore sat on the floor of Grand Central terminal and watched as commuters "like a stream of ants, began to literally climb over our bodies. ACT UP had created the perfect metaphor for AIDS in their country—normal Americans were willing to literally walk over our bodies while ignoring AIDS" (Moore, 2004, p. 142). While some questioned the utility of blocking access to public transportation, Moore viewed the action in aesthetic terms. "ACT UP at that moment had crossed into the realm of art," Moore reflected. "Day of Desperation had ceased to be about tangible activist goals: it had become a huge performance, a theatrical event designed to express desperation and rage. It will remain emblazoned in the memories of all those who participated" (ibid.). For Moore, that was a moment when his generation achieved something of a transcendent art. "It was, in fact, the first moment in my life when I felt pride rather than shame" (ibid., p. 143).

ACT UP and OutRage were by no means the only queer groups to integrate cultural activism and organizing. "I was one of the founders of a lesbian and gay gospel choir," recalled Lidell Jackson.

> I kept saying to them, "Every time you go out on stage to sing gospel, no matter how much you enjoy it, and no matter how much the audience enjoys you, and no matter how great it is, remember you are making a political statement. You are a lesbian and gay gospel choir. There has never been a lesbian and gay multiracial gospel choir, so you are making a huge political statement. Don't just sing because you love gospel music, sing because you are proud that you can do it."

Such performances overlap with mechanisms of cultural resistance, which have long propelled movements. Part of their efficacy stems from the joyful sounds, rather than the shrill tones which typically accompany social protest (Duncombe, 2002a). Such forms of resistance help actors to play with issues and reimagine social discourses (Shepard, 2005). They would remain a vital tool in the activist toolbox, even as AIDS activism overlapped within a struggle for the most basic of human needs: to find a place to call home.

SQUATTING, BUILDING, AND SUCCEEDING

Queer activists have long recognized that AIDS was a housing issue. Housing was often the difference between living and dying. Members of the ACT UP Housing Committee came from a wide range of direct action projects, some in harm reduction, others in the squatter movement in New York. A thread which runs through these movements, of course, is the desire to change the rules of the game of urban life so the poor and the marginalized do not constantly face the brunt edge of the system. A digression into the struggle for housing situates a larger struggle to find solace in a neoliberal world. Here, activists have long battled to create alternate social relations where use is favored over exchange and regular people can access places to live and thrive (Holtzman et al., 2004).

Cities as diverse as Hamburg, Amsterdam, and New York City have all had contemporary squatting movements (Abu-Lughod, 1994; Smith, 1996). Seth Tobocman was one of the many artists who brought their aesthetic sensibilities to the squatter movement in New York City in the late 1980s and early 1990s. He worked with the December 12th Movement and with the ACT UP Housing Committee to target the Department of Housing Preservation and Development. He also worked with squatters to help bring art into the DIY push for housing. "That made the building more imaginative," Tobocman said. "The meaning of the phrase 'direct action' was right there."

Throughout the years, art and even play found their way into the Lower East Side squatter struggle. The atmosphere became quite tense throughout these years between riots and ensuing battles over the remaining squats in the city in the late 1980s and 1990s (see Patterson, 2007; Tobocman, 1999).

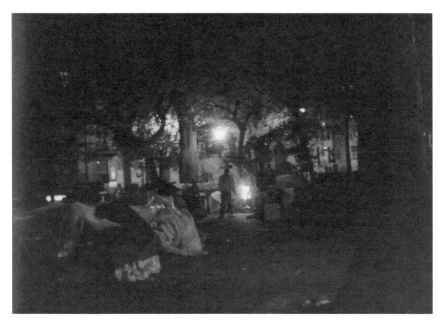

Figure 3.4 Tompkins Square Park Tent City 1990. Clayton Patterson archive. After years of underfunding for social services, many turned to the park for housing.

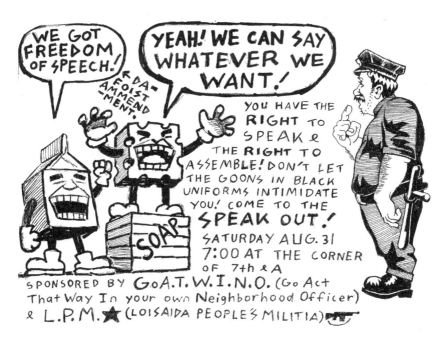

Figure 3.5 Seth Tobocman and Jordan Worley, Milk and Cheese speak-out flyer.

According to Tobocman, it was 1995 when the city had just evicted three squats and mass arrested a group of people after a speak-out. "No more demonstrations," the police told demonstrators. Yet, no one wanted to back down. Still, some of the squatters understood that things needed to chill out a little bit. Nonetheless, they still wanted to do demonstrations. So, Tobocman and fellow squatter/garden activist Michael Shenker came up with the idea of a joke protest under the theme "A Speak-Out with Milk and Cheese." These were two comic book characters, like the Three Stooges. "The kids understood they were violent characters," Tobocman explained. But, to everyone else, they looked like harmless comic book characters. The police were drawn to the call for the action, sketched by Tobocman, listing a wild range of outlandish groups, including the "LPM—Loisaida People's Militia." The police arrived in force. What they saw were two puppetlike characters carrying signs with the words "A Slice of Spite and a Carton of Hate." Shenker led the speak-out, dressed up as one of the characters. The performance seemed to disarm the police, who realized they had been played. "It allowed us space," Tobocman reflected. And the demonstrations continued.

Still, only some squatters considered play a part of the struggle. "There wasn't a lot of it," argued squatter Michael Shenker, who took part in the Milk and Cheese speak-out. "Our survival was not dependent upon it. I think it's a very brief phenomenon. I don't think it's going to make much of a difference." Shenker's answer speaks to the complex interplay between play and more conventional organizing. "We did a lot of art," he would explain, acknowledging the ways elements of culture—music and cultural production—wound themselves throughout the movement. "Visual artists were particularly effective," Shenker acknowledged. "We did a particular amount of propaganda, which was influential for people. It opened up people's minds. So visual arts were effective [with] concerts." The ludic dimension was less a part of his activism. "[T]he spirit of levity, which often accompanies play, was diminished by the seriousness of the endeavor," Shenker noted. "Some people died. Homelessness kills." The stakes were often extremely high. "[O]ur struggles in the buildings sometimes came down to physical confrontations, beatings; cops got beat; it wasn't something to rejoice about," he continued. "The result of a failed action had a direct impact, which was that people were in the streets. Sometimes they go to jail and when they get out all their belongings have been taken out of their home. So, it wasn't too joyful." Paradoxically, "We had a blast the whole time. It was like fun," recognized Shenker, acknowledging play was actually a part of this life-and-death struggle. "Yeah, it was a pain, but the other side of that was great joy and pleasure." When asked about his best experiences with the use of creativity in his work, Shenker smiled and noted: "Incredible culture, too, smoking parties and stuff like that. So there was a great deal to this. It was a great time. The stakes were incredibly high. You could lose your apartment if you had a bad demo."

Throughout the period, groups around the city joined the fight for housing. Some built on the lessons of ACT UP; others the squatter movement. Stand Up Harlem built on both. This direct action housing group was founded by longtime harm reduction activist Louis Jones. As we sat to talk, Jones, whom I'd known for years, looked me in the eye. He'd lived with HIV since 1986 and hepatitis C since 1999, he explained as we began. Fear of death had long stopped being part of the picture. "But then you find yourself still alive . . ." Jones ruminated.

Like Panama Alba, Jones was mesmerized by the Black Panthers. His influences ranged from Martin Luther King to Louis Farrakhan and the revolutionary books he carried to school. His first organizing was squatting a building on Sixth Street between Avenues A and B in New York's East Village. Coming out of this experience, Jones was "hooked." Yet "it all came together in East Harlem." Here, ideas intersected with action as he opened a homeless shelter for mothers at 144th and Lexington. "That to me felt so incredible. You talk about emotions. I just felt such pleasure. Everyone thinks about pleasure in terms of decadence, but there was more to it than that. I was moved." After a lifetime of searching, he had found something really meaningful. "It brought fulfillment. I felt animated. We were living together, sleeping together, and working for change. We were part of something very global, a global movement. Yet our take was from the local view, as the cliché goes." The DIY ethos of the housing movement proved thrilling. "Give us the resources and we can do this," he explained.

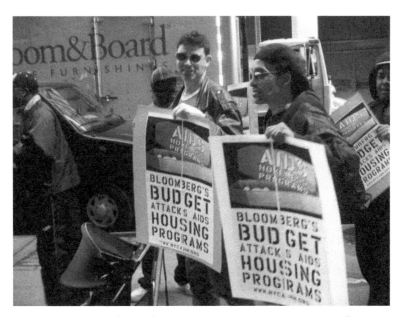

Figure 3.6   The author and Louis Jones at an AIDS Housing Rally 2009. Photo by Sean Barry/NYCAHN.

As the HIV/AIDS crisis set in, Jones was forced to cope with the looming catastrophe. "In the beginning, it was primarily a homeless movement. We marched from New York to DC. The Center for Non-Violence organized that in 1989." And still, "my colleagues, compatriots were dying. It was very scary. Yet I could not break my denial or speak out about having HIV myself . . . And I was angry," Jones explained. "That was one feeling I was in touch with." He'd recently come into contact with ACT UP.

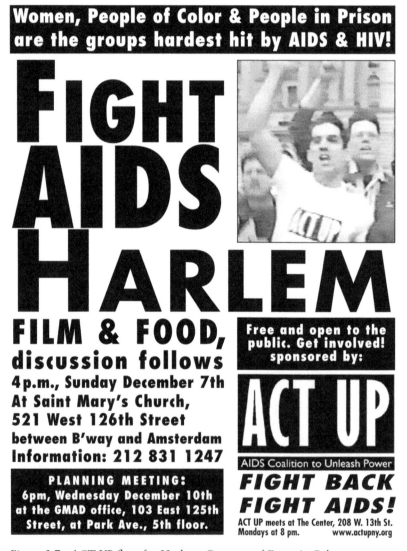

Figure 3.7   ACT UP flyer for Harlem. Courtesy of Emmaia Gelman.

So many people living and dying with HIV. Yet no one was saying anything. At a memorial for yet another lost friend, "I was moved to stand up and break the isolation." Stand Up Harlem was born of that moment.

The founders of the group lived, worked, and played together. "Somewhere along the way, we did find ways to deal with the tension 'cause we were living together at 160 West 120th Street," Jones explained. "We'd just get out of the house." Faced with illness and death, the group members required an outlet. "One of us would say, 'Let's get out of here.' So we got out of the house and walked." One day stood out. "We just started out, not knowing where, and ended up in a school yard, where we played on the swings and seesaws. And there were some tough guys, just out of the joint, acting like children . . . feeling good." It was pure play. Everyone needs to play. Not just children. After telling this story, we paused for a minute. Jones broke from the narrative and looked right at me. "Thanks for letting me remember that, 'cause most of those guys are dead now," he said, feeling the memory of the play and work, meaning and human solidarity of the movement.

"In the struggle, we had a philosophy of common living: 'Not for everyone, but something for everyone.' We would never refuse anyone." This low-threshold approach to serving everyone who walked in the door anticipated elements of the harm reduction movement that would emerge as a best-practice approach to providing services and care for people with HIV/AIDS. "We acknowledged that there is drug use, and tried to integrate it. Our view was there is a time and place for everything. So let's reduce the risks."

I asked Jones about the notion of harm reduction as pleasure activism. "We were not all work. We were play, pleasure people too. But we were not all that balanced," Jones explained. "We worked hard but we also played hard. Sometimes it was just to go out in the country and breathe. That experience of pleasure was so essential." Jones noted, "[Y]ou have to understand, we were dealing with our mortality here. There is the old expression, 'drink and be merry for tomorrow we die.'" The full expression is, of course, "we should enjoy life as much as possible, because it will be over soon" from the books of Ecclesiastes and Isaiah. The point that one should enjoy whatever of life one has in a given moment was not lost on Jones or others in the nascent movement. "I don't think we do acknowledge the pleasure, though, not as much as we should," said Allan Clear, another ACT UP veteran, now active in the harm reduction movement.

Here, drug use was viewed as part of a continuum of options, which ranged from seeking pleasure to stopping pain to sometimes just "getting normal," as Jones explained:

> Using was dying with dignity—with dignity because it was my choice. No one was making it for me. For those I knew who chose drugs when they were facing death, they would want to cop in the midst of all that pain. For some it was just to get that old familiar, this old feeling, relationship, lover, what have you. This pain relief that the doctor

might not give or it might not be enough. And this was not from a pharmacy. It was on your own terms. The liberty was what I was elated about—the choice without shame. The idea was I had choice. That was what I was doing. . . . And culturally, that was another thing. It was always part of saying good-bye at the funerals. As they say, doors close and open. The New Orleans thing. Drugs and pleasure were part of it even with recovery folks. 'Social rec' was another notion I really liked, the idea of social recreational drug use. It was about connecting with someone else, taking a bag, listening to music or watching a DVD, to get the full range of experience with no regret.

In this way, pleasure was part of an affirmation of self-determination; it was a rejection of shame.

I asked Jones about the notion of risk and risky play, themes which came up in several interviews. "Risk was always a part of it. I loved the risk, the hustle of getting my way into housing when I had nothing else," he explained. For Jones, a willingness to take risks was part of changing the rules of the housing game in New York. Like the Situationists, Jones recognized he could borrow from established rules and turn them upside down (Lasn, 1999; Vaneigem, 1967/2003). Doing so, Jones contributed to a movement which shifted the patterns and policies of everyday life among drug users and housing providers. In the decades to come, harm reduction would become an increasingly accepted model of service provision.

Throughout our interview Jones talked about the film *The Spook Who Sat by the Door.* Part of the late 1960s "Blaxploitation" genre, the film explores the fictional life of an African American FBI agent, Dan Freeman, who uses his training as a spy to support a Black revolutionary insurgency. Louis Jones's work with Stand Up Harlem echoed Freeman's approach. Having witnessed the workings of the housing game, Jones felt comfortable making use of these tools to procure housing for those most in need: "I would talk my way into places, bluffing, get the keys, and then the money would show up at the eleventh hour." For Stand Up Harlem, the point was to use direct action to get housing for those with few other options.

"[W]hat we wanna create is a new nation," Freeman declared toward the end of the movie. "In order to do that, we gotta pay a different kind of dues. Freedom dues" (quoted in Fuchs, 2004). The "freedom dues" for Stand Up Harlem were that virtually all of the original members are dead, with the exception of Jones, who has lived with their memories for the last two decades. I recall standing with Jones, with tears running down his face, as names of members of the group were read at World AIDS Day in 2001. Yet, the memories of the group's work and play continue to drive Jones, who today works with the New York City AIDS Housing Network/ VOCAL. One day the group members would get arrested or fight for housing. "The next day we'd lie in the grass in the park," Jones recalled. "There is this photo of us all laying in the grass with the light shining on our faces.

If ever there was a group of people who needed to live it was us, a group of people who were dying." By the late 1980s, the squats such as those organized by Jones would increasingly become the subject of attention by the NYPD. The housing game was changing. No one was sure if it was for the better.

RIOTS AND OVERLAPPING INFLUENCES

August of 1988, the New York Police Department cracked down on the homeless people staying in Tompkins Square Park in the Lower East Side. January 1990, they evicted the tent city in the park. Shortly after the eviction, members of ACT UP held a demonstration in support of the arrestees (Patterson, 2007). Throughout this period, conflicts between the park users, the homeless, and the police only increased (Mattson and Duncombe, 1992).

In the years to follow, ACT UP spawned a generation of direct action groups (Shepard and Hayduk, 2002). And approaches to dealing with this challenge overlapped. Some, such as Jay Blotcher, remained active members of ACT UP and its Housing Committee spin-off Housing Works, which was located in the Lower East Side. Others, such as David Crane and Steven Duncombe, joined the Lower East Side Collective, the subject of the following chapter. Squatter Bill DiPaulo participated in ACT UP's actions with an eye toward learning something from a group which never asked for permission to take a street. "I think that that was sort of the genius of ACT UP, that they were and continue to be so theatrical, but it's combined with a lot of organizational discipline," explained Lower East Side playwright and activist Jason Grote. Like Jason Grote, Bill DiPaulo was in awe of ACT UP's organization. "They did these marches; they did direct action. For me, there was no group even close to the efficiency of how to organize." DiPaulo attended countless ACT UP demonstrations. "I tried to support them with technical stuff, but mostly I studied them."

Building on these lessons, DiPaulo would start his own group.

> Around twenty years ago, I started a group called Time's Up! And I didn't think there was enough direct action. And I saw a niche. It was like, Time's Up!, what a great name. So with that a lot of the activity and the community was in the East Village, which was really important. A lot of what we were going to do was like the Lower East Side Collective where there was a decision-making process that would be much more like a community decision-making process. And I knew that people couldn't get paid so I knew they would have to be volunteers.

In order to attract people to his new group, DiPaulo tapped into the ludic spirit he'd seen within ACT UP and later with the Critical Mass bike rides taking place in San Francisco. "I was doing parties. The thing is the people who are activists are usually, I hate to say it, are really boring, people who are brainiacs." This would have to change if more people were going to get involved. "So, early on, I was always very interested in whatever event we are doing, making it fun." Yet, if people stood behind barricades or walked in a circle screaming, then street protest lost any sense of a feeling of freedom or vitality; activists became targets. DiPaulo explained: "The police were trying to harass people at events, I was at these animal rights events, everyone's screaming behind the barricades at us 'get a job,' so I realized that to make it fun it should be moving." For DiPaulo, the problem with a lot of activism of the era was: "It just was too stationary. It was behind a barricade, and it was too intense for people, and so I realized that the whole idea of motion and fun would be probably something that I was very interested in developing." In the years to come, DiPaulo injected this approach into his work with countless groups—including Lower East Side Collective, Reclaim the Streets, and Time's Up! And activism started to be more fun.

David Crane left ACT UP after the Stop the Church action. For him, ACT UP's work was done. "I've been on AZT for a decade and it's fine for me. And the fact that other treatments came out there, there were treatments that were getting into people's bodies early. So that battle had been won," he explained. "So I started looking for things that I could do that were more local."

In the following years, the cultural impacts of ACT UP found their way into countless movements. "I think the whole world's sort of going queer. Gender is no longer a big issue with most people, especially young people. I'm amazed at how open they can be. There's a certain joy in seeing someone gender-bending in pop culture," Crane reveled. "I never expected that would happen. Some people love it."

By the late 1990s, the yearnings for joy and justice, connection and pleasure seen with ACT UP found their way into any number of new movements. Here, activism looked to: "music, dance, sexuality, and humor to decommodify pleasure and liven up resistance" (Yuen, 2004, p. xii). Much of this ethos took shape in a nascent struggle for public space extending from old growth forests of the West Coast to the community gardens of the Lower East Side of Manhattan.

4   Play as Community Building
From Gardens to Global Action

> Basketball players of the world unite; you have nothing to lose but your coaches, your bosses and your landlords.
>
> —Bertrell Ollman (2005)

> [T]he spirit they share is a radical reclaiming of the commons . . . As our communal spaces—town squares, streets schools, farms, plants—are displaced by the ballooning marketplace, a spirit of resistance is taking hold.
>
> —Naomi Klein (2004, pp. 220–21)

Years before rumblings about a Global Justice Movement, New Yorkers found themselves entwined in struggles over housing, land use, public space, and community gardens. Born out of the vacant lots and rubble of the fiscal crisis years in the mid-1970s, community gardens in New York had long been playgrounds for creative expression and community building. These were spaces for people to come together to share a moment without paying an entrance fee. They were spaces for BBQs, performances, and conversation; here use was valued over exchange (Holtzman et al., 2004; Merrifield, 2002). And developers hated them.

For New York activist Brad Will, they were a place "for a fresh mix of direct action (with puppets) and lobbying with love for the land" (Notes from Nowhere, 2003, p. 136). They were also places for play.

One of the groups which championed the gardens was the Lower East Side Collective (LESC), the subject of this fourth chapter. "The fight over community gardens in New York City in some ways was a very local community fight, with purely local relevance, and yet it was more than that," explained LESC member L.A. Kauffman (2004, p. 377):

> From 1997 to 1999, that campaign pulled a lot of new people into activism and, as far as the East Coast was concerned, was a real incubator for the kinds of creative political energies that were expressed in the Seattle WTO protests, and in the big trade summit protests. Many of us who were working on the garden fight took inspiration from ACT UP and a lot of other direct action movements that had come before us.

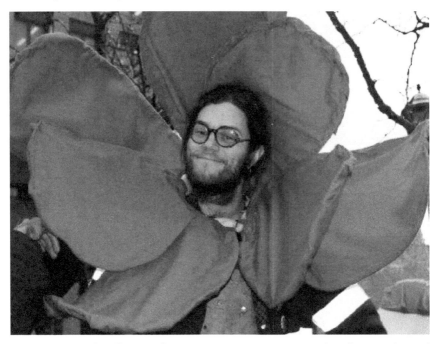

Figure 4.1   Brad Will as Sunflower. Lower East squatter Brad Will was a devoted garden activist and devotee of Emma Goldman's "If I Can't Dance" ethos. Courtesy Aresh Javadi of More Gardens.

Here, a new movement connected battles over public space, including vacant lots turned green spaces on the East Coast with Earth First's struggle to save old-growth forests on the West. "There were people who shuttled back and forth between the New York City community garden fight and old-growth forest blockades in remote Oregon," Kauffman (ibid.) explained:

> The New York City community garden fight was one of the first times that Earth First!–style blockading techniques were used in an urban context . . . And they worked really well here, putting the gardens issue onto the agenda, making the controversy something that everyone knew about, and helping transform what was a very small movement into a relatively large movement.

The campaign Kauffman refers to brought people from Brooklyn to Eugene to use every tool they knew—from play to civil disobedience—to defend these green spaces. Those involved sat in the street, linked arms, and sang as diversity and democracy intermingled in an image of what a better world could look like. "These spaces, like the carnival itself,

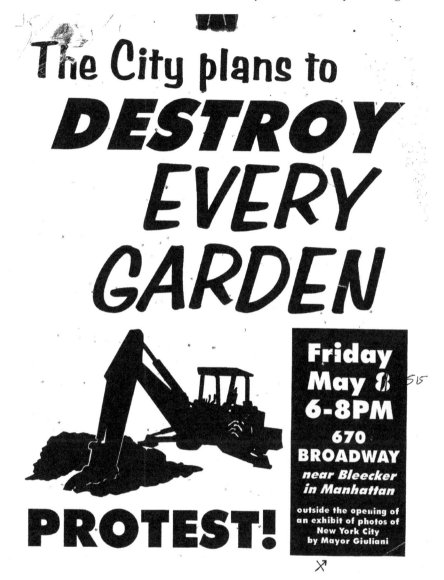

The City plans to **DESTROY EVERY GARDEN**

Friday May 8 6-8PM
670 BROADWAY
near Bleecker in Manhattan

outside the opening of an exhibit of photos of New York City by Mayor Giuliani

PROTEST!

Figure 4.2   The city plans to destroy every garden. Courtesy LESC.

function as spaces where activists create an image of an affirmative possibility, a space where creativity and democracy thrive," explained Kauffman (2004, p. 381). Simultaneously, a model of protest as carnival attracted audiences to a distinct struggle over spaces recognized as breeding grounds for creative play. Within these spaces, activists challenged the rules of consumption at the heart of organization of urban space,

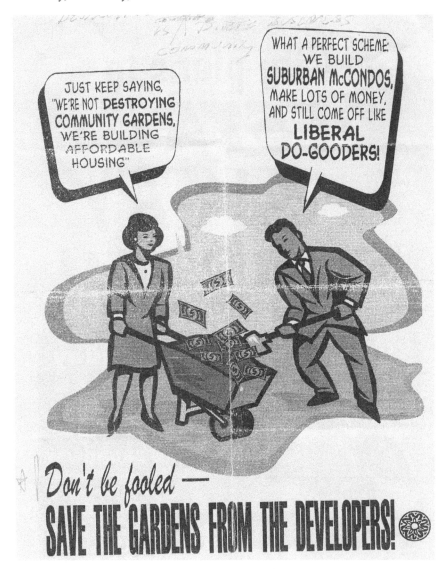

Figure 4.3   "Don't be fooled—save the gardens from the developers!" Courtesy LESC.

emphasizing connection and community rather than commerce (Holtz-man et al., 2004; Merrifield, 2002). And it is no wonder they became tar-gets. For New Yorkers, community gardens functioned as directly lived "representational spaces" (Lefebvre, 1974/1991, p. 39). They were spaces which spoke to a prefigurative immediatism which propelled a range of movement practices.

PREFIGURATIVE COMMUNITY ORGANIZING

Throughout the interviews for this project, I asked interviewees about notions of prefiguration. One of the best answers was provided by Ariane Burgess, the daughter of a community organizer from Scotland, who talked about her own history as well as ambitions to realize an image of a better world in her organizing:

> I think in terms of my work in the city, it was 1997 and it was a rent stabilization rally down at City Hall. And it was the classic flatbed truck with all the speakers. And there were hundreds of people there and you were getting tired and bored. And I was thinking this is insane. We should all be dancing. We know the issues. So why don't we get together and celebrate our relationship with each other?

Notions of prefiguration have only gained credence over the years. "Protests gain in power if they reflect the world we want to create," L.A. Kauffman (2004, pp. 380–81) elaborated. "And I, for one, want to create a world that is full of color and life and creativity and art and music and dance. It's a celebration of life against the forces of greed and death." Rather than "the angry shouting shrill position," which simply offers opposition, "having a carnival is a way of saying yes."

Burgess recalled the end of the rally that day:

> At the end, a bunch of the crowd left and Ron Hayduk was there. And Eric Drooker had a big drum and somebody had a bell. And so we started playing all this music and dancing before the police started to come. They weren't too into it. So they were trying to push us out. And I remember we walked back up to the Lower East Side and various other improvised instruments. And the police just kind of followed us along the road as we went. So then it evolved into the Lower East Side Collective.

LOWER EAST SIDE COLLECTIVE

LA Kauffman, David Crane, Steve Duncombe, Kelly Moore, Alice Varon, Alex Vitale, and this writer, among others, were part of this group, as were organizers involved with the local Reclaim the Streets chapter, the Billionaires for Bush (or Gore), United for Peace and Justice, ACT UP, SexPanic!, Time's Up!, Women's Health Action Mobilization (WHAM), and solidarity movements with El Salvador. Group members participated in some of ACT UP's most memorable moments, including the Stop the Church action and the Operation Ridiculous theater of the absurd described in the previous chapter.

Before LESC, David Crane had had a hard time finding a way to get involved with local politics. ACT UP was a tough act to follow. And organizing meetings in the neighborhood had become difficult after the Tompkins Square Park Riots. "But then when I overheard that they [LESC] were going to be doing wheat pasting, I was like, Wow, wheat pasting! I haven't done that since ACT UP," recalled Crane. "I latched on and kind of talked Leslie's ear off that afternoon. And then we became close after that, and I became a part of LESC and all."

Longtime Lower East Side resident Ron Hayduk was deejaying a party at the Brecht Forum when he heard about LESC. His prior experiences with organizing, including solidarity work in Latin America, informed his work in the Lower East Side.

> And part of what we saw our mission to be, aside from bringing material aid to the folks in Nicaragua supporting the Sandinistas, was to do education in the Lower East Side . . . The same reason that we needed things here in the Lower East Side was the same reason that our country was waging war. Okay, so things that people really need in this country are underserviced and underfinanced, and the Sandinistas were trying to develop a regime in a country to help their country develop independently from the United States and sort of corporate capitalism . . . It was empowering people who were previously stomped down. And here we are in a stomped-down community in the Lower East Side and we're going like, Oh, yeah, you know we should do some shit right here. And ultimately if you want to help anybody in the world in the twentieth century—or the twenty-first century now—you gotta do something about what the United States is doing foreign policy wise. So all politics is local and so let's get local. We got global understandings and global experience, but here we are, so what can we bring to this community?
>
> Bringing their story here, and saying, Hey, there's a reason the schools are underfunded, the reason the housing is dilapidated, the reason crack is epidemic, the reason that AIDS is debilitating, the reason that the health care system isn't available to help people, the reason you don't have a fucking well-paying job is because our country is spending billions of dollars to undermine regimes that are trying to help their own people.
>
> So here are some folks who come from a lot of different experiences and find themselves going, Well, what can we do here? What can we do to stop the gentrification of the Lower East Side? What can we do to help buttress the onslaught? What can we do to make this space a community, save it, what exists of the community and help build community? How can we community build? So it went from saving gardens to fighting for affordable housing to fighting to help support the squatters to think about commercial rent control. And all of that was serious political work but it was done with lots of fun and creative style.

From the very beginning, LESC helped local actors see the interconnections between their own worlds and global forces (Shepard and Hayduk, 2002).

In its four years of existence from 1997 to 2000, LESC contributed to campaigns to save the community gardens, support undocumented workers, and connect neighborhood activism with a global movement via one of its project groups, Reclaim the Streets. And we played. "Since forming in 1997," LESC "initiated several projects and targeted a number of issues," its literature declared.

> We're fighting for affordable housing, while defending community gardens. We're involved in local electoral campaigns for progressive candidates who answer to the people, not money or the party machine. We're making sure that everyone who works in our neighborhood gets a living wage. We don't think you should have to work on Wall Street to live in the Lower East Side. We're tired of seeing small businesses forced out by chain stores and pricey restaurants. We believe 'quality of life' means enjoying our neighborhood. *We believe politics can be fun.*

While other activist groups of the mid-1990s asked participants to play the timeworn role of the selfless activist, LESC sought a lighter path. It did so by allowing people to personalize how they participated in campaigns. "Participation didn't just mean more people to make more phone calls; it meant opening up our organization to new voices and tailoring our tactics to make use of individual personalities and proclivities," explained LESC cofounder Steve Duncombe (2007, p. 86). As a result, many new members developed a feeling of ownership of the project. This allowed participants to connect with the group at the point of their own insights and passions, which infused the group with energy and creativity, as well as a connection among various issues. A key element in this strategy was allowing engagement to feel good. Rather than write grants, the group put on huge dance parties. "We goofed around and socialized while tabling for causes, we prided ourselves on our cleverly worded signs, and working with groups like Reclaim the Streets and More Gardens!, we turned our demonstrations into festive carnivals. In brief we enjoyed ourselves" (Duncombe, 2007, p. 71). Through a vibrant process, a broad critique, and respect for pleasure, the collective brought a distinctly ludic perspective to its work. Yet, as with ACT UP and OutRage!, the group connected this ambition with clearly articulated goals and a coherent organizing model and ethos.

Much of the LESC work was informed by an optimistic reading of both Marx and the world around them. Marx's view that the world was always changing, transforming, and coming into being informed the way members thought about their endeavor. Such a perspective meshed well with the LESC disposition toward play as well as the sensuality of material life, connecting people to streets, struggles, and the environment. People make sense of the world through their senses. Here, we connect our physical experiences, our work with our play, intellectual, and cultural development. Our labor satisfies more than our mere means of necessity, it helps us realize our fullest development as people (Hendricks, 2006). LESC worked out of its context, learning from the world as opposed to an ideal- or identity-based model, which had been the predominant ideas of organization in New York City since the 1960s (Duncombe, 2007).

All the organizers in LESC were serious veterans of activism who were disgusted with old models. Those models were not delivering. LESC was not interested in ideology or identity position. What members were interested in were material positions, gardens, streets, labors; members favored direct action rather than discussion of ideology. Activism had to be fun (Duncombe, 2007). The previous Left was not (Isserman, 1993). Members of LESC were clear: we need to have fun. And gradually, LESC developed a theory of action born of lived, material existence. "All successful theory is lived theory," LESC's Steve Duncombe (2003) suggested. For Marx, theory only gained vitality "once it gets a hold" of people's lived experiences, influencing their world and actions (Ollman, 2003, p. 32). Throughout its short existence, LESC developed a distinct lived theory, which combined an ethos of direct action with an analysis of neighborhood life and pop culture (Duncombe, 2003, 2007). The result was a new kind of activism.

A close look at LESC's propaganda highlights its emphasis on flexibility and practice, rather than ideological rigidity.

> We do demos. We do street theatre and art. We do direct actions and civil disobedience. We do tabling and education forums. We do phone and fax jams. We do pestering. We do parties. We do picnics. We—with healthy skepticism—do electoral campaigns. We do whatever works.

LESC thrived within a lived theory which combined a critique of capital with a lusty sentiment that there had to be more to urban life and experience than going to and from work. This theory was deeply informed by the life and culture of the city and its thinkers. In 1999, Marshall Berman, who taught several of LESC's members at the City University Graduate Center, described his fondness for a Marxist Humanism which influenced activism. "Some people think Marxist Humanism got its whole meaning as an alternative to Stalinism," wrote Berman (1999, p. 16). "My own view is that its real dynamic force is as an alternative to the nihilistic, market-driven capitalism that envelops the whole world today." Rather than a fixed ideology, "Marxist humanism can help people feel at home in history, even a history that hurts them. It can show them how even those who are broken by power can have the power to fight the power; how even survivors of tragedy can make history" (p. 17). Conjuring up images of festive Marx puppets at a parade, Berman suggested that a century after the *Communist Manifesto* readers could imagine the different voices of Marx, the young and the old, dancing rather than sparring. "Finally, they are coming together in an activity that's expressive, *playful*, even a little vulgar—an activity that would have been considered most un-Marxian not long ago." Berman's musings seem to hint at an 'if I can't dance' Emma Goldman–like sentiment, which so inspired LESC. "We always were quoting

Emma Goldman," explained LESC's David Crane. "Almost everyone held her up in the pantheon." "Today's Marxes have kept in touch with their youthful romantic visions of politics as dancing," Berman continued (1999, p. 20). In many ways, Berman could have been speaking of the direct action group of his former graduate students, who linked dancing and pleasure within their praxis. Their dance was a celebration of caring social relations and pleasures. For LESC, play was part of the ends and the means. It was also a critique of a militant approach to politics, a Bolshevism, which had extended over a bloody century. Here, play was part of an embodied approach to politics which rejected rationalist dead ends in favor of a politics which combined dreaming and fantasy with a highly creative, humanist attitude to organizing (Duncombe, 2007).

LESC's approach to organizing anticipated the Global Justice Movement's dynamic focus on creative expression and engagement rather than ironclad ideological certainty (Notes from Nowhere, 2003). Through LESC, anarchists worked with liberals, AIDS activists organized with environmentalists, and great things have happened through the savvy deployment of multiple approaches to defending the neighborhood. A multi-issue politics, those with different approaches of action collaborated, as theory was subordinated into a form of activist practice—informed by shared projects rather than one ideology privileged over another. So people with differing political views found a place to organize together around very specific actions and campaigns. It did not matter that some were Marxists and others were liberals or ecologists or sex activists as long as they were willing to work together around specific campaigns which favored direct action. People in the group actually reveled in these differences in perspective. "We're proud of the diversity and cultural vibrancy of our neighborhood. We're upset by its gentrification, commercialization, and homogenization. We're organizing to do something about this," LESC propaganda declared. The story of LESC serves as a case study on play-based, ideologically flexible, multi-issue activism.

More than the previous chapters, an observing participant perspective informs the story of LESC, its affinity groups, and related offshoots which comprise the remaining chapters of this book (Tedlock, 1991). At various times I was involved with its project groups involved in garden activism, public space, community labor, street parties, and its group cohesion ministry from my first meeting with the group in March of 1999 through the summer of 2000 when the collective peacefully disbanded (although the affinity groups kept working together through 2004. Many continue to participate in a monthly salon which continues to this day). Work and play vacillated within the LESC experience. Some days it involved spending more than thirty-six hours in jail after defending a community garden; others it wound into a sweaty spiral dance at a benefit party in an old synagogue or at our old community center. It was all part of an organizing effort mixed into a community-building cavalcade at a time of rising radical political tides.

I became involved with the group shortly after working on sexual civil liberties activism with ACT UP and SexPanic! Many of us had been involved in the Matthew Shepard political funeral, which resulted in mass arrests in October of 1998 (Shepard, 2009). Yet, the core organizers for the Matthew Shepard political funeral, the Fed Up Queers (FUQ) stopped having open meetings (Flynn and Smith, 2004). And some, such as myself, were left out. So when FUQ started pulling together a coalition of groups that had been targeted by Rudy Giuliani—ranging from schoolteachers to green-gardeners—a sympathetic activist from FUQ invited me to the organizing meeting. FUQ reached out to many of the activists who had coalesced to give Giuliani a black eye over his defense of the police officers who had shot ninety-nine bullets into unarmed Amadou Diallo. Daily acts of civil disobedience had taken place after the event. On March 31, 1999, I attended my first meeting with the Stop the Mayor Coalition as an unaffiliated participant with others from ACT UP, the Church Ladies for Choice, Youth Education Life Line (YELL), SexPanic!, Circus Amok, FUQ, NOW/NYC, as well as four members of LESC—L.A. Kauffman, Alex Vitale, David Crane, and Todd Muller.

After the meeting, Muller told me about the next LESC meeting and let me know I would be welcome to come. Crane and Kauffman were equally friendly. Muller specifically asked that I try to make it.

Muller, who published his own online zine (or blog) about basketball, was an iconic presence in Lower East Side organizing circles. While many in the Lower East Side were interested in a militant brand of activism, Muller was more interested in a different kind of political game. Todd Muller was a basketball enthusiast. He had his own website, which he bragged covered the ins and outs of the college game, the pro game, and the political economy of hoops. If you plugged in the words *politics* and *basketball* into an internet search, his site was the first to come up. Muller played in the neighborhood league, where he was painfully aware that his group of scruffy anarchist buddies never seemed to be able to beat the Wall Street teams, despite their lack of talent. "We were never as devious as them. That's their job, exploiting people," Muller explained. What went on in the outside world simply could not be abstracted from what took place on the basketball court and vice versa; it could not be separated from the game (Ollman, 2005). Here, "play was a device that both dramatized existing social divisions and promoted the formation of new groupings centered on the playground" (Henricks, 2006, p. 18). In this way, "play permitted the negotiation of social identity" (ibid.). It opened a kind of "public dialectic in which people try to advance their own personal, cultural and social positions" (p. 19). Rather than cower at the power brokers, Muller and other LESC members attempted to reshape the way the game of urban life was played in the Lower East Side. Here, basketball and politics overlapped in any number of ways.

"Conceptually, it's good to think about basketball as invention," Muller explained, noting that it was originally conceived as a means to give workers playtime. "It was also a form of muscular Christianity, to make Christians seem tougher, healthy body, healthy soul. It was also a way to uplift unwashed masses." At the time, wave after wave of new immigrants were pouring into the United States, many settling in the Lower East Side of New

York. "If someone said, 'Have you seen my friend, a basketball player?' you'd think he was Jewish. It was also a socializing force," Muller elaborated, laying the framework for a theory of basketball as politics. "Conceptually there is no sport as close to Communism, from each according to his ability, to each according to his need. I think if society was as goal orientated, basketball would be community." In this game everyone is working toward the same goal. "If I'm Jordan, I put more in, 'cause I have more ability. But I still need something from others. Jordan didn't win a championship without a future Hall of Famer. He still needed something from his team—defense, keeping the goons off his back." Here, basketball offers a core lesson about play, social connection, and competition. "This is especially true in pickup ball. The most fun part is when the worst player scores. That can be a make-or-break moment. You're still going 'how the fuck did that happen?' And that's when you've lost."

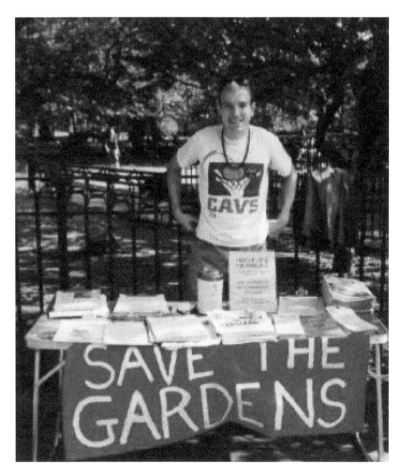

Figure 4.4   Todd Muller tabling for the Lower East Side Collective in Tompkins Square Park.

Summer 1999, I started regularly attending the LESC meetings held every three weeks at the Botanica Bar on East Houston Street between Mott and Mulberry. The back room of the bar was a dark dingy space. Half the group drank beer; most everyone joked; and in between jokes, the agenda churned forward at an efficient pace. The first event I helped organize with the group was a summer dance party/fundraiser held at the Charas El Bohio Community Center, a former public schoolhouse off Avenue B which had been occupied by squatters in the 1970s. "LESC is an activist group based on the Lower East Side," announced an advertisement for the LESC's "Radical Love" benefit dance party:

> We have been fighting for community gardens, defending community arts centers, disrupting City auctions, organizing immigrant workers, unfurling guerrilla billboards, jamming phones and faxes, demanding affordable housing, sponsoring poetry readings, holding fabulous parties, working for real 'quality of life' in the Lower East Side, and generally making life miserable for landlords, bureaucrats and developers since 1997.

The flyer for the event served as an invitation to a new sort of political ethos: "Come celebrate the neighborhood's vibrant political culture with some of its most unruly elements."

For years since the legendary Tompkins Square Park police riot in 1988, people had suggested that the battle against gentrification in the Lower East Side was lost. Yet for others, the long history and culture of activism in the Lower East Side presented an opportunity. One of the members of the group was the daughter of one of the organizers from the Up against the Wall Motherfucker, a notorious 1960s Lower East Side anarchist direct action group (Neumann, 2008). With this legacy in mind, the group looked to the neighborhood's history as a source of inspiration. While the Motherfuckers had been described as "a street gang with an analysis," LESC maintained a less militant disposition, carefully picking and choosing its battles. For many, the group and the model of organizing represented something of a break with past generational conflicts.

At an early LESC retreat, Todd Muller reminded everyone that our parents were not there. No one needed to speak to or against them. "For our generation, the Oedipal thing isn't there," Muller explained when I asked him about that moment. "We're not fighting with them or apologizing to them. There is nothing we have to take to them. They are gone. So we don't have to do anything in relation to them." Without a family tradition to live up to or to reject, those in the group looked to each other. "I'm going to do what's best," Muller continued. "It's about all that I got from my friends in school. It's about us living a better life together."

Rather than the dourness which often accompanied activism, block parties, barbeques, and picnics were as much a part of the group's attitude toward community building as demonstrations. Playwright and LESC organizer Jason Grote recalled:

> I moved to New York in 1997 and I was walking around the Lower East Side and found a flyer that LESC had put up in Blackout Books, an anarchist bookstore. And from what I heard, I was the only one who responded to the sign. It was a moving sign but the joke was 'Moving Left? Go with LESC' with a picture of a truck on it with little phone numbers that you could tear off. Supposedly, a lot of people called because they thought that it was a mover. I think it was just a convergence of things. I had wanted to get involved. I'd just moved to the city. I had gaps in my social schedule. And I was just really excited.

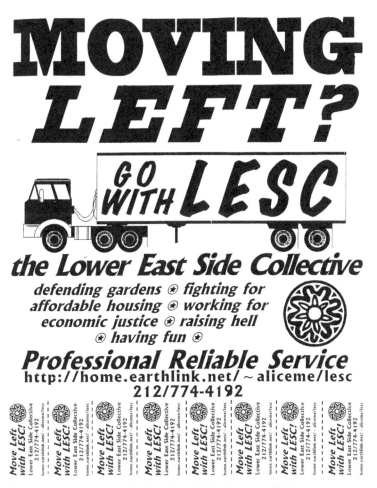

Figure 4.5 Moving Left? Go with LESC. Courtesy LESC.

Part of the appeal was its organizational model. The project groups within the LESC worked together in campaigns based on a model which recognized the importance of data and research, legal advocacy, fundraising, communications, outreach, direct action, and street mobilization. Therein policy and planning overlapped with direct action within a framework for organizing and community building. While rationality may be part of such a framework, the group managed to avoid the means–ends inversion which often accompanies organizing. Rather, lighter social friendship bonds helped shape the collective. This spirit of social connection among minds, as well as bodies—social eros—fostered a transformative context for organizing (Katsiaficas, 2002).

For longtime Lower East Side activists, such as Bill DiPaulo, the group offered a new opportunity for neighborhood organizing after years of heat from the police. DiPaulo explained: "And after that [the Tompkins Square Police Riot, August 6–7, 1988] it became very difficult to organize in the Lower East Side. The police were sabotaging the meetings. There was a lull of organizing coming out of that." DiPaulo was particularly concerned with police infiltrating meetings. So he left the neighborhood for a while. "I felt it myself. What they would do was they would drive around the neighborhood and if they recognized you, they would harass you, they would let you know, 'look, we know you are involved in this or that.'" Yet, DiPaulo had a girlfriend who said he could move in without being on the lease. So, he moved back:

> And so I could exist for a while and see what was going on. And that's when I discovered the Lower East Side Collective was forming. And I was like, how are they going to have a meeting when you can't have a meeting in the Lower East Side because every meeting is hostile whether it's organized or not. People get upset. For at least two years, there were no meetings because of this whole thing with the park. There was so much anger and hatred . . . There was so much craziness.

Recognizing this "craziness," LESC formed committees so the real activist work could take place outside the public meetings. "At that point, LESC had a number of different working groups on different issues," Grote explained. "And it was an interesting combination." Committees included: a community and labor coalition, a police and prisons project, a public space group, an environmental justice group, Reclaim the Streets, and the Ministry of Love. David Crane, who had experienced similar difficulties with the organizing culture of the Lower East Side after his years with ACT UP, took part in several LESC working groups.

> It was a group of very media-savvy, creative, fun people who would do work, rather than sit around and have meetings. It wasn't about three people with sort of dueling proposals trying to run some pseudo

Robert's Rules of Order meeting to grandstand. It was work session. . . . We had a project structure. Under the LESC umbrella you could have several projects, and that project would be funded through the LESC parties or whatever—the fundraisers. As long as we were effective I don't think any group actually got shot down.

One of the most distinct groups was the Ministry of Love. "The idea of the Ministry of Love, that was such an important thing," Ariane Burgess explained. Through the Ministry, each new member received orientation materials as well as an introduction to the work of specific project groups, and a follow-up call after their first meeting with the group. After I received my first phone call and was welcomed at the next meeting, my impression was this was about the most pleasant organizing group I had ever been around. If there were problems within the group, the Ministry of Love would try to address them, so they did not get in the way of the work. The meetings ran like a rambunctious sonata; yet, things got done. "Within a year of our founding we had more than fifty activists working with us and were engaged in six simultaneous campaigns," Duncombe recalled (2007, p. 91). And the Ministry of Love was a large part of this success. Ariane Burgess described the rationale for the group:

> We set that up because people were coming into the group continu-ously. LESC was really drawing a lot of people. And how to handle new people coming in and the human tendencies to get cliquish. And so it was this effort to stay open. And there was a buddy system and that came out of the Ministry of Love. And we also had the parties. If this is going to be our lives and we want the world to be different then we need to be living it, somehow in a bit toward the direction that we want. And so the Ministry of Love was a way for people to socialize outside the meeting context.

Organizer Brooke Lehman explained how this esprit de corps translated into the work of the project groups: "I think there has always been an element of playfulness." For Lehman, "The best actions that I have been involved with have been ones that have been satirical." Lehman explained how this ethos contributed to an organizing campaign:

> I don't think that this movement is sustainable unless people have a sense of humor. I think part of the strength of the playfulness has been to bring joy into people's experiences, but in countering the other ex-treme which is as alluring, but not a useful way to do mass organizing, which is to create a militant and even militaristic-seeming direct action organizing skills. I think when you are looking for energy, those are sort of the two poles that people get pulled into. And I'd much rather get pulled into the silly, creative side, even if it's regarded as cheesy and

sort of less serious. I think the more serious tends to mimic what we are fighting against too much.

Throughout her interview, Lehman alluded to the concept of prefigurative community organizing (Epstein, 1991). Members of LESC built on this ethos to create a thoughtful, democratic meeting culture. Yet, they were also critical of the pious Quaker roots of the practice which assumed a spirit of God actually moved through the meeting. Instead the meetings were much more tongue in cheek, as well as brief and immediate. Meeting minutes were written with self-deprecating jokes and nicknames, crazy fonts, and references to parties and social gatherings as much as to political events. Grote was immediately appreciative of the humor and play of the group's meeting culture:

> Well, I think it was also a very subtle part but it was being in a room full of people who had a sense of perspective and a sense of humor about where they were at. I think there was a lot of accessible stuff that was going on and it was humor that initially brought me into LESC. There was a lot of humor at the time. Leslie had the sign, 'What Kind of Worm Would You Like to Have in Your Neighborhood—a) a warm figure, b) a real estate developer.' And of course, there are lots of reasons to have a sense of humor, but at the end of the day, you attract more flies with honey than with vinegar.

Kauffman's "What Kind of Worm Do You Want in Your Neighborhood?" was designed specifically in specific reference to ACT UP's "Know Your Scumbag" sign from the Stop the Church action. "We do build on each other, you know," Ann Northrop from ACT UP noted when I told her about that sign.

Probably the most secretive of the LESC project groups was the Strike Team, the LESC propaganda arm, which met at Todd Muller's house. Meeting minutes from the March 22, 1999, meeting report the group had been busy. "The strike team noted that someone had redecorated billboards and ads on bus shelters on Houston and Broadway with what appeared to be paint-filled eggs and a bucket of paint." In addition to challenging the consumerism and homogenization blandifying much of the neighborhood, the team was concerned about a number of international issues. "[A] previously blank billboard on Bond and Lafayette now has an anti-Iraq war message on it." Not only was the group contributing to the culture-jamming anticonsumer ethos that was simmering throughout much of 1999, the group seemed to revel in the secretive, clandestine elements which Huizinga describes among affinity groups who play together. The minutes continued, "By the time you receive this, a group calling itself Public Works will have hung several dummies carrying shopping bags that say, 'Whose New York?' followed by a statement related to important political issues (gardens, prisons . . .), on scaffolding" on Houston Street near the group's regular meeting location at Broadway.

At its peak, LESC won an award from the Abbie Hoffman Activist Foundation for innovations in organizing, as well as criticism for being too frivolous. That's when Duncombe (2007) felt LESC had succeeded in shifting the terms of community organizing from "sacrifice to pleasure" (p. 92). Duncombe had long been weary that much of the Left had become overly professionalized or ideological. Their "game isn't much fun to play," he would suggest, speaking of the Left in general (p. 65). One reason for this lack of fun was the systematic process of professional advocates, policy analysts, and lawyers demobilizing American politics. Political scientists Crenson and Ginsberg (2002) describe this process as the "downsizing of democracy." For Duncombe, the process demarcated the ends—life, liberty, and the pursuit of happiness for all citizens—from the means: an insider's game of reports, lobbyists, briefs, and bills. "It has taken the game away from the very people for whom it is ostensibly being played," Duncombe continued (p. 65). When politics emphasize "privileged efficient ends over participatory means, the ends become totally unattainable" (p. 76). "The great strength of democracy is that it depends on its players," Duncombe mused (ibid.). Yet, the people can only be treated as spectators for only so long. Eventually, inevitably, they will want to play. But how can they do so? Duncombe pondered. If the only democratic arena is sterile and sleepy, the necessary participants will go play elsewhere. Hence Duncombe's gaze on the increasingly popular arena of video games, DIY culture, and popular culture where lessons about fantasy, agency, and entertainment are unending. Throughout his work with LESC, Duncombe would argue that the lingering legacy of the hair shirt left prevented organizers from learning from such lessons. While movements from Gay Liberation to global justice had sought to render the pleasureless Left a thing of the past, old habits died hard. "It is not the job of progressives to condemn popular fantasy and desire," Duncombe explained. "It is our job to pay careful attention to them, learn from them, and perhaps—God forbid!—even enjoy them, ourselves. Then carjack these fantasies and drive them someplace else" (2007, p. 77).

Throughout its short life, the group built a sense that social change was possible; conditions felt mutable, especially with an invigorating rich array of new types of targets on which to set their attention (Wood and Moore, 2002). "It also could have been this feeling among everybody that neoliberalism was destroying the world," Grote explains. "I felt in my gut that that's what was happening. And I remember Stephen (Duncombe) and Leslie (Kauffman) saying you are never going to get people marching against neoliberalism, which was so obviously disproved in Seattle." For many such as Grote, "there was a sense of something happening." As an antidote to systems of work and capital, play would become tremendously important for a burgeoning anti-neoliberal disposition and movement (Henricks, 2006; Yuen, 2004).

In the years to come, it would become a vital ingredient in a new recipe for organizing. "I've spent a lot of time organizing huge meetings over the past years. And when I'm picking out a facilitator, they have to have a sense of humor," noted Brooke Lehman. Moving out of LESC, she helped organize the New York City Direct Action Network after returning from the Seattle WTO protests. "You have to understand process and move the dialogue along, but if they can't get the whole room to laugh every five minutes, it's excruciating," she explained. "I think that is really necessary in terms of security culture and getting people to take what they are doing a little less seriously."

Many in LESC turned to a post-identitarian, task-based organizing model. Jason Grote described why he was attracted to such a model:

> I remember going to other activist meetings. I was working on the Charas campaign, and nobody was speaking on behalf of Charas and I had to sit in the room and listen for hours to people talking about how the dynamic in the room was making them feel based on their identities. It was not what you needed to get something done. There comes a certain point where you have to swallow your own ego if it's an important enough cause and say let's figure out how we are going to get this contract or this garden landmarked. I think a tangible goal is really important.

In response, LESC members discouraged any long discussions about philosophy or ideology during a work session. Meetings were "really tightly controlled, which was necessary because there were people on the Lower East Side who could be difficult to control on a social level," Grote explained. "It's just a risk that goes into it in general. You want a certain amount of selectivity without being elitist. But at the same time you don't want people ranting about the Kennedy Assassination." In Lower East Side parlance, the group was trying to reduce the "wing-nut factor," which could weigh groups down with endless paranoid debates about pot, the FBI, AIDS conspiracy, COINTELPRO, etc. (see Sanders, 2004). "In LESC, there were certain rules, such as you could not talk about ideology," Grote recalled. "I think the agreement was that it was a waste of time. You could get sidetracked into a discussion with purely academic debates." Grote continued: "You get people who are really married to anarchism or Marxism or the lifestyle traits. And the fact is, it was immediate goals. It was a typically American way of looking at things. Theory doesn't matter, what matters is results."

DiPaulo described the focus on thought and action in the LESC meetings:

> I attended some of the Lower East Side Collective meetings. And sure there were wing nuts who tried to get in. And people like Leslie

Kauffman, she was so on top of them. In the beginnings of the meetings, you were almost so scared to speak that you were almost thinking in your head, what you were going to say. I knew that they, the people in the meetings, knew about some of this wing-nut factor. And they knew about how people were just going to make statements in the meetings. And so they structured the meetings in a certain fashion that this could not happen at all. And it was just amazing to see this structure . . . I was there to learn what they were doing. I guess people like Leslie Kauffman were very intimidating to me at the time. And [*laughs*] still are actually. The idea that you better have your idea together before you start.

Every three weeks, the LESC project groups would meet to present their work in five minutes or less. As a result LESC—and by extension Lower East Side activism in general—was infused with an immediacy that focused attention on projects, not personalities. Ideas, tactics, strategies, and themes intermingled at each meeting, forcing activists to grapple with how their issues overlapped and how they could share resources. Along the road, the group was able to articulate what protest and community building were for as much as what they were against. Some of these things included: green space, affordable housing, a dynamic mix of cultures, living wages, and public space.

Yet some rejected the group's disposition. "Even Yuppies need their own group," Susan Howard, an early LESC member recalled a neighborhood squatter dishing when the group started. Another dubbed LESC "self-satisfied socialists."

Throughout the period, observers would suggest that displacement had robbed the Lower East Side of its character and that all that was unique about the neighborhood was lost. Former Lower East Side activist William Sites (2003, p. 101) theorized that "cities no longer produce successful movements because, in today's globalized 'space of flows,' places no longer serve as a basis for social power." Those in LESC would argue that globalization also spawned a revitalized mode of activist engagement which linked Lower East Side activism within a global context (Duncombe, 2002a, 2002b, 2007; Kauffman, 2004; Ness, 2002, Patterson, 2007). While Sites argued that "the community mobilization in the Lower East Side represented an unsurprising failure" (2003, p. 101), others would suggest that globalization, like modernity itself, was pregnant with contradictions and openings for action (Merrifield, 2002; Shepard and Hayduk, 2002).

The notion of being able to imagine a better world and then strive to create it was a cornerstone of this organizing approach. "If you want the utopian ends, you gotta find the means that work and that's the inside-outside. You gotta start here, where the people are at. That's where the play comes in. . . . It's where you can engage people," explained LESC member Ron Hayduk. "You gotta be willing to see where they are at. It's an experience of learning how to play. Part of the fun is the dance. You aren't going to go anywhere unless you try to imagine it." For Hayduk, "you gotta have a positive vision of a utopian future so we can try to create it." Such an ethos gets to core questions of play, process, and community building.

When asked which she was trying to do, create community or win external changes, Brook Lehman explained: "I think it's both. Ideally, we'd be working to create both challenges to the state within state power and outside of it by creating alternatives. This is an ideal vision of going after power from the outside and the inside." Here, Lehman echoed Hayduck's sentiment:

> I think there is value in having progressives in government and there is value in having people doing street pageantry. What I'm most against is people throwing things out with the bathwater constantly. When they find out something wasn't the be-all and end-all, they want to throw out whatever they have been involved in or the little others have been involved in. I'm looking for the ways for those different strategies to work together.

Here, utopian thinking and dreaming intersect with the impulse to organize: "If the civil rights folks had listened to those who said, 'You can't overthrow Jim Crow,' history would be far different," mused Hayduk. "Same thing with apartheid. If they didn't imagine another world, they would have given up to the naysayers." He continued:

> If they hadn't imagined a positive alternative vision and believed it and worked for it and made trouble for it, the world would be a different place. It's the bridging of the inside/outside strategy. If you hadn't heard of Ella Baker you wouldn't have heard of MLK. All those local activists made it happen, bridging the local to the global. Janet Abu-Lughod said globalization is the big problem and the Lower East Side is lost and we're defeated. LESC started from a perspective that globalization exists. And low and behold, they won some things—the gardens, the community labor coalition, the squats—despite the naysayers. If people had believed the naysayers—Sites (2003) and Abu-Lughod (1994)—you couldn't have had those wins.

Moving forward, it is useful to consider some of the issues LESC members "made trouble for," won, and lost.

PUBLIC SPACE

David Crane described the work of the LESC public space working group:

> We were providing propaganda for the defense of public space movement. We called ourselves the Public Space Project. It wasn't just

gardens, it was community centers. And what other kinds of public spaces are under attack at this point? How can we defend them? How can we help groups that are trying to defend them get together and see that they've got common interests?

"Charas, Other Public Lands Auctioned by NYC"—this was the subject head for the e-mail from gardens@cybergal.com (aka L.A. Kauffman) on July 23, 1998. The group was particularly concerned about the *El Diario* news story from July 21, "City Sells 'CHARAS/El Bohio' Cultural Center." Charas was a central part of the East Village of Manhattan, which stretches north from East Houston Street and eastward from Broadway toward the East River and up to 14th Street. Since the late 1970s, this area has also been referred to as "Alphabet City," due to its lettered avenues (Mele, 2000, pp. xi–ii). Charas/El Bohio was a former public school building that functioned as a community center on 9th Street between Avenues B and C. Between its founding in 1979 and its takeover by the city of New York in January 2002, Charas offered affordable classes, studio space, tutoring services, after-school activities, a recycle-a-bike program, and meeting space for community groups.

Charas's origins can be found in the squatter movement of the 1970s and 1980s. Charas/El Bohio began when directors Armando Perez and Chino Garcia moved their group, Charas, into the then-abandoned school building in 1979. At the time, the building was in disrepair and functioning as a "shooting gallery" for heroin users. Charas rechristened the building "El Bohio" (the hut) and renovated the building with sweat equity. By 1982, their efforts were so successful that Community Board 3 recommended Charas be given a lease on the property. The New York Department of City Planning, the City Planning Commission, and the City Council all upheld this request. But in 1998, the building was sold to real estate developer Greg Singer for $1.71 million (Moynihan, 1999).

"Dear Garden Defenders," the July 23, 1998, e-mail from Cybergal aka L.A. Kauffman began. She went on to suggest that "with the City land auction behind us":

> We do not yet know who bought the building that houses CHARAS/El Bohio Community and Cultural Center; whoever it was has very deep pockets . . . Needless to say, as soon as we do find out who the culprit is, I'll be sending you their phone and fax numbers so that you all can do what you do so well.
>
> The directors and supporters of CHARAS have vowed not to give up: They are pursuing a lawsuit to block the sale, and some in the community are already talking openly about a grassroots occupation of the building.

Once LESC members found out the name and fax information for the developer, "the culprit," they began a working group devoted entirely to what would amount to a near decade-long campaign against developer Greg Singer and those who sought to support the sale. Charas supporters sent faxes, placed personal calls to prospective buyers, heckled those who came to look at the space, tied the space up in a protracted legal battle, and borrowed from a wide range of tactics to make life untenable for those who considered renting or renovating the space.

The group used any number of techniques to defend the space. Shortly after the sale, LESC members disrupted a movie shoot on the Lower East Side. Brooke Lehman recalled the scene: "In the East Village there was a movie shoot. They were throwing glitter balls. And it would completely dismantle anything they were doing 'cause the glitter deflects off all their lighting." The point of the action was to compel the theater union to come out in support of Charas, which they eventually did. "They did that because so many of the actors have gotten their start in community theater supported by Charas," Lehman explained. "I thought it was a really good successful action."

GARDENS, CRICKETS, AND A DIFFERENT APPROACH

"There was another group that was involved, which was the Lower East Side Collective, which played a really crucial role in it," explained Lower East Side squatter Michael Shenker, recounting the rise of the Lower East Side community garden movement. "And they were very, very effective." Here, he specifically referred to Kauffman: "One of the architects of that group [LESC] kind of brought in what you are describing, which is a joyous aspect." Shenker recalled one of the most notorious of the garden direct actions . "Its first manifestations were with the crickets and Charas," Shenker elaborated. David Crane explained the rationale for the action:

> Well, Giuliani then decided he was going to sell all the gardens, and we started hearing that this was a possibility through people that we knew, insiders, that this was bubbling up and that there was quite likely going to be a wholesale sell-off of the gardens at public auction. And so Charas, annually it came up on the auction list and then was removed at the last minute. But when it was clear that it was not going to be removed then a group called the Cricketeers, I think it was actually twelve people who actually risked arrest by releasing ten thousand crickets into the auction where they sold Charas a couple lots before Charas came up. If they didn't remove Charas from the lot we were going to stop that auction, and do it by releasing crickets into One Police Plaza.

Here, members of LESC and other garden and Charas supporters disrupted a city auction of public land, which included Charas and many community gardens, by releasing bags full of crickets which set off a panic (Patterson and Rensaa, 2009). The action took place July 20, 1998, the same day

Charas was sold. Its aim was to prevent the sale of Charas and other community gardens.

In a monumental statement that they were not going to sit by and watch the corners and edges, bits and pieces of their neighborhood auctioned off, LESC borrowed a page from ACT UP's book. ACT UP veteran Steve Quester explained why he admired what the garden activists were doing during this period:

> Well, first of all because they plant gardens. But also because all these carrots and snap peas got arrested blocking the streets. Tomatoes lobbied Elliot Spitzer. There were a couple of tens of thousands of crickets released in some hearings. . . . Of course we need carrots getting arrested blocking traffic. How else is change going to happen?

Quester's question—how else is social change ever going to happen?— echoes through the thoughts and creative gestures of freedom which propelled action during this period.

Tim Becker, who took part in the cricket action, recalled:

> Yeah, with the crickets. I met that guy who writes plays—Jason Grote—I had never met him before. They were having some meetings at Charas and talking nonstop. And Leslie Kauffman was there and David Crane. So those meetings were going on and then Leslie pulled me into this back room and whispers, "We're planning something with crickets. Do you want to be part of it?" I said yeah, so she invited me. I went to a couple of planning meetings.

Grote described the theme and context for the action:

> A bunch of gardens had been auctioned out before and it caught everybody off guard. Nobody was expecting it. But the next time around people were like, we have to prevent this somehow and bring attention to it. I think nobody really knew about this. And I think urban environmentalism and environmental racism were ideas people were talking about. So there was this idea of creating a media stunt at an auction. I think they were going to do it at One Police Plaza so there would be little bit of intimidation and this idea that anybody who decided to disrupt this auction would be punished extra in the heart of the beast. One of the people in this organization had this idea of doing this crazy stunt that would get media attention, would be somehow newsworthy.

As far as the mayor was concerned, either you were for the redevelopment program, which included the sale of the gardens and Charas, or you were a supporter of the urban decay. The point of the cricket direct action was to shift story lines. Since he was elected in 1993, Rudy Giuliani had talked up the storyline that New York, nicknamed the "Big Apple," had become a "rotten apple." According to this view, New York was a city in decline before he entered office. This story line positioned the mayor as the city's advocate for regeneration over decay (Beauregard, 2002). For Giuliani, hyperdevelopment was the most appropriate antidote to decline. Those who opposed it were "dangerous anarchists," "reds," "jerks, idiots, morons," as the mayor was prone to describe them in press conferences and on his radio show (Kifner, 1999; Lederman, 2001). "Giuliani was such a grim man," Dana Beal reflected after his group was targeted by the city. Garden advocates sought to advance a different story line. Healthy neighborhoods need homes, gardens, and public spaces. Part of the effort was to demonstrate that garden supporters had neighborhood interests in mind when they did what they did. They were not violent nihilists.

"The idea was in keeping with Jiminy Cricket, who was Pinocchio's conscience. This would be the conscience of the city," explained Jason Grote. He continued:

> The idea was that it would be an act that was funny and bizarre and really disruptive but also not necessarily harmful, but like an act of sabotage that wouldn't really leave any lasting damage. And we also wanted something that was sort of silly. The part of it—also the narrative that was happening even before September 11—was that people who do civil disobedience are dangerous. We were going to do something silly just to say obviously we're not violent. And if I think back even the judge thought it was funny.

There was also a theatrical point to the presentation style of the garden advocates (Goffman, 1959). "It was pervaded with silliness so that its ridicule would break down the idea of authority was being deadly serious," noted Grote. "You could kind of paint a smile on it. It's more complex than many think." Here the gardeners made use of humor, as well as ridicule (see Bogad, 2005a). "There is no way to really win under those circumstances, so ridicule becomes like the only take," Grote explained. "One thing about power is, they do not know how to be funny. You look at Rush Limbaugh and Fox News, it's totally lame. You don't even have to be political to think that.." And lots of people agreed.

The cricket action built on the new resources made available with the Internet, as Grote explained:

> You could pretty much order anything from a pet supplier. We ordered ten thousand crickets. They were kept in storage. And a few people kind of feel bad for the crickets and I can understand that, 'cause they were not kept under the greatest conditions. So the person who was

organizing this tried it out early, she made an envelope with airholes and swept it through the metal detector early and she tried to take one through security and it worked. So, then we all went in. And the idea was we were going to go incognito.

For Tim Becker, the sight of all his scruffy Lower East Side buddies dressed as developers before the auction was both absurd and ridiculous:

Then the morning of the auction, everyone I knew from the Lower East Side was out waiting to get into the auction. And it was the only time that I have ever seen Seth Tobocman in a suit, before, after, or since. And it was obviously a borrowed suit because the pants legs were at least 40 percent too short. And he had stolen the tie. [*starts laughing*] It was some polyester number that he had gotten from somebody and it looked really bad. And I said to myself, the police are going to watch the TV in the back and they are going to know that something is going on. This guy is not a developer. It doesn't say money to me. If you call this guy money, it doesn't work. [*laughs*] Seth in a cheap suit. And then the women I knew, well. When you go to midtown people have the corporate look. The clothes say I can hang with the rest of them. Well, the neighborhood girls were this mismatched, half-power, half-mismatched. [*laughs again*] I don't know who we were fooling but it was early enough that the police were not on their toes. It was just like a little fly, a gnat buzzing around. It looked more like the people who showed up for the free teas, But the police let us in to the police auction. Ten people have crickets in briefcases. The people who put together the idea of the crickets somehow knew that crickets are like a skeleton. They don't show up under X-ray. You can get them in. You just walk in. There are people who do a lot more of the planning than me . . . I just show up. But they had it already planned out. I have no idea what it was. [*laughs again*] As far as that demo went, I wasn't in on the talking points.

Like Todd Muller, Tim Becker's self-deprecating humor made working with him a great deal of fun. Becker laid out the terms for the action, "Well, how bad do we want it? We're like in the belly of the beast—right at Police Plaza." The police could just take those arrested straight downstairs without them even seeing the light of day. They did not even have to leave the building.

Grote, who was "completely terrified," had similar forebodings when he arrived. He kept his eyes on the exits during the entire action.

We got together at someone's apartment at like six in the morning. And we were going to go down together. It was terrifying. We were all really scared. I made it there like only an hour late. I did make it there before everyone left. We were in this auction hall and I was in the bathroom when someone else took this spot. And I ended up with like the worst spot. I wanted the one with a view of the escape route. So the plan was we were going to sneak in, in suits, and go incognito. But of course, nobody else was dressed in business clothes. There were a lot of people that wanted to buy real estate that were from like Russia or Korea that were wearing T-shirts and jeans and polo shirts. And so we were kind of out of place. And no real estate developers go to these little tiny auctions. We went in and were totally sticking out.

Dressed in Salvation Army and Sears's finest, the garden defenders fanned out throughout the audience. Clayton Patterson was there filming. Tim Becker watched nervously as the auction began:

[I]t went on for a while and then there was a symbol when we were actually going to unleash them. And all during that time, there were two ideas that were going on: release the crickets and have false bidding. You had like Michael and Seth and they had their action. They didn't do the cricket action. They were doing false bidding. So you had developers bidding like a million two. And you had Seth going a million four. And [*laughs*] Michael going a million six. And developers coming in at a million eight. And Seth going "Two Million!" And it went into the stratosphere. Even the real developers were looking around like, "What's going on here?" We're talking about little patches in the Lower East Side. Maybe five hundred thousand? But

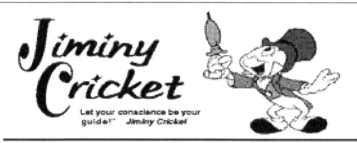

Figure 4.6   Jiminy Cricket press release.

not two million. And so that got out of control really fast. The guy with the gavel was just beating on it and couldn't figure out what was going on. And so at some point they made a ruling that said that you had to show that you were good for part of the check. You couldn't just start bidding. It was all very civil back then. But all the guys were outbidded.

False bidding was long a part of the repertoire, noted David Crane:

We had been warned at that one that anyone who did this false bidding would be arrested, yadda yadda yadda. But we didn't obstruct by participating in the bidding. Oh my God, it was so funny, the auction before when Leslie Kauffman, when they came around for her, whatever, $38,000 down payment that had to be in cash, she starts emptying out her pockets, and then she says, "Oh, there's a $1.50 left on this Metro Card!" And then the woman threw it on the ground, "Disqualified!" And we were escorted outside.

While it is easy to theorize the disruption of the mechanisms of power, the process can be excruciating. "It's horribly nerve-wracking. It's not fun. It's fun when it's over and you can say, 'Wow, that was great,'" mused Cindra Feuer, an ACT UP veteran. Still, the anxiety followed by release is part of what Huizinga characterizes as play.

Grote was not of the "I do not care if I upset you" ilk:

I'm sitting there and I'm waiting. We had one lot that after it was auctioned, it was a garden, that was when we would unleash the crickets. And I'm looking around scouring the area and I'm looking at the escape routes. The young woman who was sitting next to me was dressed really artsy. . . . Somebody screamed to call attention to it. That was our cue and I started dumping them . . . I was one of ten people then trying to dump this bag of crickets out . . . But it was sort of like one of those old dishwasher commercials where you drop the dishwasher into this little bowl of dishwater and all the oil kind of evacuates to the side away from the soap. That's sort of how it was with me. The arty woman next to me saw the bugs, screamed immediately, jumped on the chair, and then immediately there was like three feet between me and everyone else.

"Adrenaline was definitely high when you were ripping open that envelope and dumping your allotment of a thousand crickets onto the floor," recalled David Crane. "The poor crickets hadn't had enough water, it had been a hot day, and so they weren't as lively as they could have been."

"The crickets just spilled out on the floor and created a lot of eee eee eee, created a lot of noise," recalled Ron Hayduk.

Becker described the scene:

There was just pandemonium. It was just like a Sunday-morning cartoon. People were jumping up on chairs. You know, we're talking about crickets here as if it was a subway rat or something. But it was just crickets. But everyone was up on chairs and pandemonium was ensuing. People were yelling and the guy was beating on the gavel.

The activists eyed the exits and tried to get out. But: "Instead of just leaving immediately, I was worrying about fingerprinting or something and I was trying to stuff the envelope back into my bag," Grote confessed.

And then I'm pushing my way through the crowd and one guy; you are always going to find one guy who is enthusiastic about siding with authority, said, "him, him, him." And then I ran and all of a sudden I was eye level with this big barrel chest with a badge hanging off of it. And I just immediately just put out my arms like you got me.

Becker was also apprehended:

And we were all supposed to head for the exit and get the hell out of there. Well, it was just crazy and everyone was just rushing to the exit and trying to get the hell out. I got all the way to the X-ray machine. I mean I could see the promised land—the pavement. I could see it, and all of a sudden this arm came and grabbed my arm. And I was sitting there in a suit with a really old briefcase. And that's when I met Jason Grote. But there was screaming and screaming. And I remember Margarita Lopez came up to me and said, "What did you do?" I said, I released some crickets. And she looked at me like I was out of my mind.

A few other activists, including Tompkins Square Park Riot videographer Clayton Patterson were also arrested. "I ended up spending the night in jail," noted Grote. "They put us through the system. At that time it was like a special punishment. I made friends [and] met a lot of people . . . I felt I was in good hands. Ron Kuby's office was representing us."

"I was trying to get out of there" Becker mused.

When I got arrested I got put in a closet briefly with Jason, briefly. I don't have any idea. We were put in a small room in the cleaning closet. And crickets were coming out of Jason's pocket. I felt like I was getting arrested with one of the Three Stooges here. [*laughs*] He has things coming out of his pocket. How can I plead innocent now? It was like we were useless crooks; they were crawling out of his cuffs and his pants legs.

Before being moved to the Tombs, New York's central booking area where Becker and Grote spent the night, the two were locked in a cell at One Police Plaza. There Becker stayed up most of the night. "The lights were on. The floor was hard. I wasn't into it. It's fun telling the story now. But at the time, I'd rather have been at home in my bed."

For Jason Grote and the others, going through the system was an exercise in slow futility.

> It was a night full of encountering just all sorts of characters. It was not the adversarial relationship between cops and activists. I mean there was the Tompkins Square Riot, but back in the early 1980s they had the big antinuclear marches and the cops were kind of a model of cooperation. We sat in the holding cell forever. There was this weird fingerprint machine and nobody could figure out how to work it. And I suspect a lot of the arresting officers were trying to milk it for overtime. I don't know. But we were just there forever. And finally at the end, we found out we were going to the Tombs for the rest of the night.

The arrestees were welcomed as heroes when they were finally released the next day. For Grote, the release was a distinct part of the play experience:

> We were kind of greeted by people. I felt a little like we'd accomplished something. I called up a couple of LESC people, Vicki and Rachel. I couldn't get into my apartment. All my personal possessions were locked up as evidence. I had cash on me and they cut me a check for that. I was walking around, my shoes were flopping, I had no belt, I had no keys. And I called them up and said, "Can I stay with you guys?" They were very sympathetic. It was kind of a great bonding experience. It was kind of an example of the traumatic experience as play.

Ron Hayduk reflected on the action's message and impact:

> Think about it people. If ten thousand crickets in the middle of an auction are released and people are very serious about their bidding, it would be a very destructive thing. But a very ironic and like odd, funny moment to see crickets running around the floor and people sort of shrieking. But it's very symbolic in terms of the gardens that are being auctioned off. And these people that helped to organize this, and I was honored to be among them, were savvy enough to not only conceive of it, find out how to get the crickets, dress up like we were playing the part, and sneak past the guards to get there, but videotape it and get it to the media stations within the several hours that it occurred so that it was on the evening news. And it was that kind of fun, creative activity that was great to be part of. It was energizing. It was exciting; it was fun. It was ultimately effective at sending a message

and getting lots of people involved and aware of the gardens, and ultimately some of the victories.

As activists spent the night in jail, the city's newspapers wrote sympathetic
descriptions of the action. "As the crickets hopped about, hundreds of onlookers scrambled to avoid the swarms," began a report by the *Daily News*, "Activists Bugged by City Land Auction" (Cauvin, 1998). Most of the LESC story
line found its way into the press reports. "We're hoping he gets the idea and his
nose stops growing," the *Daily News* reported Wendy Madison, a supporter,
saying of Mayor Giuliani. "Ten people left a larger group protesting outside
Police Headquarters . . . carried the insects in manila envelopes with mesh
air holes . . . The arrested activists were Timothy Becker, 39; Dennis Griggs,
52; Francine Luck, 55; Clayton Patterson, 49, and Jason Spiegel" (who later
changed his last name to Grote). "Auction Disrupted, but Charas Is Sold,"
Anderson (1998) of the *Villager* reported. "Cricket Invaders Turn an Auction
into 'Madness," wrote Waldman (1998) for the *New York Times. El Diario*
put the action on its cover (1998b), while *Newsday* and others reported the
cricket action and the Charas auction simultaneously (Associated Press, 1998;
Vega, 1998). The activist message came through loud and clear. Rather than
the Giuliani rotten-apple narrative of a city of decay in need of a savior, the
reports clearly sided with the story that the community was losing something
precious. "Community Group: 0, Real Estate Interests: 1," announced an *El
Diario* editorial from July 23.

July 23, 1998, Cybergal sent out an e-mail reviewing the action. "The
Giuliani Administration did succeed in selling off CHARAS and some
250 other pieces of public land—but only with enormous difficulty, and
at a high public relations cost." She noted that a neighborhood perspective
found its way into a larger citywide political debate.

> The coverage of the auction and accompanying protests was sympa-
> thetic to our side. The TV coverage was especially good, with NY1 and
> Channel 11 as stand-outs, casting the issue as community use versus
> luxury development and presenting our call for a moratorium on the
> sale of public land pending the development of a democratic plan for
> open space, low-income housing, and cultural facilities.

In these early dispatches, Cybergal identified the rumblings of something
very powerful. The garden struggle was taking the shape of a burgeoning
social movement:

> Most encouraging of all, this movement is clearly growing in both size
> and strength. Five months ago, the City land auctions weren't even an
> issue; public awareness has increased enormously in a short time, and
> more and more people are coming forward to fight not just for com-
> munity gardens but for democratic control over public land.

Remember, too, that 18 Lower East Side gardens have now been saved as public community space. This is as many gardens in one neighborhood as have been saved in the rest of the entire city—a testament to the enduring political fact that action gets results.

We're going to have to fight another auction in three months' time, and we're going to have to keep pushing if we want any more gardens saved. But for the moment, take heart in what this movement has accomplished so far—and go spend some time in the gardens!

Gardens had always been a place for kids, families, friends and neighbors to share space and play; but they had also become a part of a new political movement, with echoes reverberating around the globe.

5 Play as Street Party
Reclaiming Streets and Creating More Gardens!

> The magical collision of carnival and rebellion, play and politics is such a potent recipe and relatively easy to pull off that anyone can do it. Even you . . . reclaimthestreets.net. (Notes from Nowhere, 2003, p. 61)

While play was a central ingredient to the LESC mix of activism and politics, there were those, such as Ariane Burgess who wanted more of it. "For me even Lower East Side Collective wasn't playful enough. I was kind of looking for something." While searching, Burgess stumbled upon a mix of cultural experimentation and politics in a LESC project group called Reclaim the Streets (RTS). New York's RTS "was kind of an offshoot of the RTS that grew up in Southern England," she explained. "Motorways were being built on land that was pristine forests. So these huge rave parties would happen." Most took shape as makeshift street parties, which served as blockades of bodies, many locked to the streets. RTS actions were characterized by festive images of bodies in motion, which formed a sort of temporary autonomous zone (see Bey, 1991). Here, the interplay of gyrating bodies replaced cars moving to and from work as pleasure superseded commerce. For many, reclaiming streets was an appealing strategy for challenging a neoliberal assault, privatizing public spaces the world over. To disrupt the process, those in the new movements sought to break down the lines between art and life, while injecting "creativity, imagination, play and pleasure" into the game of social change (Jordan, 1998, p. 129). Here, an ideology of a playful revolution informed a new brand of activism (see Chapter 5 of Shepard and Smithsimon, 2011).

I spoke with John Jordan, a veteran of London's RTS, about his experience with the group. For Jordan, activism began with the arts. The two concepts, art and activism, mix in much of Jordan's work. "I had a notion of social sculpture and/or the expanded context of art, which was really an amalgam of ideas of Marxism, anarchism." Here, "everyone had the potential to be artists, the artist's work was to bring out everyone's potential to transform the society," explained Jordan. "I came to direct action

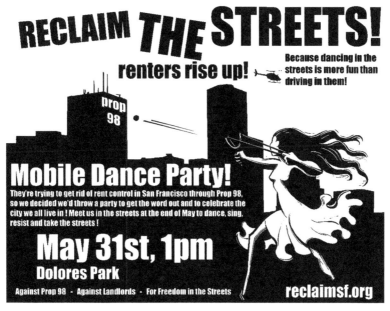

Figure 5.1   The first RTS action in the United States took place in Berkeley, CA. Courtesy RTS.

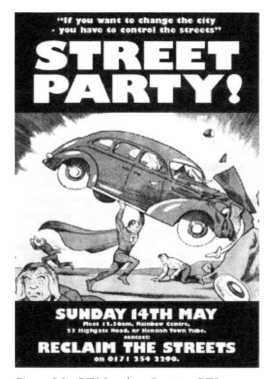

Figure 5.2   RTS London. Courtesy RTS.

very late," he confessed. "My background was very much performance art, or what is called live art here." As the Thatcher years progressed, Jordan became increasingly radicalized. "I sent a postcard to the Earth First! address. And I never got a reply. This was pre-Internet. And I got involved in the anti-roads movement." Jordan paused. "That was the beginning of my involvement with direct action." There, Jordan witnessed a social movement inspired by the thinking of Dada, Surrealism, and the Situationists. Jordan read them all. "The joy of getting involved in the direct action was seeing the extreme creativity, especially in the M11 campaign, and that's when I got involved with RTS."

THE ANTI-ROADS MOVEMENT

The campaign that galvanized the anti-roads movement in England was M11. Like the garden struggle in New York City, the M11 Campaign was ignited by a threat to a significant public space. Jordan explained:

> There had been a plan to build this road that began in the early 1900s. There had been the Twyford campaign, very rural campaign, but it really brought a lot of publicity. And from that came an urban campaign, the M11. The road was going to wipe out entire neighborhoods and houses, for six minutes (in commuting time) . . . This had generated a local community campaign and it became extraordinarily creative. To me the question was always how to have space to connect the transformation of politics and the poetics and imaginary space of the arts. And then I went to this space and it was like, oh my God, this was happening. None of these people were calling themselves artists.
>
> For me, it was an absolute moment made up of stories and beautiful acts. The whole campaign began with an absolutely beautiful act. There was a tree on the common, and it was a 350-year-old chestnut tree. And we were told it wasn't going to be knocked down. And, of course, as it turns out it was going to be knocked down. And the parks department boarded it up. One day we decided to have a tree-enclosing ceremony. And we opened up the space. And all these kids went down and pulled the boards off and reoccupied the tree. And they actually built a tree house. And of course this had been happening on the West Coast of America with Earth First! but it had never happened here. And the papers wrote about the tree house. And lots of people wrote letters. When the postman arrived with letters, they had marked the address to the 'tree house.' And the postman [treated] 'tree house' as an official address. And lawyers on hand realized that once the place had a letter box and an address, then it become an official dwelling place and could therefore be categorized as a squat. Then the whole process of evicting it would have

to go through court. So there was a beautiful combination of collective creativity, with group creativity, with people writing letters, lawyer creativity. We then created this model of tree house that grew throughout several years. I really got involved as we got into the way of machinery; people got into the way of the cranes. For me it was actually very performative. For months, the arts and crafts and performances really held off the construction of the road. And it cost them hundreds of thousands of more pounds then they would have spent before the tree was actually bulldozed.

In *All That Is Solid Melts into Air*, Marshall Berman (1982) writes about watching his childhood neighborhood in the Bronx razed in order to make room for a highway. The chapter that is not included in this monumental story is what might have happened if the neighborhood members had stayed and defied the bulldozers. This is what the citizens of Claremont Road did when they created a blockade of forty-five buildings, homes, slated for development. Jordan recalled the campaign's origins and creative efforts to defy the bulldozers.

They claimed use of forty-five houses to build this road. They sent people letters saying you have to sell your house. Most all of the houses were empty except one by a lady who had lived there all her life. She was actually an actress and she said, "I am not leaving. I have never lived anywhere else. Fuck it. I'm not leaving." It was pretty much her and several hundred activists living in the street. In blocking off the road to traffic, they transformed it into this extraordinary zone of play and creativity . . . It was just an extraordinary laboratory of techniques of resistance—from lockdowns, to tunnels in the country. Basically, there were several tunnels. There was a tunnel that went under people's houses and another that actually went through the side walls of people's houses without going out onto the street. They also broke down the kind of isolation of the individual living unit.

Lesley J. Wood, a Canadian activist who for many years was part of New York City's Direct Action Network, witnessed the Claremont Road blockade.

I went to England in 1993–94 . . . There was a road blockade in the far East End of London. A whole row of houses had been taken over in order to protest this new highway going through a poor area. And some of the original residents stayed in their homes on Claremont Road. It was a place which was friggin' magical. They had nets strung over the trees and across the houses. And there'd be people climbing over your heads all the time. And things like music, raves on weekends, and jam sessions.

I don't want to always say temporary autonomous zone, but it felt like a temporary autonomous zone for about a year. And it was there that a lot of seeds that became RTS were really formed. At the same time Critical Mass had arrived in the UK. And so there was an increase in thinking, like, gee, protest can be a lot more fun.

As public spaces were cordoned off, privatized, and sold to the highest bidder, an ethos of resistance seemed to be taking hold around the globe. Yet instead of waiting for a leader, regular people looked to their neighborhoods, friends, gardens, parks, and public spaces to find support to reclaim their commons (Klein, 2004).

RTS NYC

"A few people here were inspired to try to create an aspect of that here," Ariane Burgess explained, referring to RTS London and the Anti-Roads Movement. "It was a beautiful idea." This spirit inspired the formation of New York's group (Duncombe, 2002a, 2002b).

This new resistance movement built on any number of political trajectories, including the sense of wonder and fun, as well as the "play and creativity" Jordan described. Emma Goldman's ethos of an unrepentant pursuit of joy and justice would provide a huge inspiration for the street-party style of protest of RTS (Duncombe, 2002; Jordan, 1998).

The first RTS action in the United States took place on Telegraph Avenue in Berkeley, right off the People's Park, where the Free Speech Movement took root in the 1960s. New York's chapter of RTS was born when a young philosophy student named Louis read an article about the UK group and was inspired enough to invite people to come talk about the idea. A group of Lower East Side activists, crustie punks, anarchists, a DJ, bikers, gardeners, as well as LESC's Steve Duncombe and Bill DiPaulo gathered at Blackout Books on Avenue A for the first meeting (Duncombe, 2002b). Todd Muller and Duncombe connected the group with LESC propaganda and recruited new members at Blackout Books. Like the self-photocopied zines and manifestos clogging the collective bookshop where the group held its first meeting, New York's RTS chapter was inspired by a DIY philosophy. This ethos propelled the group to organize the first RTS event in New York for the fall of 1998.

An RTS communiqué situates RTS's struggle as a battle over both "Quality of Life" politics and public space.

Community gardens bulldozed throughout the five boroughs; community centers auctioned off to profit-driven developers; aggressive police intrusion into peaceful assemblies; thousands of cyclists and pedestrians hit every year; parks rigged with police video cameras; rents soaring (which profits whom?); sanitized chain stores and remote corporations reshaping every neighborhood in their own image . . .

The Mayor carries a "No Dancing" sign and hangs it wherever he goes. Corporations buy "You can dance if you pay" signs and hang them wherever they go. Fundamental democratic ideals are being squeezed. If there is no place to freely assemble there is no free assembly. If there is no place to freely express, there is no free expression.

Observing this pattern of events Barbara Ehrenreich (ibid.) notes, "conflict over public dancing has a long history—one that goes all the way back to the ancient world." So do efforts to resist this brand of social control. The RTS broadside continued:

Reclaim the Streets is at once a unifying symbolic action and a movement to reclaim public space and reinvigorate inner-city public life. Our definition of "quality of life" does not mean conventional, homogenized, capitalized life, working 80 hours a week to pay the rent. Why must New Yorkers aspire to the least common denominator? We want real, eclectic democracy . . .

We demand great feasts of public space. We demand our freedom to express. We demand our freedom to express. We demand clean air—as if the basis for democracy were not the ability to breathe! . . . Reclaim the Streets! Let the vibrations of our dancing feet rumble like subway trains.

Like many in the city, the group openly worried that the Quality of Life campaign of then mayor Rudy Giuliani was homogenizing communities' differences while robbing much of the colorful pulse from the streets and clubs of New York. "Dancing to music is not only mood-lifting and community building; it's also a uniquely human capability," writes Barbara Ehrenreich (2007a, p. 14). "This is why New Yorkers—as well as all Americans faced with anti-dance restrictions—should stand up and take action; and the best way to do so is by high stepping into the streets." Like many, RTS was aware that efforts to sanitize the city meant pushing out the poor so the city was more amenable to business interests (Flynn and Smith, 2004; Logan and Molotch, 1987). "The Mayor's homogenizing 'Quality of Life' campaign is fast privatizing scarce public space, squeezing the pockets of diverse communities, and stealing our freedom to express," the flyer concluded.

I first heard about RTS when Katherine Walsh, the founder of the Lower East Side Bluestockings Bookstore who had worked with the queer direct action groups SexPanic! and Fed Up Queers, gave me a flyer promoting the first RTS action during an anti-queer-violence rally in Brooklyn. Attacks on communities of difference had become a common byproduct of the cultural apparatus known as the Quality of Life Campaign (Ferrell, 2001).

In reponse, activists across the city pushed back (Flynn and Smith, 2004; Shepard, 2009).

The first RTS action took place on October 4, 1998. I came with Bob Kohler, Chris Farrell, and a couple of other members of SexPanic! The flyer Walsh gave me instructed us to meet at the Cube sculpture at Astor Place in the East Village. While I knew several of the activists there, the scene and the people felt different than the usual protest.

It was William Etundi's first street protest since moving to New York. He heard about the action from a card someone gave him which he remembered declaring: "STREET PARTY PROTEST. It's not a revolution if I can't dance to it." It was audacious to think one could stop the everyday flow of traffic and by extension the commerce of capitalism, with a simple street action. Yet, that was the goal. The group planned to do it with many of the people who usually spend their nights dancing in clubs closed away from the public. I had never seen that crowd in streets in the light of day. Yet, here they were mingling with the usual village vagabonds and hipsters at the Astor Place cube. And then out of nowhere, a horn blew and everyone started screaming for us to run west. "I can remember at the Astor cube, there were like two hundred, maybe three hundred people, there was this spontaneous moment of running. Myself and my roommate, Gabino, at the time we didn't know anybody," recalled Etundi. "We didn't know what to expect. We were just right there, just ready to take the streets." As the group completed its short sprint to Broadway, we filled the street with dancing bodies. The sound system blared dance tunes into the air. Louis sat some twenty feet in the air atop a tripod. The NYPD stood scratching their heads as Broadway transformed into a street rave. "Being there taking the streets, and being there holding the streets, the fire spitters. It was just exactly what I felt like so much of my life had pointed to," mused Etundi, "being a party person, a politically conscious person, it just made so much sense. It was fun. People wanted to come out and join us."

"By filling the streets with people freely expressing themselves, RTS not only protests what it is against, but also creates an experimental model of the culture it is for," mused Steve Duncombe (2002A, P. 347).

"It was just exactly the mix of party culture, fun culture, and protest culture," Etundi had wanted to support, "exactly what I would want to be involved in. I went and it was transformative, absafuckinglutely. I can really trace a lot of what I've been doing to that day." The simple gesture opened a space for a new way of looking at a relationship between individual and public space, for an entire cohort of people. Yet, it all begin with the simple invitation to holding a street party.

"An RTS action is like a potluck dinner," Duncombe (2002b, p. 220) later wrote. "RTS secures the space and provides the music (and post-protest legal support), but what happens at the action depends upon what people bring with them and what they do once they are there." For Duncombe

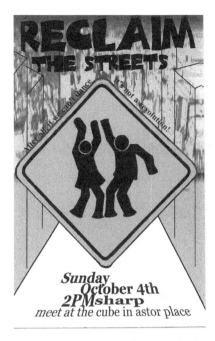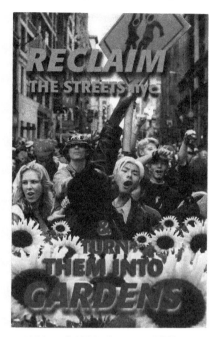

Figure 5.3   First two RTS New York actions 1998 and 1999. Courtesy RTS.

(2002A, p. 347), RTS was an embodiment of a model of prefigurative politics: "RTS reclaimed more than a style of protest—they popularized a model of political action wherein the protest itself is a living, breathing and *in this case, dancing*, political message." This model invites spectators to be part of a low-threshold, highly participatory form of social change practice. Here, spectators are encouraged to be performers (Bey, 2003). More than a protest, at their best, such actions draw people into the experience of creating a community of their invention (Duncombe, 2004). And draw people in they did.

Many were intrigued with the notions of activism as a gesture of pleasure. "My favorites were the early Reclaim the Street actions back when the police didn't know how to handle it or if they should be stopping it," recalled Jason Grote, reflecting on his favorite moments in Lower East Side activism:

> It seemed so harmless at first. I remember the first couple at Astor Place and on Avenue A. It almost seemed as if the cops were amused by it. But the threat wasn't. After a while they started using the terrorist or anarchist black bloc hysteria . . . But when you look at those early protests. And they saw what they were seeing with their own eyes. They saw a bunch of people dancing and laughing about it . . . And there

was this tremendous feeling. Aside from the question of the effective-ness, the interesting thing about play as a political force and these kind of micro-level revolutions is there is something incredibly immediate about dancing on a city street with blocked-off traffic and music, and taking it back.

Etundi reflected on the ethos of the action:

> There's a lot of organizing that goes into those events. But I think the idea of making protest enticing and fun is the core value of what Reclaim the Streets was both locally and internationally. Making it attractive, making it interesting, making it intriguing, making it exciting, I think that was a real sea change in the way people see movement-building.

There is grainy black-and-white film of the early RTS London actions. Speaking over images of cars, congestion, and pollution, the narrator explains that he had always loved cities. But now they were dying. People were killing them. Facing a world which felt like it was crumbling in front of their eyes, activists hoped to cultivate a generative ethos which sup-ported the cross-pollination of bodies and ideas, as well as gardens, com-munities and public spaces squeezed within the concrete jungle. For public space activists, social eros among dancing bodies helped combat the mate-rialism strangling, overdeveloping cities, polluting waters, and bulldoz-ing community gardens. And the movement for public space overlapped between street actions, auction disruptions, and garden blockades.

THE LOSS OF THE CHICO MENDEZ MURAL GARDEN

Squatter Michael Shenker reflected on some of the early garden struggles during that fall of 1998. "We interfaced very effectively with the Lower East Side Collective, with Leslie Kauffman." While the cricket action had given the movement some momentum, the movement was still fight-ing the capital that moves New York City: real estate. Yet, the LESC pro-paganda continued. "[S]he was very creative and very dedicated, and [she made] fine posters too, great posters; and they really did get those posters up," Shenker reflected. "The first campaign was to save Chico Mendez Garden," Shenker recalled. "It was a beautiful garden. The campaign got everybody warmed up. But I liked the ones when we actually won. Chico Mendez was a great sacrifice."

The garden had been the centerpiece of Tim Becker's social life.

> I came to New York 'cause I'm an artist. I've been in the Lower East Side the whole time. There was always a huge social element in getting

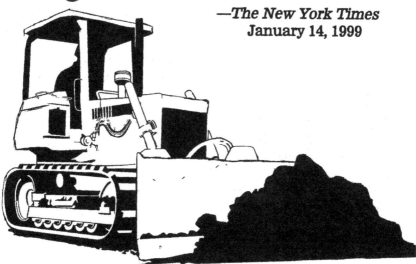

"Bulldozing a working garden is an act of neighborhood violence."

—*The New York Times*
January 14, 1999

Community gardens are publicly owned green spaces that provide New Yorkers with places to relax and play. These beautiful gardens were created by your neighbors for everyone to enjoy, on what once were dirty and dangerous garbage-filled lots.

But now the Giuliani Adminstration wants to sell these neighborhood treasures to private real-estate developers, to build whatever they want — without community input.

Don't let the City destroy our public spaces — speak up for gardens!

New York *NEEDS* community gardens!

Figure 5.4   LESC gardens in danger flyer. Courtesy LESC.

involved in Lower East Side craziness. I didn't have tons of friends when I got here. I'm only in New York ten years. And how I started to meet people was through the art world. But also I started going to garden meetings in Chico Mendez Garden. It was on 11th Street between A and B. And it was right on the eve of the storm clouds on the horizon that the city was going to start taking gardens. It was one of those early meetings and all these people from the Lower East Side were getting it together.

Becker described the feeling in the space.

> I was a member. Before it was bulldozed in the Christmas slaughter of 1998, it was a really nice vibe in the garden. It was mostly a lot of artists. There were murals around the edge of the garden. Jeff Wright, he was really the maître d' of that garden. And he was the MC . . . There was food too. And so that was a hub. And another artist had done these rock gardens. It was an off-the-charts garden.

Storm clouds started brewing that summer and fall. So activists started having emergency meetings. "They were getting word from Françoise, the little French lady who was plugged into what was happening in City Hall," explained Becker. They tried to put the word out to the neighborhood. David Crane and L.A. Kauffman worked closely with Françoise, who had been a member of the French Resistance to the Nazis decades prior. Her very presence helped link the garden movement with a larger ambition of freedom of space, self determination and autonomy. And the movement to save the gardens started gaining momentum. Felicia Young helped organize a procession to the East Village community garden's called Earth Celebrations. Members of groups such as Time's Up! as well as RTS started showing up. "So then all of a sudden a lot of the people from the neighborhood who were not 100 percent gardeners but who were activists, they got wind that Chico Mendez Garden was the hub," Becker explained:

> So Bill DiPaulo from Time's Up!, he showed up with this English dude. He showed up with these big tripods; in England they were using them in the middle of the streets. And you'd put a person on top. So he built two tripods. And then we fortified the fence with furniture and futons and stuff that was around the neighborhood. And it became this sort of organic sculpture and it got weirder and weirder and wilder and wilder. And at one point there was a rooster flag. And a chair. There was, like, pictures of the Pope. Anything that people had found from the streets, they would put on the barricade from the fence. So, it became this really wild decoration, like something that you see down in the Caribbean or something. And it got thicker and thicker. Gotta keep [Donald] Capoccia back. Well, I guess the siege probably lasted about two months there—all through the fall. And that's where I first met your friend Leslie [Kauffman]. She was doing Lower East Side stuff then. Time's Up! was helping and then the Shenkeristas came in too. Michael and a guy named Rooftop Rob and of course Seth Tobocman, they all started showing up and lending their expertise. And they started teaching classes about lockdowns and nonviolent civil disobedience.

This flurry of activism kept Capoccia back for most of the fall of 1998. Art and cultural resistance were vital tools in the movement to defend the space. "We stepped up all of the arts evenings just to have people in the garden. There was a lot of bands playing and a lot of performance going on," and more people started coming by Becker explained.

> And then we started meeting every weekday morning from seven to nine in the garden. And we would have coffee. We figured if there were going to be developers snooping around, that would be the time—at the beginning of the day. Before we all went to work and did our thing, we would come to the garden for two hours. And MaryAnn Gold showed up with cookies. And we would hang there. And then we had Rooftop Rob sleeping in the garden. And then we started a bike patrol. This was real high-tech. [*laughs*] My grandmother is rolling over in her grave now. You're doing what? You're a grown man. And Hugo,

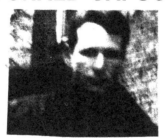

WANTED

DONALD CAPOCCIA

FOR
BULLDOZING THE
COMMUNITY GARDENS
FOR PROFIT

LAST SEEN IN BED WITH PAGAN.
IF YOU SEE THIS MAN, MAKE HIM EAT HIS CELLPHONE.

DO NOT CONTACT THE AUTHORITIES: THEY ARE JUST AS CORRUPT AS HE IS.
TAKE ACTION YOURSELF.

Figure 5.5 Wanted: Donald Capoccia. Courtesy http://times-up.org.

he was a real lefty from Columbia. He was doing bike patrol too. Well, we were trying to see whether the police were staging anything. Before they demolish the neighborhood, they would get a staging area. They would set up the bulldozers; they would set up the paddy wagons; they would do all that kind of stuff.

The structure used to blockade the bulldozers functioned like an open-ended, highly democratic art project. The blockade included the RTS tri-pods, which the group had used to block traffic during the first RTS action. Neighborhood kids made most frequent use of the garden. Most of those defending the space would have little but concrete and highly dense urban space if the garden was destroyed. "It was a lot of fun building the tripods. That was really fun 'cause I remember someone saying this was like a bunch of kids playing in a garden. Kids were climbing up and down like they were on a jungle gym," Becker recalled.

And there were also parades around the neighborhood to let the neighborhood know what was going on. And there were three boys who lived next to the garden. And they hung out in the garden all the time. And a few politicians even came to speak at the garden, including one who won by like 120 votes with our support . . . And the wall grew and all that went on until Christmas week.

Only a few garden activists were there the day Capoccia's bulldozers arrived. Many of the supporters were out of town for the holidays. A small group was there to watch it disappear. "[W]e all watched them bulldoze it," Becker mused. For Becker, the space connected multiple pieces of his life.

It was a good time getting to know everyone in the neighborhood. You know, Chico would come by, the guy who does all the murals in the neighborhood. He had a mural in the garden, a lot of young artists. People came out of the woodwork. There was performance art. Penny Arcade, she was there a lot . . . To see a part of my neighborhood taken away. It was such a big part of my social life. I was there every Friday night. 'Cause Jeff had started the Molotov Cocktail Hour. It was every Friday till whenever. Artists would show up. And you could kind of, it was a good way to network and connect. You had people who were writing plays who were connecting with people who did sets and stuff. And it was really perfect . . . It was such a big loss.

IF YOU LOSE ONE GARDEN, BUILD MORE GARDENS!

For many gardener supporters, the loss of Chico Mendez was a wake-up call. Garden activists realized they would need to do a great deal more reaching out to other stakeholders. "Everyone realized that a lot of dominos would fall if we did not get a lot of people involved, a lot more than just the Time's Up! people and the Shenkeristas and artists from Chico Mendez," Becker noted. Afterward, "They had to get all the gardeners from throughout the city. We started sending out information to all the gardeners throughout the city to let them know what was coming down."

But they realized a more coherent response was necessary. Michael Shenker recalled four tactics used in the garden struggle in NYC: direct action, a judicial strategy, fundraising, and a legislative approach—"a real snake pit," he explained. Direct action combined with a defiant, disruptive approach played out through tactics including a "sing-out" disrupting a public hearing, as well as a model of organizing that compelled countless actors to participate in the story themselves. The aim was to convey their messages and engage an audience without being excessively didactic. Activists made use of a range of approaches aimed at engaging and lulling audiences with stories that seduced rather than hammered. This theatrical mode of civil disobedience had a way of disarming people and shifting the terms of debate.

More Gardens! coalition organizer Aresh Javadi explained this successful approach to tackling the looming crisis facing the gardeners:

> Theater has always been a method. It opens you to all sorts of possibilities. Again, when you see a plant or a vegetable, you automatically come back to a world of childhood, cartoons, something that is not like the "there is a protest and they are against us." Rather the reaction is "That's so magical. That's so amazing on top of concrete." It brings you a recognition of why it is that people care so much about green space when you can't actually take them to the garden. Did you see this over here—what it meant to this woman, to this grandfather, this granddaughter, how much it's improved their health, their life? You can do that by having a flower dancing with a giant tomato and then there is the action of someone trying to take that away from people and people are willing to step up and move that. It allows people to really engage and question their own intents. It's a very, very powerful thing that I will say again, Bread and Puppet and other groups have utilized . . . We are just like, this is fun, it's loving, and you are going to see how passionate we are about that.

Ariane Burgess put on her own play about the gardens, which she held on the streets downtown. "A bunch of us did the garden play, *Cherry Tree,*" she explained. The play was a Japanese play so a few of the activists adapted it to make it about the community gardens. "We all dressed up and put white paint on our faces and went to different places and performed it. Theater was part of getting the message out to people that the gardens were in trouble." "People on their way to work would stop in their suits and their briefcases. And people who had fifteen minutes," explained Tim Becker. "And they would watch the play and get some idea of what we were talking about with the gardens. And it sunk into them in a nonthreatening way. Regular people started getting interested in the gardens."

The other vital ingredient of the More Gardens! coalition was an open invitation for people to engage. What many appreciated about More Gardens! was that the barrier to participation was nil. If someone wanted to do something, they were welcomed in with a simple "hello, what can you do?" and a suggestion to go give it a try. With other groups, there was a higher threshold to participation. Unlike many others, the MoreGardens! approach was inviting. "That's an incredibly empowering thing," Shenker explained. "Even if you can only do it for twenty minutes a week. The barriers were reduced to the point that anybody could participate and lots of people did. It felt very empowering." The point was to help people feel part of something to which they could actually contribute. "People need to have that feeling," Shenker continued. "It's rooted in us as a species. A lack of empowerment means you might die in the forest. Our survival is contingent upon it." Becker described Aresh: "He had a soft touch. He didn't yell and scream at people." Instead, he created activism with a very low-threshold model of engagement. "Aresh really brought that spirit way into the garden movement," Shenker concluded.

JKtheCat, another longtime member of the More Gardens! coalition, recalled the first time she met Aresh:

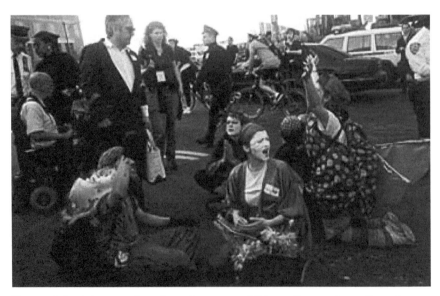

Figure 5.6 Ariane performing. Courtesy of Diane Greene Lent (http://www. dianelent.com/).

I met him when he was compost man at Earth Celebrations. I met this strange and delightful creative. He was dancing with this woman. And he had unlimited energy. It turned out to be his mother and she looked like his peer. And she had unlimited energy too. Every time I'd see him at Wetlands, I'd say, "Hey." And he always invited me to get involved.

"More Gardens!," muses Becker. "They got onto the scene a little bit later than the Lower East Side Collective garden group. But Aresh . . . saw that the regular gardeners should have their group."

Shenker described the ways the organizing strategy fit together:

But really the fundraising, the judicial, and the direct action components of that front worked synergistically. And it's always important, when you are dealing with a guy like Giuliani. The way we did it was with a lot of great civil disobediences. We took over City Hall. And sixty-, seventy-year-old people were doing it. Gardeners from all over the city were getting involved. The very first civil disobedience where we did our CD training was a sing-out. . . . I think it was Rector Street, where it was one of these things where it was going through these moribund administrative committees. And this guy has a little placard which says he stands for the mayor and he sits there and they are going through the necessary steps in the legal process of disposing of property. There was this wonderful woman named Lisa, who went to Casa, and she wrote the More Gardens! songbook. And it had things like "The Battle Hymn of the Republic," and we rewrote the thing to be a garden song. We went into the hearings and we distributed the songbook. And people at key moments would just sing for long periods of time, which brought the hearings to a halt in a very, very unthreatening way. And it kind of got people's feet wet to challenging authority. And it began to give them that feeling of collective empowerment through that collective challenging of authority and also was spiritually inspiring by joining together in song. And we began to say, "Aha, if this works here then we can make it work there in such and such a way." And it wasn't such a stretch to ask people to go into City Hall and not leave. And City Hall has great acoustics. There was a hearing at the legislative wing and people took over the lobby. There were like forty or fifty people arrested in that.

Becker was there as well:

We went to City Hall many times. One time, Michael [Shenker] had this idea that we should go to City Hall and we should sing. So, we got about thirty people and we practiced. And we got this twenty-part harmony going that people could join. It's really loud if you have twenty people. So we went to City Hall and they were having just a full body of the City Council. And we of course sat up in the balcony. And they were down there doing some planning. And we started singing. They have pretty good acoustics in there. And so all of a sudden they hear this really beautiful harmony coming from the balcony. And the council meeting stopped. And they all got out of their seats and they looked up to the balcony. It was as if the Martians were landing. They had no idea what was going on. They had probably had protests of many descriptions. It's usually someone yelling or throwing something. They were mesmerized by some harmonic, beautiful song. They didn't know what to do. They just stared there with their mouths open. And then of course security came and bum-rushed us out the door.

Yet, Becker and company kept on singing: "It was an oooom. People were singing higher and lower. You stay with one harmony and then someone else stays with something else and it just becomes very powerful and forceful."

Adding to the mix, Aresh noted, "The other aspect was that even during the civil disobedience, we would have hats and colorful things. The police sometimes didn't even know what to do with the puppets. And they would be like, 'We can't arrest a flower. [*laughs*] That's not a person that we can arrest.'" This lighthearted approach offered a counterbalance to the increasingly heavy handed efforts to control public space and protest. "It's very disarming. When you're dressed like that, you're not perceived in the same way," JK explained. "You kind of get to people through the other side of their brain. And you get to the officials 'cause you've got a trail of children with you. Children pulling a wheelbarrow full of flowers." And the dynamic changes. "They have kids too; they can't bear to treat you like you are dangerous."

For activists such as JK and others in the garden movement, this lighter approach was a refreshing alternative to traditional models of organizing and politics. "It's consistency and open-heartedness and a refusal to play a game of backbiting." JK, for example, simply will not work with "no" groups. "I can't stand that dreary stuff. It doesn't work," she explained. "It turns people off. If you are standing in the line and you are protesting fur, which I do, and you are just screaming at the people going by, they're not going to listen to you."

William Etundi concurred:

The politics of play is all about creating a political movement that is enticing, engaging, intriguing, fun, engaging. I mean, there's been and there still is so much political action that is opposed to everything. It's sitting down and saying no; it's alienating people; it's pushing not only what you are fighting against away but anybody who's doing it. Like the self-righteous, "we're right and everyone else needs to change to what we're doing." And there's no invitation. And locking down in front of a store. Not to make fun of any one group. But the fur protests that happen on Buy Nothing Day, the day after Thanksgiving, outside of Macy's [Fur Free Friday] are a perfect example of something that is actually destructive to its own movement.

With such actions, Etundi and others argue the message gets lost within the shrill tactics. "They stand out there and they scream at people on the street, the consumers, and show them bloody pictures with the fur. And I really believe people buy fur coats just to spite those self-righteous kids screaming in the bull pen."

Several interviewees noted they are acutely aware that no one wants to be lectured to; conversation and dialogue are much more engaging. Most agreed a more affirmative politics offers solutions and new ideas. Aresh explained: "To me it was just like, how can we be a 'yes' group?" To be such a group, activists focus on articulating what it is they want rather than emphasizing what they are against. Ariane Burgess explained:

> What I aim to do is to articulate a vision and live in the world in a way that I want to as much as I can. If I go to that "NO, No, NO!!!" Then that's the way I'm living my life. And that's the feeling in my body . . . If we spend our time going against the system and the machine with our fists in the air, that's what we are doing. But as we go on over here with planting the gardens, growing our food, and being aware of how much waste we create, instead of waiting for the government to regulate how much recycling we need to use, we can start making those choices ourselves. And if people do it, "When the people lead, the government will follow." That's what it's got to be.

The More Gardens! strategy was always to advance images of healthier communities. "Sustainable, healthier communities . . . they've always had spaces where people can gather and be part of nature," Aresh explained.

To articulate this sentiment, More Gardens! looked to mix activism and art. Joe Tuba, a musician, recalled getting involved with the garden struggle in 1998. He would go to Casa Del Soul, a community space in the Bronx. "On Sundays, they would have these puppet-making workshops. . . . Aresh would be there and he would guide us through this puppet making . . . And I had no idea what the fuck this spade was going to be used for." To Joe's surprise he started seeing images from these workshops throughout the city. "I started seeing this shit cropping up in the newspapers."

"The visuals enhanced the words," noted Aresh.

> We didn't try and overstate it or get wordy, saying, "Oh well, housing versus the sunflower. Do you want a house or do you want homeless

children?" We said, there it is: ten thousand vacant lots and they are being given away to rich developers, while the community gardens that could be there next to real housing are being bulldozed. We were not against real housing. Why not have these two balanced? And keep both of them. We want both—real housing as well as real green spaces. The point is opening up spaces that are communal and cultural.

After losing Chico Mendez Garden, the garden movement escalated. Here, absurdist defiance became intricately entwined with the playful garden struggle—both in the courts and the streets. For Tim Becker, there were many funny moments:

I can see certain moments with crystal clarity and with others it's blurs. There was stuff happening every week. There was More Gardens!. The people from Casa Del Soul up in the Bronx were coming down. Bueno was for some reason dressed as an Indian chief, getting arrested at the tip of City Hall. And they arrested him and Harry Bubbins. They put him in the squad car. And Bueno, even though he was handcuffed, got out and was running down Chambers or something as a handcuffed Indian. And the police were chasing him. It's like going down a rabbit hole. It just gets wilder and wilder. [*laughs*]

Throughout this period, activists dressed as parts of gardens and converged on City Hall. They interrupted hearings with songs; they released crickets; they lobbied the state attorney general dressed as tomatoes. And at one point, a garden activist wearing a giant sunflower outfit climbed a tree in City Hall Park. "Matthew Power climbing a tree in front of City Hall. That was like a big moment," Joe Tuba remembered. If there is one iconic moment when activists and the general public alike seemed to sense that the garden movement had come of age, it was the moment when twenty-four-year-old Matthew Power brought his defiant love of the gardens to the city's most public of public commons, City Hall Park. He would not leave until the city agreed to save the gardens. It would take hours for the police to coax him out of the tree. "This is a real war; it's just like Chiapas. We're going to see Giuliani out of office," insisted Power, still wearing his sunflower headdress before the police took him away (quoted in Ferguson, 1999). This story comes up a great deal. There was something about the smiling garden creature, the defiant sunflower, comparing this battle for gardens with the Zapatista struggle. Here, the theater of delight of the garden movement made it to prime time. The police didn't know what to do. Can I arrest a flower? Can I arrest a tomato? Combined with the puppet shows and the songs and the other theater, the garden model succeeded in creating a new ludic model of disruptive protest.

One of the most popular themes of the monthly Critical Mass bike rides was the ride that called for activists to create a garden within the streets of

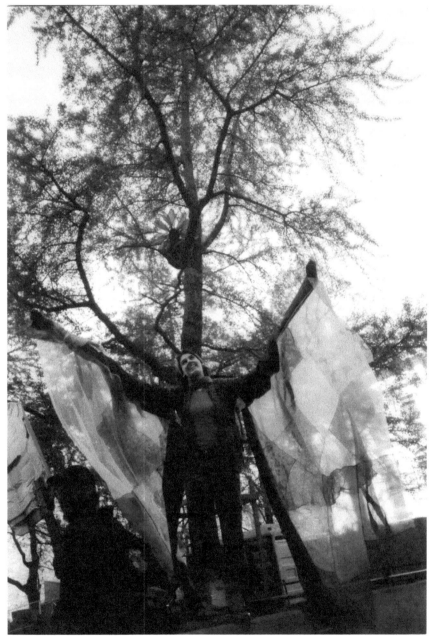

Figure 5.7 Matthew Power in tree in City Hall Park. Courtesy Aresh Javadi of More Gardens!

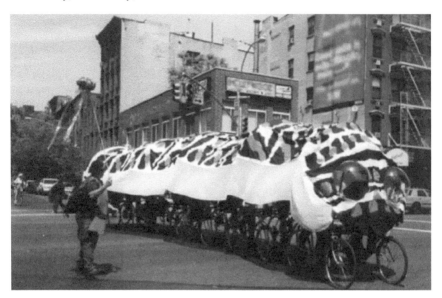

Figures 5.8   Image of caterpillar bike. Courtesy Times-up.org and More Gardens! Coalition Collection.

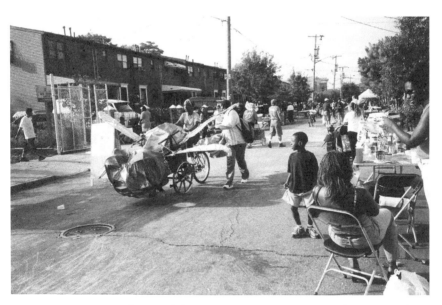

Figures 5.9a   Image of insect bike. Courtesy Times-up.org and More Gardens! Coalition Collection.

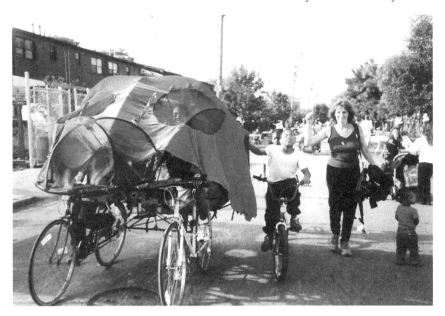

Figures 5.9b Image of tomato bike. Courtesy Times-up.org and More Gardens! Coalition Collection.

New York City. This call offered a challenge to the imagination. In response people did different things including creating a dragonfly and even a cater-pillar bike made of six bikes welded together. The wings of the dragonfly bike moved as bikers inside pedaled.

On another occasion, More Gardens! and Time's Up! built a tomato bike at Charas, with two bikes welded together. "First they had the tomato. And it was two bicycles and welded together. And it was a huge monster tomato," Tim Becker explained. And they rode the creaky contraption from the Lower East Side to City Hall. "And it was the most fun I've had in my life. You know, we were going down Allen Street. And of course the thing was held together by wires. It could move but it was a little shaky." Most loved the hilarious contraption. "But people's jaws were dropping. They couldn't believe a tomato was going down Allen Street. It was big. Two bikes, as big as your couch and eight feet high. People loved it and they couldn't believe it."

RECLAIM THE STREETS AND CREATE A GARDEN

Throughout the peak months of the garden struggle in early 1999, activists tried to generate more creative ways of highlighting the call to save the gardens. After all, another auction was around the corner. Throughout the campaign, Giuliani had a harder and harder time demonizing his opponents or playing on the rotten-apple narrative. Instead, he was drawing criticism. San Francisco mayor, Willie Brown, not known as a preservationist, is said to have called Giuliani to ask what he was doing and to remind him that gardens help community members. "Giuliani created a problem for himself there," Shenker recalled of the days before the 1999 garden auction. "He set himself up by trying to bite off more than he could chew, by trying to take four hundred some gardens at once. Before that they were effectively taking a few gardens from small numbers of gardeners."

The New York RTS group, which by this point was functioning as a project of LESC, started to plan a solidarity action to draw attention to the plight of the gardens. "Reclaim the Streets and Create a Garden," declared RTS. The RTS broadside for the garden action situated the garden struggle with a larger story about the need for a public commons to be part of a healthy democracy:

> The American public, like the Florida panther, faced extinction largely because the American Government tends not to respect its space. The sustenance of a well-informed citizenry—which most would agree is essential for the sustenance of democracy—is impossible without a forum in which citizens are both enabled and encouraged to freely exchange their ideas and more accurately articulate their wants and needs. Rarely, however, the government has been using all its power to actively discourage citizens from participating in the democratic process. In New York City, community gardens are being bulldozed by the dozen, community centers are being auctioned off to profit-hungry developers, and obscure ordinances prohibiting the posting of information on city-owned property are being enforced at a seemingly unprecedented rate.

Without a civil society intermediating between the market and the government, American democracy is thought to crumble. Without a strong public, democratic engagement recedes. RTS sought to create new ways for activists to find a way back into the process.

The action was to take place shortly before the next garden auction. William Etundi attended his first RTS meeting shortly before the auction. He recalled:

> I wanted to get involved and months later ran into someone from the action at a party. This little underground club on Monday night. She says, there's gonna be another meeting next week at the Hub. And I'm like, I've been wanting to be involved. I'll check it out, absolutely . . . We get there. The meeting is big—like sixty or seventy people. It's like a couple of weeks before the action. A lot of the groundwork has already been done. But they need a couple of key roles filled;

one includes climbing on the tripod. Definite arrest, definite physical risk. Louis, the gymnast, climbed the last one. [*laughs*] No one else was willing to do this. So I volunteered. It was my first meeting, my first real political action activist meeting in New York City, and I was like, "I'll climb the tripod." And that was it.

Action speaks louder than words. Etundi's quiet gesture would make him a bit of a hero for the group, and by extension cultural resistance political circles and networks.

Ariane Burgess recalled the garden demo fondly:

My favorite action was the Reclaim the Streets Garden Action. It was about the garden struggle. And what was so beautiful about that struggle was that a lot of people were doing different actions . . . And Reclaim the Streets thought, okay, we're going to do a Reclaim the Streets with a theme of the gardens. And so we decided to do it on Avenue A. And it was amazing because people really dressed up for it. They really took over the street. We planted the grass. It was an incredible operation.

You know Brooke Lehman, Torolf, and I were responsible for the main production of that. We worked really well together, planning everything out, deciding where we were going to meet, deciding how we were going to get there. Who was going to be bringing in different music and different elements. And I think the advantage was that we were in a more local community and the other ones we did were in Times Square and Wall Street. A lot of people dressed up for it. It was very powerful. And it was part of the leading up to the larger auction action, which was incredible.

Garden activists, RTS members, and the burgeoning Hungry March Band all met in a community garden in the East Village the day of the action. Someone gave me a bass drum and the action began as a parade poured out of the garden into the streets. As we arrived at Avenue A, between Seventh and Eighth, activists started dancing. The tripod team jumped out of a sidewalk café where they were sitting, stalling, ordering food until they got a signal, and they threw Etundi up into the tripod. Aresh brought out heaps of grass and placed them all over the street, and for a small hour or so the group really had reclaimed the street and turned it into a garden. Throughout the decades, activists have viewed Seventh and A, where cohort after cohort of scenesters have converged, as the most pulsing street corner in the country (Neumann, 2008). It certainly felt like it was that afternoon.

It was Joe Tuba's first street action with Hungry March Band. "It was great. I went in and I was used to playing in the orchestra in school. Now I could just fart around and it was great. And I just basically had no idea what

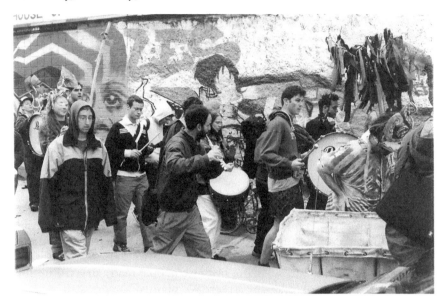

Figure 5.10   The author playing base drum on the way to the RTS garden action. Courtesy Times-up.org.

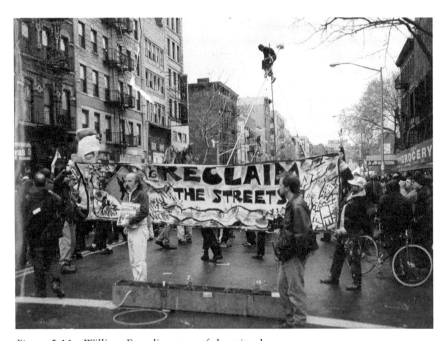

Figure 5.11   William Etundi on top of the tripod.

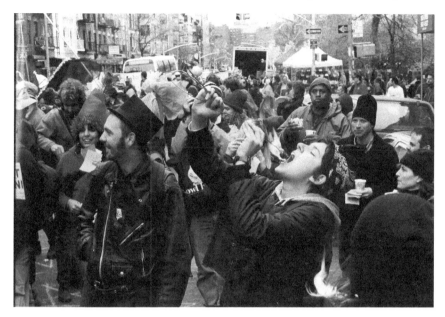

Figure 5.12   Kathryn Welsh eating flames at the RTS action/ street carnival. Courtesy Times-up.org.

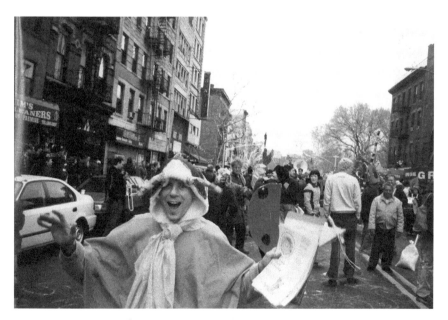

Figure 5.13   RTS garden action. Courtesy Times-up.org.

was going on around me." While the political theme of the action drew him in, the hook was the open-ended participatory dynamic of the action. "The reason it grabbed me in the first place was like, hey, this is really fun and exciting and crazy and stupid and you don't have to have some pedigree like in Marxist theory to do it or understand it," he explained. "It's just very personal and immediate."

For many, the concept of reclaiming the street and creating a garden conjured up a world of possibilities. This was the case of Jason Grote:

> One of the very exciting things was not so much putting out this idea that you could have a different world, which is important too, but the fact of actually doing it. And then there was the other sort of thing of memes. Reclaim the Streets starting in London and moving to New York and popping up in all these different cities. That was really exciting too. It must have had some impact, because universally all these governments all over the world were threatened by this sort of thing. I think in this sort of ontological way, I was really baffled when I first got involved as to why Giuliani would be opposed to community gardens, first of all, why anybody would and then thinking from this libertarian perspective. It's not people seeking money for their program as much as doing it on their own. Who wouldn't agree with this? And then I started realizing that stuff like this is a real threat to any entrenched power. And real genuine play, not hyper-regulated consumerist play.

As a form of authentic, unregulated play, the RTS and garden actions built on a highly subversive dynamic. Here, the networks in which RTS was involved were engaged in a project of direct action aimed at a politics of neoliberalism transforming the globe, privatizing everything in its path (Harvey, 2005). Yet, this social capital was growing and growing. Before he joined RTS, Tuba had heard rumblings about anarchist groups actually willing to fight the neoliberal assault. He had heard about an economic conference in Toronto. "They stole all their food. It totally grabbed my attention," Joe Tuba recalled. "I felt like I had no idea how to get involved with stuff like that. Then stuff like RTS started happening and More Gardens! I felt like More Gardens! was the local manifestation of the kind of stuff RTS was talking about."

The DIY spirit of RTS helped Joe and many others find a language and means of action. With these tools, they were able to identify and challenge social forces propelling a politics of sameness thought to be necessary to support a better business climate (Logan and Molotch, 1987). "It's a kind of a neocolonial thing," Tuba mused. "If Starbucks wants to move into the neighborhood, they are part of something that is determining that this lot is where this garden has to go. It is this kind of colonialism."

Yet instead of analysis, RTS offered an alternative. "It was just very refreshing that the approach to it was let's go have a big weird fucking party," Tuba explained. He reveled in participating in a group which both knew what it wanted, not just what it was against, and was willing to act on this desire. "That was really important for me," mused Tuba. "That was like one part, and the other part was like, God it was such a fucking turnoff to see people walking in lines with fucking picket signs. It's like, nobody wants that. It's really counterproductive and boring." The play of RTS served as a counterbalance, injecting energy into an expanding campaign for public space under assault.

THE AUCTION

One of the core goals of the community garden movement in New York City is the aim to make streets and neighborhoods healthy places for multiple forms of social experience. During the fiscal crisis of the 1970s, neighborhoods, such as the Lower East Side, were lined with abandoned vacant lots and garbage dumps, with tires, rusty needles, and trash. Over the next three decades, neighborhood members cleaned up the spaces, changed the soil, planted seeds, coordinated networks of volunteer urban gardeners craving access to even a few inches of green space, and turned these spaces into a network of community gardens. Gardens make urban neighborhoods healthier greener spaces, they are outlets for various forms of free play, planting parties, and BBQs. They thrive outside of the world of buying, selling, and capitalist exchange. Paradoxically, this made places where gardens thrive more valuable and attractive. By the mid-1990s economic resurgence, developers were beginning to recognize this. And so the city arranged for multiple land auctions to sell off plots of city spaces, which had been transformed into gardens. They were being auctioned as anonymous lots, not the gardens they had become through decades of hard work (Ferguson, 1999).

I came into the gardens direct action movement in March of 1999, during the organizing to stop the auction of 114 community gardens. My field notes from May 2, 1999, are on the civil disobedience training at the Charas/El Bohio Community Center. L.A. Kauffman facilitated the meeting attended by many members of LESC, squatters such as Brad Will, first timers, and so on. After introductions, the facilitator asked everyone in attendance if they had ever been arrested. Many had not. Some talked about the Matthew Shepard political funeral from the previous October. "The mayor has been after gardens for years," Kauffman declared. "Stop this and future auctions. Stand up and say no! He's already planning another auction. Bottom line. CD works where other more traditional models have not worked. We have written letters, lobbied, called people, etc. . . . . Check in with your body."

Aresh recalled the weeks before the auction:

> During the organizing to save the 114 gardens, we had moments where we were in the gardens that were like a week away from being destroyed or given away to some developer. And the children came and took the puppets and automatically told the story. They would tell the story of the garden. And they would say, "So why do you think we shouldn't have housing right there?" And the other kids would say, "Look at that house across the street. That's not for us." And I had nothing to do with that scene. Yet, these kids represent a future of why New York is going to be such an amazing space.

Shenker described the political context:

> Well, they're not stupid. But then they tried all of them and he [Giuliani] thought if he demonized the gardeners, called them Communists, he could succeed. And so he tried to take everything all at once in a big handover to real estate. And basically, it was like a thousand different groups got involved with it. One of the groups that I was particularly involved with was More Gardens! I'm a founding member of More Gardens! More Gardens' original members were: Harry Bubbins, Michael Shenker, Rafael Bueno, and Emily Nobell Maxwell. And really what motivated the formation of More Gardens! was that on that list of four hundred gardens was Cherry Tree Garden. That was the garden next to Casa Del Soul. It's always a great motivator to movements when they are directly impacted by the outrage which was occurring.

A civil disobedience action was scheduled for May 5, 1999, the day before the auction was to take place. The city had invited prospective buyers to take part in the following day's auction. The training took place at the Borough of Manhattan Community College. Ariane Burgess and members of More Gardens! performed their play, called *Cherry Tree*, for the lost garden. "[We] performed it on the corner of Chambers and Washington," Burgess recalled. "There was a groundswell of people coming. And sixty-four were going to get arrested outside." And the streets were filled with bodies of those committed to being arrested. City Council member Steve DeBrienza and future Council Speaker Christine Quinn were standing chit-chatting with all the activists sitting in the streets. "Sit down Christine," someone asked her. "Not today," she smiled. "We're here to make sure you are treated okay."

After blocking the street, we were all eventually carted away.

Many members of LESC, including this writer, Steve Duncombe, and others, were arrested. That night was the first time I met Burgess, while we were waiting to be booked at the precinct. Burgess was leaning over with

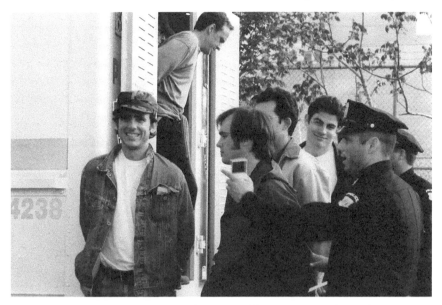

Figure 5.14   Image from right to left, police officer, Benjamin Shepard, Steve Duncombe obscured, Mark Read, and Tim Becker and others getting arrested after garden action. Courtesy Aresh Javadi of More Gardens.

her cuffs behind her back, silent, with her white paint still on her face. I asked her about her pose.

> I was staying in character. We did the play and some of us walked down to the West Side Highway and sat down there. I had a big bunch of peonies in my hair. I think I was quiet like that because my cuffs were too tight and my character was someone who had walked away from the world because he was fed up with what was going on so he got involved with this garden . . . It's fun to do things like that.

We were let out in a relatively short period of time, maybe five hours. On the way out of jail, a short person dressed as a caterpillar approached, congratulated me, and asked that I sign up for future mailings. That was the first time I met Aresh.

"And then we did the auction, with like eighty arrests [at the pre-auction action], and I think we'd already won by that point," Shenker recalled. "And that was to drive home the point that you'd better make sure that we've won."

"That was probably the peak of the movement because it involved real gardeners, not just activists," Tim Becker recalled. "They were doing a seminar on buying city property for developers. . . . There were so many

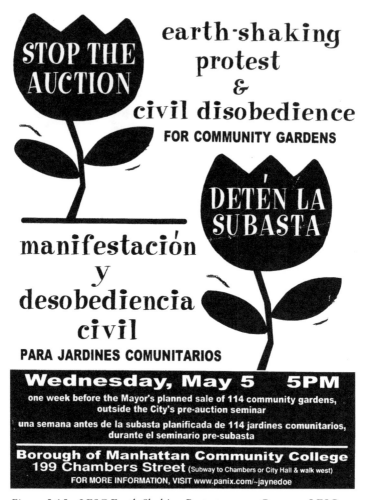

Figure 5.15   LESC Earth Shaking Protest poster. Courtesy LESC.

people arrested that they put people on city buses. I was out blocking the street. But a lot of people went inside. And yelled and screamed." One activist with LESC said she was working on a big fart concoction with sulfer, which she would release, to stink up the precedings. But it wasn't even necessary. "The developers freaked and ran out," Becker remembered. "They went out down the back door and they were hailing cabs down the West Side Highway, getting out of there." The auction was eventually canceled.

"Gardeners Plant Selves in the Street," the *Daily News* reported the next day, noting that sixty-two activists had been arrested the night before (Rein, 1999). After countless acts of civil disobedience, gardeners were able to celebrate a victory. On May 6, Bette Midler and a group of garden supporters paid over $4.2 million ($1.2 by Midler alone) to put the gardens in a public land trust. This action saved 114 gardens from redevelopment (Barry, 1999a, 1999b). "The end result of this organizing was a compromise, which helped preserve the community gardens in New York City," Aresh explained.

Shenker reflected on this moment: "So direct action has done its job. And the state's got a dilemma. Holy mackerel, people express popular support and look what power they have." The More Gardens! strategy includes fundraising and judicial strategies. "So on a parallel track we have the state attorney general, come to the rescue. And all the various City Council people are lining up. Lawsuits are filed in Brooklyn. And this is happening simultaneously to all the direct action." The fundraising included outreach to supporters. "I talked to people and they said, 'Bette Midler saved the gardens.' But that was part of the strategy, which was fundraising with the Trust for Public Land, New York Restoration Project, that there would be opportunities for funding institutions." Shenker credited Raphael Bueno for coming up with the strategy. "And we discussed this strategy before. So Elliot Spitzer and these people who had standing brought suit to stay the bulldozing through the courts. All these things worked in synergy. My job was to do the direct action component." Both controversial and flexible, anarchists collaborated with liberals out of mutual interest throughout the campaign. Here, a desire for results trumped ideology and activists collaborated in effective and pragmatic ways. The East Coast mix of activists struggling to preserve public space was simultaneously matched on the West Coast. There a similar liberal radical alliance of activists took shape as Earth First! blockaded, while the Sierra Club sued. And Earth First! delayed the cutting of old growth forests until the cases made their way through the courts. The inside-outside strategy thrived on the East Coast.

And in terms of the gardens in New York, the play of the actions contributed to a larger organizing strategy. Components of this model included mobilization, fundraising, legal advocacy, mass communications, and direct action. Tim Becker described the ways play helped contribute to the campaign. "I think it was just tailored to the moment of the gardens," he explained. "For something like community gardens, it was great to have people riding down the street dressed as tomatoes. It was just the right level of protest."

RETURN OF THE HAIR SHIRTS, REVENGE OF THE BLUE MEANIES

In the weeks after the victory, Kauffman designed a poster that proclaimed, "WE WON," with the words superimposed over the image of two flowers. Text followed:

> After a two-year direct action campaign of protest and education, we stopped the Giuliani administration's plan to destroy our community

gardens. The auction was canceled and the 114 gardens slated for sale will be permanently preserved. There are 600 other gardens that remain unprotected. Join us in this ongoing battle—we fight to win! Lower East Side Collective.

LESC members wheat pasted the poster all over the Lower East Side. And immediately the group received criticism for "taking credit" for the gardens success. Members of LESC chalked up the complaint to a culture of incessant bickering, grasping defeat out of the jaws of victory among the Left. David Crane recalled:

We used the same dancing flowers image we used on the earth-shaking protest. It was explicit, we thought, that we were trying to credit the community . . . And whatever, the Blackout Books was Bill Brown? Oh my God, what an insane person, who's now completely discredited, and for all I know doing time somewhere for molesting little girls. But, We

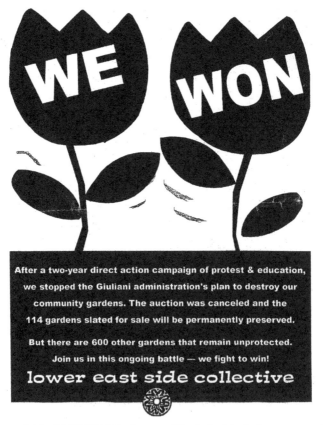

Figure 5.16   LESC 'We Won' poster. The hair shirt Left was never far behind the play of Lower East Side Collective. Courtesy LESC.

Won, oh brother. We did win. The people did win. And we were trying to reclaim it, like, We, not Bette Midler. And then for someone to use this divisively and to say, well, "we" is actually a restrictive thing. Please. *We* was plural, as opposed to *she*, Bette Midler. But we didn't want to attack Bette Midler, we wanted to make people realize what they had done.

The point of the LESC poster was to inform people that there was still a great deal of work to do to save the rest of the gardens.

Further, members of LESC had the next action to plan for: a June 18 Group of Eight (G8) street party organized by RTS. The idea was to throw a street party in the heart of the finance capital of the world. The idea was that the transparent democracy of dancing bodies would counter the secrecy of the G8 model. "Don't Let the G8 Control Your Fate!" was to be the slogan of the day. An RTS London action happened hours earlier. The windows of London McDonald's were smashed, as the action dissolved into a riot. In response, the police adopted a zero-tolerance policy for the New York action. They shut down the street party before it began; arresting most of the organizers, thirty-seven total arrests.

Yet even if the police had not been there, many tried to get the hundreds of regular people to take the streets themselves. The RTS core philosophy was, after all, that the true action of social movements happens when people step off the sidewalk. "[W]hen you come to challenge the powers that be, inevitably you find yourself on the curbstone of indifference, wondering, 'should I play it safe and stay on the sidewalks, or should I go into the street?'" claimed RTS London (quoted in Duncombe, 2002b). Yet, unlike the past RTS actions, few people actually stepped off the sidewalk. "I think that's an internal limitation—a fear of authority that has been drummed into us from a very young age," explained Ariane Burgess, who took part in the action. Wilhelm Reich (1970) suggested these internal checks often result in people feeling too inhibited, too alienated to participate in gestures of personal freedom or actively participate in social movements that might create more liberatory conditions for their lives. In contrast to this, forms of civil disobedience offer space to counter such restrictive social relations, to put one's body on the line, to act with it, to live, and to participate.

Walking home from Wall Street, I felt dejected. The police had successfully arrested the organizers and dismantled the event. I felt like I was being told to just go watch TV. Later that night, I had an e-mail conversation with Stonewall veteran Bob Kohler, a friend from SexPanic! In response to an e-mail headed with the words "Not Too Fun," Bob, who had taken part in the action, responded:

> Guess what? I thought it was a good demo . . . I am never happy about arrests and it looked to me like a couple of very first arrestees were treated badly, but, in all, I was very pleased with the anger and the enthusiasm. . . . I must say some of those cops were ready for us! So—I

think we had a good crowd, we tied up traffic, we made some points. I was glad I went.

Shortly after the June 18 action, Stephen Duncombe sent out a press release announcing the number of arrests and providing follow-up information for the action. The press release stated: "The protest party was organized by Reclaim the Streets/New York City, a local chapter of the international protest group Reclaim the Streets." Like Kaufmann's "WE WON" poster, the press release provoked a small but vocal reaction. "Finding this press release to be full of the very same combination of misinformation and self-promotion that marked the LESC garden group's 'WE WON' poster," Bill Brown issued a short response. In it Brown noted, 'The protest party was organized by RTS NYC, AMONG OTHERS, including [only laziness, or a total lack of interest in anyone else but your own group, prevents you from filling this in].' The egocentrism of certain activists is appalling" (notbored, 1999). Within the next few weeks, LESC was asked to stop volunteering, posting outreach information, or doing outreach for the group through the Blackout Bookstore on Avenue A. Midway through his interview, Jason Grote suggested that the "hair shirt Left" never quite left the scene. A reactionary, dour side of community organizing never disappeared.

Members of LESC did their best to shrug off the conflict over the June 18 action press materials and the difficulties with the action itself. "Your first two actions, you had home-field advantage," the ever-amiable Todd Muller explained at the next LESC meeting, offering a sports analogy for the first two RTS actions that had taken place in the Lower East Side. "June 18 was your first away game." Many members of RTS would travel for the rest of the summer. Some would work on SexPanic! Garden activists would continue to struggle to secure a winning settlement for the rest of the lost community gardens later that summer. Throughout the summer, the stage for organizing felt like it was opening in countless ways.

BUY NOTHING DAY 1999

By the end of the summer, RTS started meeting again. The first meeting was held sometime in August in an East Village community garden. By the end of that meeting, plans and a date for the next action had already been established. The action would take place the Friday after Thanksgiving on the biggest shopping day of the year, the day known both as Fur-Free Friday and International Buy Nothing Day. A couple of people in the group had also been hearing about an action planned to coincide with World Trade Organization (WTO) meetings that were scheduled to happen the week after in Seattle. Buy Nothing Day could be a Seattle solidarity action.

For many involved, the challenge was to bring a spirit of DIY color back to the public sphere and public space, which felt increasingly homogenized by the ongoing Quality of Life crusade. Two weeks before the RTS Buy Nothing Day Action, LESC members worked with SexPanic!, RTS, and the Church of Stop Shopping to organize a civil disobedience action in the heart of the sanitized beast, the Disney Store in Times Square.

TAKING A BUST AT THE DISNEY STORE

It had been a year since Supreme Court Justice Ruth Bader Ginsberg rejected an appeal of the XXX zoning law case, which supported the Times Square cleanup (relating to the 1995 New York City Zoning Text Amendment N950384 ZRY). The zoning law was the cornerstone of the Giuliani 'Quality of Life' campaign. As part of the campaign, Giuliani has resurrected New York's Prohibition era cabaret law to restrict dancing (Ehrenreich, 2007a). While supporters of the campaign suggested it was about quality of life for everyone, activists were quick to note that XXX zoning would shut down adult businesses and push the poor further out of the city (Flynn and Smith, 2004). Activists from SexPanic! to LESC had been battling this pattern for years (Shepard, 2009). Others suggested XXX zoning sanitized urban space, subordinating other perspectives to the imperatives of capital (Harvey, 2005). That August, SexPanic! looked to organize a legal topless march through Times Square to mark the anniversary as a day of infamy. As outreach, I took the idea to the LESC. It was suggested I contact Reverend Billy and the Church of Stop Shopping.

The next day I received a phone call from Bill Talen, a local actor and instructor at the New School for Social Research, who had created the alter ego Reverend Billy. Over the next two months we planned an action. An affinity group from LESC, SexPanic!, RTS, and the Church of Stop Shopping staged a sit-in at the Disney Store on November 15, 1999. Our goal was to bring attention to a series of Disney's offenses in the new Times Square. "We're here to protest the inauthentic . . . the use of entertainment as ideology . . . the celebration of the bland," declared our propaganda. Riffing on Benjamin Barber, we concluded: "Whose world do you want this to be—Disney's or yours?"

The day of the action two or three activists at a time trickled into the store. Ron Hayduk and I tried to buy some Disney stuff and haggled over the price. When the cashier turned down Ron's offer to haggle, the line to the cash register got involved in the dispute. After making a scene, we all sat down, locked arms, and blocked traffic to the cash register. We distributed lyric sheets to everyone in the store before leading the crowd in a resounding rendition of Disney's classic, "Whistle While You Work . . . for 15 Cents an Hour," in homage to Disney's Haitian and Indonesian sweatshops. That was the cue for Reverend Billy to begin a nonshopping sermon which further disrupted the somewhat excited shoppers and befuddled staff. Our chants, "No Strippers! No Peace!" and "Put down the mouse!!!"

echoed through the once staid space, before police moved in, arresting six of us. "It is my civil right not to live in a shopping mall," I screamed before being escorted out to the police van. L.A. Kaufman would congratulate everyone for the absurdist defiance of the action. Bill Talen would later muse that the action had helped transform Times Square once again into a culture-making space, a theater of ideas. For those involved, the action had brought a spirit of free, uninhibited play and ritual to a place that felt increasingly restricted and colorless. Victor Turner (1982) suggests such ritual performances create in between luminal spaces, which contain the possibilities for cultural innovation and structural change.

Jason Grote was also working through creating that feeling for himself.

I think the best moments include the arrest with Reverend Billy. That was exciting in a specific way, and getting arrested in the Disney Store was a lot more frightening than getting arrested at One Police Plaza. It was as if a much more significant taboo were being broken. I felt like we'd grown up thinking that if you are principled enough you want to go to the places of government and disobey. I think that a lot of Americans grow up thinking that that's right. That's the legacy of what Martin Luther King did. That's what you are supposed to do. But I think we also grow up with a certain socialization, thinking you don't go to a store in the mall and do rebellion that isn't scripted. You do the teenage mall rat thing, and even though you may have confrontations with security, it is still part of the script. Whereas doing something that was in defiance to a really powerful hegemonic thing . . . You go to the Disney Store, you quietly browse. You buy something, you don't . . . What you *don't* do is make noise. What you don't do is get in the way of the cash register. You don't repurpose the kitschy crap for anything other than what it is there for. And I think that in a way was almost more scary . . . While at the time, I thought about it as the cops being scary, but when the cops came in it was a bit of a relief. It wasn't the cops I was scared of. I was scared of violating this taboo. It was powerful, almost in a Freudian way, like violating an incest taboo. It's this thing that you don't ever question. It was surprisingly terrifying even though I could say Disney was bullshit.

Doing invisible theater with people who like a product is a tough kind of performance, especially in such an inhibiting space. Bill Talen, the actor who plays Reverend Billy, notes there are times in such a space when he starts to speak and no one hears him; no one is listening—they just go on shopping. But the disruption does eventually happen. And here the "really frightening" feeling Grote talks about becomes "really exciting." Like a high-octane adrenaline run (Mains, 1984/2002), the energy released through such actions produces a tantalizing high. This risk release is perhaps the purest form of play (Huizinga, 1950). Just as Reich (1970) suggests bodily inhibition is a key source of repressive politics, those who tap into embodied experiences of pleasure, connection, and communitas reject the docile bodies and minds which support capitalist social relations (see Foucault, 1980; Martin, 1973; Turner, 1982). Grote reflected on his interaction with the Disney staff during the bust:

> It's interesting as the years have passed and I wrote about this guy who was an employee who was kind of a really effeminate guy who was really affronted who kicked me. And I think now with Wal-Mart and the Republican Party, there are a lot more people who are a lot more identified with corporate parties. And it's a little bit more sinister than when you are in high school and someone makes fun of your favorite band. It's like your feelings are hurt. You feel like it's an indictment of you personally. Some people in that line wanted to get out and others were personally affronted, like an attack on Disney was an attack on them.

Yet the core question in such a scenario is whether play can offer a counterbalance within what was increasingly feeling like a tragic comedy. Within a quality-of-life crusade pushing for increasing controls, was play an effective response? Grote suggested:

> I think it was a moment of resistance. There were two things going on. There was this corporatized form of play with its unspoken rules that you have to obey, but then within it, if you are willing to buy your fun, you can enjoy. You have this police regulation of fun and you have this MTV version of fun, which is not spontaneous, and it's not personal. There was a movement like ours that was really based in play and liberation and dancing and humor and laughter and things like this. I think there are historic moments, where that sort of thing arises.

The days in between the Disney bust and the next RTS action were a heady period of action.

RECLAIMING PUBLIC SPACE WITH STORIES

Two weeks after the Disney action, RTS held a roving street party in Times Square on the busiest shopping day of the year, November 26, 1999. "The Buy Nothing Day Action, that was great. Just 'cause it was so much fun," recalled Joe Tuba. "It was so bad, like in a Black exploitation film kind of way. It was like we're going to take over Times Square. It was like, damn, that's so great. That's so good. That's so exciting."

The action began in Union Square. After the sound of horns, marshals led over one thousand people on an impromptu run down into the subway, away from cops at 14th Street, where everyone caught a train up to 44th and Broadway. The ride up to Times Square transformed the subway into a makeshift street party; chants echoed through the subway cars. Once at Times Square, the crowds flowed out of the subway station, following people with big orange signs to 44th where Brad Will and his tripod crew had already set up a sound system and placed it on the corner of 44th and Broadway, clogging traffic with dancing bodies. As usual, such things rarely go as planned. First the sound system stopped. "The sound system always crapped out," Tuba recalled, laughing. "Every time. That's okay with me, because I play tuba." But the group was able to hold 43rd and Times Square for about fifteen minutes. "I don't think we can even say that we held it that long," confessed Tuba. The Hungry March Band kept the music going. But I'll never forget the feeling of those fifteen minutes.

The action was designed to bring the thousands of unsuspecting shoppers already cluttering the streets into a new more authentic, participatory form of performance. Once confronted with the street party, in one grand culture-jamming moment, many joined in, as if they had stumbled onto the production of a music video at nearby MTV. Sometimes magic-realist narratives, like all stories, become reality-creating machines. By the end of the day, forty-five activists were arrested for dancing, rather than shopping, in the New York City streets. "I was hanging back a lot 'cause I had one of those neon orange signs with pointed arrows," noted Tuba. After the arrests, he and others led the remaining activists downtown. "Later I used the arrow to direct everyone to the precinct, where everyone [arrested] went [*laughs*]."

A group of some fifty of us followed the arrestees to the police station, playing drums, dancing, and doing calisthenics as we waited for the arrestees to be released. "That was fun, too. Yeah, that was a lot of fun too," Tuba mused. "I have really great memories of really fun kind of weird experiences outside of central booking downtown." Many interviewees talked about that moment of storytelling and dancing, aerobics and running around the police precinct as afternoon turned to evening, in solidarity with those inside as one of their best RTS moments. Bill DiPaulo helped organize the jail solidarity.

> We were down on Pitt Street. So part of the whole thing with Reclaim the Streets is we knew that the police were going to arrest people and make it unfun, so we wanted to continue to support the arrestees plus bring the demonstration to the police station we were down at the precinct.

I led everyone in aerobics. We ran around the block, sang, played drums, and Bill Time's Up! and Ariane Burgess helped keep everyone's spirits high. Bill explained:

The high idea was to bang stuff to let the people arrested know we were out there, but also annoy the police, putting pressure on them to let the people go. And there was all night long, the police would come out and say, That's it, we're going to arrest you! And then we'd bang the drums more. And the lawyers would then go, "We can't get the people out if you're going to keep banging the drums." There was this one point where we ran around the corner, we did aerobics, but we kept the fun going and we kept the noise level up and I really think that it really did help get people out.

The point was that when you get out of jail there's always a group of people waiting for you. Many interviewed claim that action was the most dynamic moment they ever had in activism. About half the arrestees were not let out till the next day. Bill DiPaulo and company there to greet them.

> Remember that one moment—I have it on video and it's a really great thing—is I think Will (Etundi) got arrested and Louis, and they came out of the precinct, it was in the West Village, and everybody held them up in the air as if like a basketball player above their head, and then they were cheering them, as they were the ones who climbed the tripod [with Brad Will]. And it's a great moment where you took the chance of climbing the tripod and we will raise you up as victors. And you could see the look on the polices' face, like this is not going to go away 'cause look how they're treating these people.

Throughout this period, a festive spirit of defiance combined a range of tactics, in both serious and ludic dispositions. While Brad Will led the tripod crew for the Times Square RTS action, he was also one of the activists who participated in the multiple days of jail solidarity in Seattle the following week. The mixture of bits and pieces of direct action helped create a rich mixture of activists' dispositions within an upsurge of activism. The Times Square action was held in solidarity with the following week's WTO uprising in Seattle; indeed, many RTS activists left jail for flights to the West Coast the following day. What had started as a movement about the quality of life in one urban space had become part of an international resistance effort. This movement connected the struggle for gardens, with efforts to preserve autonomy for indigenous people around the earth. It connected pranks, such as wraps of activist headlines into newspapers, with new friendships, sleepovers, as a new world of activist pleasure and solidarity transformed the streets from Seattle to the Lower East Side. The night before those in RTS left for Seattle, everyone sat around telling stories as we waited for activists to get out of jail. Aresh stood to tell the story of a garden which had not been saved the previous spring. The name of the garden was Esperanza.

THE STRUGGLE FOR ESPERANZA

In the fall of 1999, JKtheCat received a phone call:

> So, we, like many people, were under the impression that the gardens
> were saved when the auction was canceled in 1999. My friend calls me
> and tells me about a small little garden on Seventh Street that was go-
> ing to be bulldozed. I said I don't know what's going on. I thought this
> issue was resolved. I went for a walk. I saw Aresh. And he asked me to
> draw him a coqui. And so I did and it pulled me in.

JK was not the only person pulled into that campaign by Aresh or More
Gardens! The coqui, a Puerto Rican tree frog, was the organizing symbol
for the campaign. Few campaigns brought the divergent activist communities together like the campaign to save La Esperanza Garden on East Seventh Street in the Lower East Side. Like many actions during the period,
play was an integral part of the struggle.

On my way home from the holidays on December 25, a friend passed
a flyer to me as I was about to enter my apartment on Stanton Street. The
flyer declared, "Esperanza Community Garden and El Coqui need your

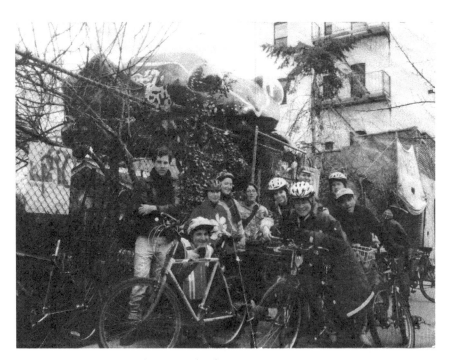

Figure 5.17   Time's Up! photo outside of Esperanza. Courtesy www.Times-Up.org.

immediately support!" The next day I walked to the garden a few blocks away and was welcomed by a group of activists standing around a bon fire, in the snowy community garden. I would stay involved with the campaign until the very end. It would be one of my most memorable experiences in activism. I was not alone.

Aresh recalled:

> That was a case where we really were able to work with the community that was being threatened by gentrification in 2000. It has the dynamic of this huge corporate developer, Donald Capoccia, buying the administration and coming after community-minded groups of people of Puerto Rican origins who had built a community, a block group, co-op housing, and green spaces around them that they were sharing with the community.

Throughout the campaign, La Esperanza—the twenty-two-year-old garden named for hope—had come to symbolize the tensions between the privatization frenzy of corporate globalization and the civic need for public spaces open to all. Despite its history as a community center, in August 1999 the city sold La Esperanza to developer Donald Capoccia—a man who had just happened to donate some $50,000 to the mayor's electoral campaigns and acquired the garden site from the city outside of a competitive bidding process. Giuliani claimed that Capoccia planned to construct "low-income housing" on the site, and that garden supporters were "not living in the real world." In reality, the seventy-nine apartments Capoccia slated to build were "80/20 housing"—80 percent market-rate, luxury apartments, with a token 20 percent set aside for low-income tenants.

In the months after the garden settlement of May 1999, the city changed tactics. It began selling off individual gardens, perhaps one or a small group at a time, but not enough to draw citywide attention along the lines of the May auction. All the while, the general public believed all the city gardens had been saved. Yet the city continued to put more Lower East Side community gardens up for auction. In December 1999, developers ripped the wall off the back of the Esperanza garden, preparing to bulldoze. The scene was a vivid reminder of how Capoccia had bulldozed the Chico Menendez Garden on Christmas back in 1998. Activists, community members, and friends of Esperanza were determined to prevent the same thing from happening again.

Garden advocates sought an injunction to save Esperanza after its sale. Little came of it. Alicia Torres was the original gardener who had planted the seeds of Esperanza back in 1977. "It was open to the children of the neighborhood. They grew up there, and their own children would play and chase each other and fight and do homework and blow out birthday candles there, and eat hot dogs," JK remembered. Adults would celebrate every holiday major or minor. "There was a gorgeous jungle rooster who lived in the garden and would hide from all the people. He is brown, red, yellow, and black, and lovely beyond description. Esperanza was always being used."

In 1999, Torres received a letter from Capoccia stating that construction would begin on the land in a week. Having traversed every legal and policy channel they knew of, activists sought alternate solutions. As Aresh explained:

> Garden activists created a magical creature—the coqui, which meant so much to their own community and the larger Puerto Rican community in the world. And then to allow the gardeners, the local residents, the artists, and activists, as well as thousands of people from all over the world, being able to connect and to share to understand this magic and to come and sleep and stay inside this giant frog—it was just so fantastic.

In Puerto Rican folklore, the coqui has long been known to successfully vanquish larger adversaries. Esperanza could use the same sort of mythology. JK explained how activists mobilized around this story:

> The story of the coqui is that there was a horrific monster in the woods. And all the other animals were terrified. And they were shivering and running away and the coqui encounters the lightning bug and the dragon fly and the mouse and they said, "What's going on? Don't you hear this roaring sound coming out of the forest? It's terrible." And the coqui said, "All right, everybody calm down. I'll take care of it." The little tiny frog hopped into the darkness. And the roaring continued. But suddenly you heard an enormous frog sound. It sounded like it was coming from an animal about ten feet high. And the monster, who could not see in the dark, figured he must be even larger than he was and he left. And the little tiny coqui hopped right out. And he told all these trembling animals that they could go back to bed. It was safe. So the coqui makes an enormous noise but is very small. More Gardens! made an enormous noise but we were very small.

Garden activists built a giant steel and canvas version of the coqui for the garden. "And the kids on the block helped make it, put the wire mesh under it," explained JK. "Eric cut out the two eyeballs, and put in these big plexiglass globes which were the eyes. And they were the windows." The ten-foot-tall frog faced the street, drawing crowds of sympathizers to the cause of the garden, as art and activism overlapped. "The day that we inaugurated it, we had all these kids come in and they made puppets together. They enacted the story I just told you," recalled JK. "They had the big pea costume. There were all these creatures running around and making noises. The adults would come over. In the morning we had breakfasts donated . . . We would have the most amazing gourmet food—croissants, espresso."

People from all over the city came to see the coqui and help support the garden. "I went down there and checked that out," Tim Becker recalled. The practical applications of the space were infinite. "The frog," as Becker described it, helped activists build on past lessons:

> They were fortifying Esperanza and that was on the hit list. What happened was the bulldozers and the police slipped into Chico Mendez before anyone could be in the garden. So the idea was to not let that happen again. So Aresh, the mad scientist that he is, said we'll build this big home there. And we'll live there before anything can happen. So, they made the papier-mâché frog, or coqui, and people started living in there and having a good time.

Activists could spend the night inside the structure, equipped with telephone lines, a heater, and materials to lock themselves down to the coqui if bulldozers were to roll in early in the morning. "[I]t was so beautiful. The coqui was just so magnificent," recalled Michael Shenker. "People's involvement and the winter and the fire pit over there and the solidarity with the Torres family, their willingness just to say 'do it.'"

Between late December and February, a spirit of play pulsed through the garden and those who both enjoyed and defended the space. Many in More Gardens! maintained a distinct philosophy of 'deep ecology.' Here, a close relationship between gardeners and their community translated into a joyous feeling of connection. "This deep ecology is a way of being in the world with an understanding that we are a part of the web of life," explained JK. "We can realize that the planet is a living, breathing being, who is incredibly wise, ancient, and conscious." And while ideologies, such as deep ecology and Marxist Humanism, tend to conflict, most involved with the campaign maintained a sense of ideological flexibility, with an emphasis on direct action. Many shared a nonchurch spiritual love of the gardens which derived just as much inspiration from the pagans and Radical Faeries as anything else. Few were very doctrinaire about politics; what they cared about was saving the garden.

It was also a space which cultivated liberatory play. "I teach a lot of kids," Aresh explained. "And knowing they can put their hands in dirt, play with worms, and be themselves. And you must play this game, wear this lipstick and these clothes. You are not worrying about clothes." This is a space where children grow via their free-flowing exploration and problem solving (also see Brown, 2009; Linn, 2008; Piaget, 1962; Wenner, 2009).

People from all over the city supported the garden. For JK and many others, social eros and play became an intrinsic part of the campaign:

> It turned into quite a scene. It was a dating scheme. People would take their lovers into the coqui. They were actually booking the coqui weeks in advance. There was lots of blankets. There was room for

two people. There was a phone. A heater. It was quite comfortable accommodations.

Tim Becker concurred when I asked him about what happened in the coqui at night. "Don't come a knocking when the van's rocking. That's what I heard." At one of the coqui slumber parties, JK was interrupted:

> One night I slept in the coqui and I was drifting off and I heard this scrambling noise outside. I looked around and it was Aresh scrambling like the skin on the coqui. And so he pops in and makes his bed next to me and the two of us. And we hear this noise outside and it's this drunk guy. And he says, "Hey frog. How're you doing?" And we say, "Fine." And he says, "What, you got a woman in there?" And so it was like that [*laughs*].

The space created room for community building. "They had a lot of fire circles too," Becker remembered. At the time, one of the garden organizers said the warmest place in New York City that winter was the fire in middle of the Esperanza garden. The space functioned as a sort of public commons. "Every night there was a fire," JK remembered. "People would come from every walk of life, every philosophy, every economic strata, and different countries. And they'd come and they'd pontificate and they'd philosophize. It was very playful, very fun." Tim Becker reveled in the fact that "they were having cookouts there and people were getting to know each other."

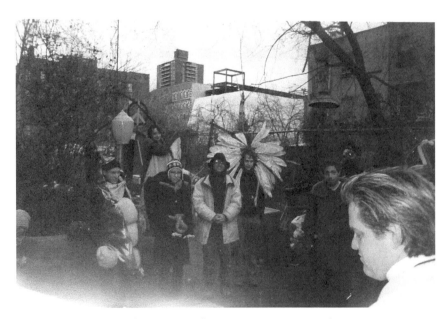

Figure 5.18   Last day of 1999 Rev. Billy at Esperanza. Courtesy http://times-up.org.

I remember on December 31, 1999, being in Esperanza with Bill DiPaulo dressed as a tomato. Those in the garden were taking part in a performance. And everyone was dressed as garden vegetables. Bill DiPaulo from Time's Up! said to Reverend Billy, "I am a tomato! I am a tomato!" "You're a crazy fuck," Billy responded, in jest. Yet, at the time, DiPaulo seemed to believe it. This was also a moment of looking at the world from other perspectives for just a minute, of seeing luminal openings for new social meanings and transformations (Turner, 1982). Organizing overlapped with poetry, within a Whitmanesque view of what democracy could be. "We're forever altered whenever anything changes on the planet," JK mused. "When a garden is sucked off the earth, we feel it." Many felt it the day Esperanza was bulldozed (see Chivers, 2000).

Valentines night, I started getting phone calls saying the next day was going to be the day the bulldozers moved in. On the day of the eviction— February 15, 2000—New York Attorney General Elliot Spitzer was filing papers calling for an injunction barring the destruction of all gardens. Garden activist Susan Howard had helped make the contact with Spitzer, pleading with him to get involved. No injunction could go into effect until 2 p.m. that afternoon at the earliest, but if activists could stall the police and bulldozers all morning, there was a chance the garden could be saved. Some activists locked themselves to the surrounding fence with bicycle locks around their necks, while another group locked themselves to a forty-five-foot-high steel tower of a sunflower and tripods. Five activists locked themselves inside the coqui. And I stood chanting with activists locked inside the fence. It was like the Gunfight at O.K. Corral.

Police swarmed the front of the garden while a bulldozer loomed in the distance at the back. The activists were locked inside. The police moved in, tearing down the fence in front of the garden, sawing off the chain of an activist who had locked herself to it. While protestors were being arrested, Giuliani restated the usual debate that the city has to decide between housing or gardens, as if it is a zero-sum game. Garden activist spokespeople retorted that with thousands of vacant lots and dilapidated buildings to rebuild in the five boroughs, there is room for both gardens and housing. While More Gardens! had successfully constructed a multicultural coalition, mobilizing activists from all over the city, this was not enough to match the deep pockets of New York's real estate industry and their influence on the city's political culture. Aresh explained:

> In terms of Esperanza, we regrettably lost the space and the coqui was destroyed. A lot of people said, "Get the frog out of there. You can save it. The garden is gone." And I was like, "This is not about a little art piece. It's about the bigger picture. The coqui is the garden. The garden is that. And the people who are there who are going to be hurt are part of this frog. And no matter what, this is inseparable." It's semipermeable. It's an art that has the life and heart of the seeds that surround it. So what became of that destruction was, to me, like, as the frog

was destroyed, there were seeds that were exploding and flying all over the city. And we have little froglets that, as JK so wonderfully puts it, have grown by hearing it, who said, "I was not part of it but I want to make sure that does not happen again. I want to make sure that there is something of this creativity and greenery and there is something coming from it."

"Of all of the sacrifices, ones that we've lost, one that I thought we kind of transcended our defeat was Esperanza," explained Michael Shenker. The *Times* quoted Shenker quoting Sophocles as he was arrested during that action: "Giuliani fooliani, the furies will be following you for the rest of your days." As with many of the other cases in this study, the activists were distinctly aware their struggle takes place on a tragicomic stage. Play was even part of the jail experience, which the police did not appreciate. When Shenker, Becker, Brad Will, and myself started to meditate and simultaneously "oooom" as part of our prayer, voices rose as the meditation grew louder and longer. More activists started to chime in. And eventually the cops barged in admonishing us: "Being in jail is not supposed to be fun." Brad Will, Tim Doody, and Tim Becker on the guys side, Brooke Lehman, Jennifur Witburn, and L.A. Kauffman on the women's side—we all did our best to make it a worthwhile experience. Still, the thirty-six hours in jail were exhausting. The cell space was crowded and the hours seemed to go on and on. I ended up calling

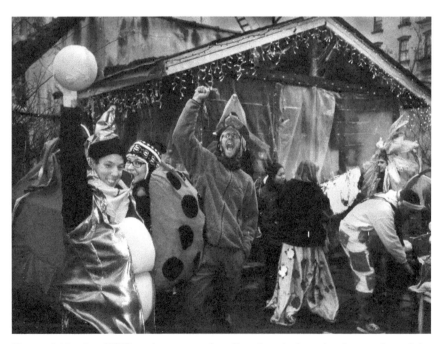

Figure 5.19   Brad Will and company howling days before the destruction of the garden. Courtesy Aresh Javadi of More Gardens!

in and missing two days of work, only to be chastised by supervisors when I returned. The gap between work and play can become a chasm.

Yet, the time was worth the effort. As we were going through the system, the attorney general issued a temporary restraining order on bulldozing gardens and eventually a settlement to protect the gardens from 2002 to 2010 (Spitzer, 2002).

"Community gardens, they are precious to me," JK explained as she looked back on her work on that campaign. "They are so important in the hope of the community."

For her and many others, Esperanza was a catalyst to act. The caring spirit of the space continued. "I think that's what really got me. A lot of people to this day identify themselves with More Gardens! because of their emotional connection to Esperanza," JK noted. "I was so enchanted that I started acting locally, at least for a little while. And you can see the results of your actions when you act locally. It's very empowering."

The following summer of 2001, members or More Gardens! worked with those defending Charas and other spaces to push for a public referendum around the garden issue. JK viewed the referenda process as part of an ongoing DIY struggle to save space. This meant "sing or make a puppet or draw a coqui or climb a sunflower—you could do that." But it also meant taking a step into New York City politics, in a slightly ludic fashion, explained JK:

> We took out all these petitions to all these concerts and the philharmonic and the gay pride parade and got our signatures. And when it came time to deliver the signatures, we had a couple of councilmen standing on the steps of City Hall. We had Norm Siegel. And we were dressed as peas and butterflies and caterpillars and tomatoes. . . . But it was so much fun, especially in that repressive moment to do politics in that playful way.

Part of the richness of organizing around the referendum was bringing a sense of pleasure to the often dour theater of New York City politics. "And then there is always the big 'you are not going to get credibility if you go on New York One [a local television station] with a big bird head,'" JK explained. Yet the group persevered.

The attorney general's temporary restraining order prevented further bulldozing in the final two years of the Giuliani administration from February 2000 after Esperanza until after he left office in 2001. Another two hundred gardens were made permanent park space in the fall of 2002 in a settlement between Spitzer and the new mayor, Michael Bloomberg, which was to last until 2010 (Spitzer, 2002). Many have argued that the legal settlement that came out of the Esperanza campaign was a profound community success. The attorney general even noted that the reason he imposed the temporary restraining order was because "a giant tomato told me to." While the Spitzer-Bloomberg settlement represented real progress, some 150 other community gardens remained vulnerable, and the agreement would only last eight years (Earth Celebrations, 2004).

Throughout the years of garden activism, much of the catalyst was regular people taking part in the process of creating change. "Around Esperanza, that was a campaign that really gelled a whole lot of people around a specific thing, a lot of specific connections between people," explained William Etundi, who reveled in the social capital created along the way. "It was an emotional everything. It was challenging. It was growth. It was building connections, networks. It really catalyzed different sectors of people around one thing." Building on these connections, the campaign connected research along with an engaging model of protest, which bridged a praxis divide between a theoretical demand for public space and a real-world struggle over land use in a global city. Other campaigns had a harder time reaching these ends. Yet, new activists joined the playful movement throughout the year.

LOAN SHARKS, TUXEDOS, AND WORLD BANK PROTESTS

While Esperanza was one of the great campaigns in the history of Lower East Side activism, it was also a tough act to follow. In the months after the Battle of Seattle, members of RTS organized a squad to go down to Washington, DC, to protest at the International Monetary Fund (IMF) and World Bank meetings in April 2000. The concept for the action was hatched during a brain storming session at ABC No Rio, a squat turned art and community arts space on Rivington Street in the Lower East Side. The group members planned to dress like "loan sharks" wearing baby blue tuxedos and to sing their own version of "Mack the Knife," comparing IMF lending policies to those of loan sharks: "the shark has pretty teeth dear."

"Who are these chuckleheads?" Amanda Hickman thought to herself before joining the group. Countless activists came into the group during this period. Matthew Roth had just moved to New York. "I think I saw you in a shark suit," he explained when I asked him how he got involved as an organizer. "I saw these beautiful people in these powder blue suits with shark wigs. It was A16, the IMF protests in Washington, DC." He continued:

> I had been working at the *Nation* as a researcher, intern, and fact-checker. And then this guy wrote an article that was going into the issue right before the April 16th big anti-IMF/WTO thing. It was a small article about RTS in London [see Ghazvinian, 2000]. And I fact-checked it. And I was like, wow, what is this? Everything about it struck me as just fantastic. It was a bunch of heretics. It was a bunch of revelers and celebrators. And it struck me as like, having lived in New York for only six or seven months, as exactly what I wanted to do in the streets of New York. I wanted to tear them up and plant trees in them. And the author

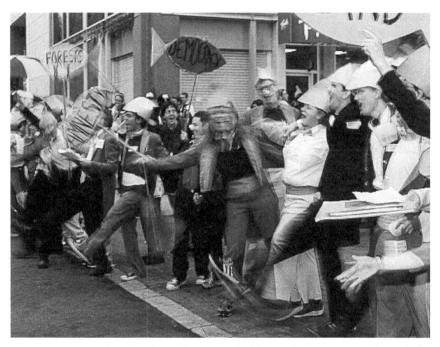

Figure 5.20   RTS loan sharks performing a kickline and their version of 'Mack the Knife' at the IMF meetings. Photo by Caroline Shepard.

came in and said, "Oh, but there's a Reclaim the Streets New York. You should find them. They are going to be down at the A16 rally."

So Roth went to Washington.

Andrew Boyd (2000), the founder of the Billionaires for Bush (or Gore) plugged into RTS New York after the Seattle protests. "Five months later, my friend Lois and I drove from New York to DC, the back of her pickup crammed with shark costumes for an RTS action." Boyd and the rest of RTS were part of a "flying squad." "Lois and I were dressed as corporate loan sharks, wearing plastic jaws, fins cut from file folders, and gray tuxedos borrowed from a South Bronx community center. With about one hundred other sharks we moved from blockade to blockade." Once there the group helped bring a little positive energy to those participating in the blockade to prevent delegates from entering the meetings. "All the while our costumes made the visual statement that the IMF and World Bank operate much like predatory lenders on a global scale." They also communicated a message about the ludic disposition of the group, "having a lot more fun than anybody else out there, really eating it up," explained Matthew Roth.

Chuck Reinhardt, of RTS, offered a narrative of the afternoon. "[A]fter the RTS NY shark flying squad, and others, had prevented

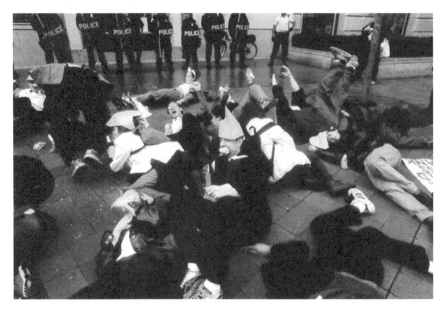

Figure 5.21 Jason Grote eating corn at die-in. Photo by Caroline Shepard.

several buses and vans from entering [the meetings], RTS moved on to the nearby Ronald Reagan trade center, the reputed headquarters of the dreaded Monsanto corporation," he explained. "The building appeared to be a dreary, cheerless, almost gloomy, depressing ugly structure. approximately 80 RTS sharks formed two chorus lines, at the building's entrance, and danced and sang the song . . . 'the twelve days of Christmas Monsanto.'"

Standing in front of the headquarters of the Monsanto Corporation, RTS members ate pieces of genetically altered corn, sang "The Twelve Gifts of Monsanto" to the tune of "The Twelve Days of Christmas," and slowly every member of the group fell to the ground in theatrical death—an homage to ACT UP's signature "die-in." Group members sang the following words:

> On the first day of Christmas, Monsanto gave to me
> A greenwash campaign

By the twelfth day, Monsanto had given everyone:

> PCBs in rivers
> Biotech potatoes
> Salmon gene tomatoes
> Deaths from Agent Orange

Hormone injected cattle
Ad campaign lies
Seed piracy lawsuits
Dead butterflies
Firefly tobacco
Gene altered seeds
New super weeds
And a greenwash campaign

The Monsanto die-in offered a lighter, more theatrical moment to what
had been a rather ominous weekend. Police had swept a group of activists off the street the night before. The following day, most in the group
were concerned we would face a similar fate. The RTS affinity group
found it difficult to establish some degree of autonomy during the action
planning and the interminable spokes council meetings. They seemed to
work better in theory than practice. One member of the group misrepresented the group at spokes council meetings, committing the group
to things it could not or was not willing to do. Compounding this, the
police had become more sophisticated at incorporating forms of intimidation at convergences such as this (see Juris, 2008). And much of the
group's play felt diminished within the attempts by some to confront
or provoke the police. For others, this confrontation was part of the
fun and the purpose for being there. Play happens in countless contexts
and frameworks, with differing experiences and meanings. For some, a
confrontation with police may feel like a lived fantasy, a riskier form of
play. Not for me. I could not have been happier to see DC in the rearview
window as we drove back to New York. Still many considered the actions
and theatrics of the weekend a success.

John Sellers of the Ruckus Society, which helped make the Seattle protests so special only months prior, described some of the silly approaches
his group took to dealing with the intense security at A16:

> During A16 in Washington, one thing we did that was super-effec-
> tive and really funny . . . that we'd seen in Seattle was a phalanx
> of storm troopers walking around and they looked like something
> out of *Star Wars*, battalions of them marching the streets and stuff,
> and I swore to myself that I wouldn't be caught again without a gi-
> ant sound system that could blare the Death Star theme (from *Star
> Wars*). And so we had this powerful backpack system for April 16
> and I remember marching up to the big barricade where the big
> tremendous standoff was and DC's brass and even some National
> Guard guys were like ten feet above us looking down and all these
> cops with their gas masks on and their whole storm trooper look.
> And we walked out and CNN was there and we started blaring
> that Death Star theme. Daaan Dann Da Na Ta DDDDAaaa Dan da

na. It was incredible. All the cops took their masks off in a couple of minutes. You could see that the brass must have been having a major conversation cause the CNN guys were just cracking up and lovin' it. If you use pop culture . . . if globalization is so good, why are there storm troopers out there in the streets having to defend it from the public?

Much of the struggle over the meaning of the IMF would take place within the public sphere of news reports, the Internet, and the press. As with the Seattle protests—which helped inform a whole cohort about the WTO, an institution many had heard little about—the aim of RTS IMF protests was to introduce a critique into discussion of another little known institution—the IMF.

Much of the process took shape as activists shared stories about what they planned to do or had done during the IMF action and why. After returning home from the action, on April 17, William Etundi posted an e-mail message with the subject head "A16 SUCCESS!" In it, he specifically talked about the links between the RTS actions and the critique of IMF policies in public discussion: "Everyone who participated in and supported the events in Washington this weekend (and continuing) should be proud," Etundi wrote. "Not only did we create a major disruption and delay in the meetings, we also successfully pushed the issue on to front pages and into social consciousness of people all around the nation." RTS's theatrical model of protest helped advance this counterpublic message. "Reclaim The Streets NYC's role in the events came off amazingly. We created festivity and disruption all over the city by dancing, singing and liberating space. Ain't no party like an RTS party," (William, 2000).

Gradually, the movement's critique found converts among notables, including Nobel laureate Joseph Stiglitz (2002), a former chief economist of the World Bank, who echoed the activist critique of the IMF.

In the two weeks after that action, members of RTS planned yet another action in conjunction with May Day activities scheduled for May 1. RTS London had planned a guerilla gardening action for May Day 2000, so RTS NYC followed suit, organizing its own gardening action for the same day (see Duncombe, 2000). When that day came, the police preemptively arrested a group of anarchists wearing bandanas over their faces under the aegis of an 1845 mask law (Bogad, 2003). The May Day action would also serve as a rally for underpaid, and some undocumented, greengrocer workers (Ness, 2002). Eventually, the police followed the group's march from Union Square through the financial center, across the Manhattan Bridge, and over to a public space under the bridge where activists had hung a banner reading "Free the Land" and cleaned up the space so as to create a garden. Many had a great time with the action. Yet, the absurd feeling of the NYPD following us

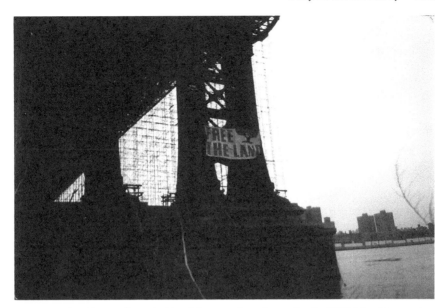

Figure 5.22 Photo—Free the Land banner drop from the the RTS May Day action 2000. Courtesy http://times-up.org/.

through the financial center over the bridge to another borough gave way to an ominous feeling of heavy surveillance. There was nothing anyone could do about it. The heady feeling of the springtime gave way to a much darker feeling the following summer and fall.

THE POLITICS OF PROTEST AND PARTY

After the garden action, many committed themselves to coming back to work in their own neighborhood. Once home, the group faced a dilemma at the center of the politics of play. While RTS had been able to get hundreds of people to their actions, the tension between those who participated because they like the street party and those who hoped to link the play with larger political organizing was only growing; it was a tension which dated back to the Situationists (Aufheben, n.d.).

Summer 2000 was a difficult time for Lower East Side activism. LESC stopped meeting that summer. David Crane described the decision:

I think the thing that swayed me was Steve's [Duncombe] speech about ending something before it became fetishized. Like okay, we can all go our separate ways and dissolve the Lower East Side Collective. But actually Reclaim the Streets had drawn away—that and the Community

Labor Coalition, it pulled apart from LESC. And certain key people had moved on. So that it might be a victim of its own success. But it had succeeded in planting a joyous brand of activism again. I was sad to see it go. I'd been looking for years for such a thing and it happened, it lasted a few years . . . But it didn't blow up and it didn't peter out, it just ended.

Certainly, there was no animosity; people just stopped wanting to go to the general meetings. "They did because there were other meetings to go to really," Crane acknowledged. Many were more interested in just attending affinity group meetings or working on global justice issues, without the overarching collective structure. After a while, LESC meetings felt like just another additional meeting to attend. Some suggested that the group had become the Fleetwood Mac of Lower East Side activism. Like the old band whose members married and divorced in between records and tours, so many of the members of LESC had connected as lovers, dated others, broken up, and so on, that it became difficult for people to continue to meet or work together. For many, it did not feel as comfortable as it once had or it felt like the group had simply run its course. A similar fate befell the Fed Up Queers, which also stopped meeting during the same period (Flynn and Smith, 2004). It was difficult to tell if a controversy stemmed from an activist conflict or a lover's quarrel. Regardless of the cause, what was lost for RTS NYC was the connection between street-party protest and a ministry of love, a labor group, and a public space group. Few recognized this as a limitation at the time, but without a concrete connection to a coherent organizing campaign, the politics of play loses its vitality as a source for social change.

That summer, RTS felt a pull from various directions and several long-time members left the group. "When I left Reclaim the Streets, I was a bit frustrated—a feeling I've since gotten over—but I had an idea of where it was going and I was not into that idea," reflected Brooke Lehman. "There was a moment when Reclaim the Streets kind of lost its politics."

During the summer a small group of RTS members, including this writer and William Etundi, went to the South Bronx to organize an action which addressed issues of environmental racism. Yet the small group was unable to generate support from the general body of the group during a crowded meeting at Umbrella House, a squat on Avenue C. After a long discussion about the politics of a mostly white group of hipsters going to the Bronx without a clear connection to that community, the group voted against continuing the action. Others thought the group was playing it safe. William Etundi recalled that moment:

That was a pivotal moment for RTS. Actually, that was my last involvement in RTS. I don't fault the group for that. But I think it was an incredible learning moment for me and I hope it was a learning moment for the group. It wasn't a matter of fault. Like you, myself and Amanda had this idea of partnering with groups in the South Bronx to work on a local issue in the community, to bring the Reclaim the Streets group out of the Lower East Side, out of our comfort zone to work on something more tangible and more meaningful and really build alliances across boroughs and across different cultural stratas of people. And it would have taken a lot more energy than we were used to putting into actions 'cause building coalitions to do actions takes a lot of energy, more energy than RTS was used to putting out. And it wasn't ready to do that. Instead it did really the most safe action it could have. And I'm not sure if there was a way that South Bronx action could have really worked well, 'cause I don't think that either sphere was at a place to make that go. And I go back and forth with thinking, do those things need to go?

While members of the group were unable to make connections with those in the Bronx, the failure to outline a strategy to do so was a clear limitation for the group. "Those were challenging moments then. And there are challenging moments when you wonder how much of this is fun and how much of this is trying to create change because sometimes it does feel like a social club," Etundi ruminated. "And it's a slippery slope. Is this just a group of buddies acting silly in the streets or is this a group that is really dedicated to making things happen?"

Instead of the Bronx action, the theme which the group approved was "Reclaim the streets for a world without cars." The action would be sponsored by RTS and Time's Up! New York. The dance party would take place after Critical Mass. The action would build on the old RTC NYC broadside that stated:

> We reprove the street as a place where cars are free to pollute air, congest the city, and ultimately upset [and] divide entire communities. As our friends in the UK say, "the privatization of public space in the form of the car continues the erosion of neighborhood and community that defines our metropolis."

The day of the action everyone met at Union Square, for a ritual destruction of a piñata of a car before Critical Mass. Police were breathing down the group's neck. Between arrests of bikers on the ride, a mass of police surrounding members of RTS, much of the coherence of the action was lost between the ride and St. Marks Church, the location for the street party planned for after Critical Mass. Flyers describing the who, what, when, and why of the action were lost along the way. "[T]here were no flyers, no nothing," Lehman notes. Throughout the months since Seattle, Lehman had been concentrating on Direct Action Network [DAN] organizing instead of RTS. "But I came to it and was like, what is this about? I didn't think that anybody had put any energy into letting me know what it was about. That was when

I was like, I don't know." Anthropologist David Graeber (2009), who was active in New York's DAN, recalled seeing flyers and talking with RTS members who noted the flyers had been left up at Union Square during Critical Mass, at the beginning of the multisite action.

Others recalled the action with fondness. Kelly Moore, a long-term LESC member and bike activist, participated in the bike ride that later turned into the street party. After the event she wrote:

> On the day of the RTS/Critical Mass action, I wrote in my notebook: Could human experience get any better than this? Playful, festive, beautiful, expressive, and diverse. I was dressed as a yellow and red sunflower. No one would call me a "sunny" sort of person; how grateful I was to be able to express that side of me. Every kind of person was there, showing off what life could be like—IS like—when people stop abiding by rules that say: be one kind of person, you are what you buy, disconnect from nature, art belongs in museums, faster is better, shut yourself off from strangers. (Shepard and Moore, 2002)

The action reminded Moore that there are moments when joining with others to say yes to possibility and justice are profoundly important choices. She brought some of that righteous indignation to the RTS action: "I decided that day that the best life I could have would be to make sure that I joined others in public and private places to celebrate life, to defy those who hate, and those who want to divide us." In this way, the hunger for caring connection was projected as a counterbalance, a challenge to systems of domination.

Police filled the streets around the proposed meeting site for the September dance party at St. Mark's Church in the Bowery. Some suggested the party should be canceled so as not to interfere with Critical Mass. RTS was already high on the police radar, and activists did not want the same thing to happen with Critical Mass. Standing in front of the meeting space, the organizers started to whisper for everyone to quietly meander out into the evening flow of people meandering through the East Village streets. Befuddled police officers, who had tried to surround those organizing the street party, failed to take notice as people trickled away from St. Mark's Church to meet down the street. And the street party began. Almost immediately, a cavalcade of riders careened into the dance party in progress. There were no arrests at the party (although police had arrested riders). Part of the success of the action was the agility of the collective body of dancers and riders. "[W]e were not the things that interfered with the movement of the automobiles that destroy the earth and speed people away from each other," noted Moore. "[W]e were not one bloc of 'protestors,' but people on foot, bikes, skates, and skateboards who moved together as a big amoeba made up of dazzling light, humor, and joy."

While many enjoyed the action, others remained skeptical of the utility of such actions. "For me, RTS was always about educating people and bringing them into politics through the pageantry and the dancing," explained Brooke Lehman. "The last RTS [action] that I went to was just somewhere in the East Village and it was very small." Some said it was not worth the effort. Others felt it was too much work for too little reward. And others felt ambivalent about the politics, especially after the fall 2000 election results. The police confiscated the RTS sound system at the end of the night. It would be the last 'old-school' RTS street party for a long time.

GROUP PROCESS WITHIN A POLITICS OF PLEASURE

At its best, the politics of pleasure, of making politics intriguing and enticing, involves a social eros between mingling minds. Another dynamic of the politics of play is an ambiguity about means and ends. Describing the meetings of the original English RTS, John Jordan confessed the group had its own blind spots. "It was never really thinking about the process. RTS meetings were the most macho, boring, unembodied, unpleasurable experiences ever. The radical culture here is way less trained in issues of racism and sexism. There wasn't a way out of it." Many had similar experiences with RTS NYC. Amanda Hickman reflected on the irony of a group that aspired to create a better world, having difficulty overcoming interruptions and conflict during meetings: "Are we trying to build a better world or a more abusive world, 'cause the abusive one already exists out there. We don't need to replicate it here."

"If you can't even play with each other, then how can a group change anything else," pondered Kate Crane, who worked with the group. She explained: "I got really tired of a couple of people. There were a handful of people whom I wanted to throttle every time they opened their mouths. And it wasn't fun for me and it made me angry."

John Jordan reflected on the demise of RTS in London:

> But when the really serious repression happened and, in all the papers, we were enemy number one, all the pictures, and we were going to bring everything that Britain held dear to come crumbling down, when all that stuff started to come down around 2000, especially around May Day 2000, post June the 18th [1999]. And then we started to get very pointed surveillance and threats and all of that sort of stuff. And we did not get together as an affinity group and discuss it. . . . Starhawk has said, "more groups and social movements destroy themselves than any number of cops." And that's exactly what happened.

There tends to be a two- to three-year life span for direct action affinity groups. Yet, RTS continued far longer. Still, "I for one do not think that direct action groups think strategically. And two, they don't include play in the process."

IN THE END

Despite the difficulties, RTS and the culture of resistance of the movement of movements churned forward. The Buy Nothing Day action, the Seattle WTO actions, and the Esperanza garden campaign that followed functioned as battlefronts in a public–private debate. In the era of globalization, there remains a need for public space for the people to meet, talk and create a public commons. The groups and struggles covered in this chapter were part of a burgeoning movement of DIY activism aimed at preserving public space and civic culture. Through radical street performance, play, culture jamming, protest street parties, and other pranks, spaces left for dead regained life, public cultures were remembered/reenacted, and new stories took shape. A few years after the May Day 2000 garden action, the space under the Manhattan Bridge where DiPaulo and Etundi had first imaged and then hung the call for the city to "Free the Land" was designated open park land by the City of New York. And the RTS's plans were cemented into the very geography of the city. Still, the police presence on the day of the action was a harbinger of things to come.

6 Playing in Topsy-Turvy Times
From Carnival to Carnage

> Carnival marks a stage in the history of laughter. . . . an especially
> glorious moment in the history of laughter because so many ordinary
> people whose voices normally would clearly not have been heard,
> participated in it.
>
> R. Rawdon Wilson (1990, pp. 36–37)

> The revolution . . . it has become a sort of carnival.
> Subcomandante Marcos (Notes from Nowhere, 2003, p. 176)

> Carnival life itself performs . . . And so in carnival life itself performs,
> and play for a time becomes life itself.
> Mikhail Bakhtin (quoted in Renfrew, 1997, p. 194)

By the year 2000, carnival had become the primary metaphor for a
new model of protest, linking the Global Justice Movement with a long
history of laughter. Here, play supported the reversal of hierarchy and
social status (Turner, 1982). More than protest, the carnival offered
a compelling image of something better. "The central idea behind the
carnival," L.A. Kauffman (2004, pp. 380–81) explained, is that protests
gain vitality if they mirror or create an image of a more compelling
world. "[I]t's not unlike creating a community garden. It's a way of
saying, we not only oppose what's happening now but we have a vision
of a different moral order, in which people are free to express their creative energies to the greatest extent." Here, "public space is dedicated
to community-building and fostering public expression, instead of given
over to commercial expression" (ibid.). Notions of creative play, community building, and carnival would become constants of the movement
between 1999 and September 2001. This chapter considers the trajectory of a movement destined to play in topsy-turvy times. Such play has
a long distinct cultural history. "The fact that play and culture are actually interwoven with one another was neither observed nor expressed,
whereas for us the whole point is to show that genuine, pure play is one
of the main bases of civilization," Huizinga wrote in *Homo Ludens*
(1950/2004, p. 120).

For those involved with the Global Justice Movement, this creative play took place within a series of social and political festivals, convergence actions, and "Carnivals against Capital." "The carnival is one of the sorts of play tools," explained Andrew Boyd. "It grew up organically, partly out of the decentralized civil disobedience model, converging with the dominant underground cultural sensibility with play and raving and all-night dance parties and do-it-yourself culture and free self-expression." Here protest merged the joyous spirit of entertainment with a political agenda aimed at progressive political change. Within this festive, revolutionary carnival, progressive politics linked with notions of social renewal, moving spectators to join in the fun to become part of the concrete action of social change (Ornstein, 1998).

PLAYING JAZZ IN TOPSY-TURVY TIMES

During most of the old RTS street parties in New York City, the DIY sound system stopped working. Yet, in the best of the actions, backup was generally provided by the rhythmic sounds of the Hungry March Band. The band accompanied much of the social and cultural activism in New York for these years.

The first time I encountered the band was in a community garden in the winter of 1999. Activists from RTS New York converged with the band for a successful parade/street party to defend the gardens. Later that fall, the band led activists from Union Square through the subway to re-emerge and take over Times Square in a solidarity action before the WTO meetings in Seattle. The following April, the band led a group dressed as loan sharks in their rendition of "Mack the Knife" during protests of World Bank/IMF meetings in Washington, DC. The Hungry March Band functioned as the catalyst for the transformation of the street party into a social movement carnival, turning "the world upside down with joyous abandon" (Notes from Nowhere, 2003, p. 175). As protest intersected with a burlesque of possibilities, the Hungry March Band was there to provide a sound track. And most of the time, the band brought its Kurt Weill/Brechtian/Weimar boogie-woogie to their actions come performances. The band combined the "harmelodics" of Ornette Coleman with the New Orleans marching band tradition to create something new; its sad yet ecstatic tone seemed to echo a cultural demise as high culture clashed with low. Their performances created stages of subway cars, concert halls, and even city beaches. Horns and drums escalated with the throbbing, yearning, frenetic quality of ska and punk shows, combined with a mix of influences from the transcendent call of street jazz to Brechtian theater.

If there is one activist/performer who has integrated the spirit of play into her work and life, it is Urania Mylonas. A veteran of the Committee in

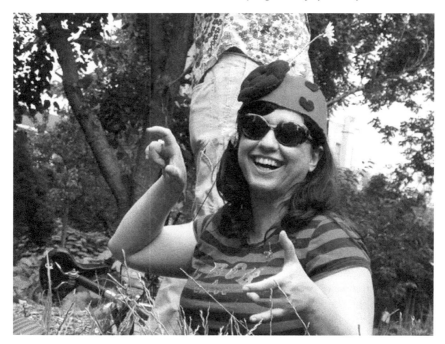

Figure 6.1 Urania Mylonas, by Gaylen Hamilton. A member of Reverend Billy's choir, the Hungry March Band, and the Billionaires, few have done more to propel the ludic turn in activism than Mylonas.

Solidarity with the People of El Salvador (CISPES) and ACT UP, Mylonas has been a member of the HMB, the Church of Stop Shopping, and the Billionaires for Bush (sometimes simultaneously). Between these gigs, she writes, sings, and performs as a twirler in New York. For Mylonas, humor and irony get to the truth of things. But the performance—that's where ludic activism generates the heat which alters social hierarchies (Turner, 1969).

The first time Mylonas saw the Hungry March Band was during their performance at the Halloween parade in New York in 1997. "[M]aybe it was 1998," she conceded. "[T]hey were playing while someone was kicking a flaming soccer ball around," recalled Mylonas. "It stopped me dead in my tracks, and not just because it had singed my sneakers. Somehow, I knew that this burning soccer ball, these musicians and their siren call, were my destiny" (Hungry March Band, n.d.). That heat would characterize many of the band's best shows. Like many in this story, Mylonas suggested these performances create change by creating communities of friends, activists, and cohorts. "My father was in a march band," Mylonas explained. Like his daughter, his work in an Eastern European marching band overlapped with political struggle. "He played bass drum and was always the one who got caught." As a baton twirler with the Hungry March Band—a band which had their own issues with police in less-than-permitted street actions—these experiences became deeply engrained.

I asked Mylonas where she found meaning in night after night of performances. "Connecting with others, such as in New Orleans," she explained in reference to the group's spring 2005 trip to New Orleans Mardi Gras street festivals—the last before the devastation of Hurricane Katrina the following summer. Those moments in New Orleans were a highlight for Mylonas. "I was also wondering how on earth the band could play, and play well, for that long."

Throughout the week, the band reveled in the almost magical realist quality of experience overlapping with technicolor reality. "Probably the best compliment I've ever heard came from a guy who said, 'You guys remind me of a John Waters film' . . . The parade organizers actually called Samantha the next day and invited us to do another parade." It was one of any number of carnival play moments. "There is a kind of quiet beauty about a parade whose theme is the toilet," Mylonas remembered. Duchamp would have been proud. The lineage of play from today's carnivals to Situationism extends back to gestures first seen with the Dada Movement (see Molesworth, 1998).

"That night there was an eerie mist in the streets, and if you looked behind you, the band was coming out of the mist, kind of like that movie *The Fog* only without the homicidal pirates," recalled Mylonas, reveling in the luminal topsy-turvy quality of the moment. Throughout the march a small African American girl danced and twirled with her, thriving in the culture of her neighborhood, which only months later would be consumed by the hurricane. That moment stood out.

For several years there, Hungry March Band shows created a participatory quality of performance, as politics swirled with sweating bodies and a cultural activism that spoke to the hopes of a desperate American landscape. Here, the improvisation of horns and drumbeats connected a music and democracy. If the call of the movement of movements was to globalize democracy, the Hungry March Band shows embodied both the failed promises as well as its possibilities of what freedom really could feel like, if only for a moment. Here, a mix of cultural play and protest offered a glimpse of what Henri Lefebvre must have imagined when he called for movements to demand a "right to the city" achieved through a new jouissance of sensual pleasure, free conscious movement, protest, carnival, theater, and recognition of the radical possibility of the lived moment (Merrifield, 2002, p. 84).

PLAY, CARNIVAL, AND COMMUNITY BUILDING

Mikhail Bakhtin used the concept of carnival to consider issues of empowerment, knowledge construction, and the embrace of social justice. This concept integrates many of the themes which run throughout this text: the liberatory nature of humor, culture, performance, and the possibility of play. By breaking down power hierarchies, carnival helps actors dream of and act on a more equitable brand of democracy than standard forms of political participation. It does so by destabilizing forms of social knowledge. "Play, considered as free play, lies beyond stable, centered structures, makes them untenable, decenters them, and deprivileges them" (Wilson, 1990, p. 16).

Much of the utility of play to social movements involves its capacity to create open spaces where new social relations take shape. Yet, it isn't just any play which does so. Many forms of play, of sports, reinforce social hierarchies. In contrast, improvisational, less competitive forms of play help shape alternate understandings and forms of community (Turner, 1982). Such transformative play takes place in open space where a range of stories and conversations thrive (Bial, 2004, p. 115). Dialogical ("open") spaces run in stark contrast to monological ("occupied/closed") spaces, where closed minds and ideas thrive (Bogad, 2005b). As Harold Weissman (1990, p. 252) explains, "An oppressive environment lowers the odds on the gestation of creativity and innovation." On the other hand, open space stimulates "collective-individual, do-it-yourself creativity" (Bogad, 2005b). Here pleasure, "play, struggle, art, [and] festival" find their rightful and "necessary" expression (Lefebvre, 1974/1991, p. 177).

Such spaces open a carnival of ideas and interactions. Here, regular people can engage, connect, play, and build their own communities. For those interested in an organized model in which there is little difference between leaders and spectators, the carnival offers useful tools. Instead of leaders speaking and followers listening, the carnival breaks down distinction between the two, allowing everyone to be a leader (Bakhtin, 1981, 1984). Joe Tuba of the Hungry March Band described his entry into the group within such a context. "I came into this band through Reclaim the Streets. The structure of it was basically show up and participate. It's kind of the antithesis of top-down. It's not even bottom-up, it's just—horizontal."

This low-threshold approach to community building is also described as participatory culture. Here, someone or a group puts out a press release, lists a time, a place, and a theme for a party—such as a call for everyone to come dressed as Santa Claus and romp around town in an event called Santacon. "I've been very inspired by Santacon," Lower East Side party promoter Abby Ehmann noted. "Participatory culture . . . where you just put out that this thing is happening. And it isn't at a specific place and it's not sponsored by anyone and it doesn't cost anything, it's just something that everyone can come and participate." The threshold for participation is very low. It is a space in which everyone involved revels in a celebration of difference, as diversity and democracy intermingle in an image of what our world could look like. And in the process, the carnival attracts audiences (Bakhtin, 1984; Duncombe, 2004).

Another form of participatory event, of this period, was the subway party. Here, members of RTS, Ransom Corp, Complacent and their offshoots announced a color for a train line (which served as a dress code), as well as a time, and a meeting place. The day of the ride, hundreds of attendees would converge on a subway platform, with drinks and party props, such as whistles, horns, and sound machines. Sometimes a marching band was on hand. Yet, almost always there was someone with drums. Once the train arrived, the group would jump on and decorate the car, as sound machines, drums, and chants transformed the cars into a traveling party careering toward an undisclosed after party lactation. Once inside, I enjoyed stepping on the seats, turning backward, falling, and crowd surfing through the standing room only group of revelers, as if in a mosh pit in a club. Absurd moments, such as chanting "Corn on the Cob" during the "Yellow" party characterized these frenzied nether rides. In between stops, revelers would sprint out of the cars, sometimes up or down the platform, before hurling themselves through open doors into other sections of the subway party. In peak moments, train parties became roving street carnivals moving through the city for hours on end. Sometimes they ended up in Harlem; other times they found their way to the ocean for a polar bear swim off Coney Island; after Esperanza garden was bulldozed, a group of revelers exited the subway only to rampage over the fence surrounding the space and tear it down (Kauffman, 2000). These unsanctioned parties opened up a space for pleasure, personal freedom, and risk. Long a part of New York City party culture and history, notorious club kid Michael Alig used to organize train parties where revelers careened through the streets betwixt and between trips in and out of New York's carnival-like club underground (Haden-Guest, 1997).

William Etundi described the feeling of inherent freedom that often accompanies these gatherings:

> Another element to New York City, which is kind of specific perhaps to this town, but the feeling of inherent liberation even if it's a semi-legal party in an alternative space, it feels liberating. If it's an explicitly illegal party on a subway or on the street, that is liberating. Just dancing in the street is a liberating moment. And we should never underestimate the power of these liberating moments. That's really self-sustaining. I mean, even if you get arrested after it, you feel like, wow, you stood up and took something. And sometimes being arrested is the most politicizing thing that can happen to a person. And hearing people's stories and having other people realize, "Oh shit, I never thought I could get arrested for dancing in the street." Suddenly a person's life has changed from that, which is interesting and exciting.

Within Etundi's narrative, the street party becomes a transformative space, capable of shifting the way people consider their everyday lives and communities (Turner, 1969).

Throughout these years, a number of activists came to actually describe their actions as rituals. San Francisco activist David Solnit explained: "As I get older, I see that there is no difference between a ritual, a performance, and an action. You are trying to shift consciousness and change reality, and change how people view reality. And communicate ideas."

At its best, the movement's carnival-like atmosphere created a space for participants to design interactions of their own invention and creation. "Carnival is not a spectacle seen by the people; they live in it, and everyone participates because its very idea embraces all the people," explained Bakhtin (1984, p. 7). Here people play with power as they break down social boundaries (Sutton-Smith, 1997/2004). And conversely, such activity takes on a revitalizing function. "It is the capricious moments in history when we can see that carnival and revolution have ideological goals: to turn the world upside down with joyous abandon and to celebrate our indestructible lust for life" (Notes from Nowhere, 2003, p. 175). Yet, social change is anything but certain.

LIMITATIONS OF THE TAZ

Through these actions, activists aspired to reclaim public space through their burlesque of activism. Aware of the role of corporate influence-peddling on government and the privatization of even public space (Dunlap, 2000; Shepard and Smithsimon, 2011), the movement aimed to alter ways to experience urban space and challenge the mall-ing of our cities (Ferrell, 2001; McKay, 1998). Yet, as the years wore on many were left to ponder whether the idealized notion of a public sphere was not just another storied space, existing more in memories and carnivals than in day-to-day experience, no different from Hakim Bey's (1991) elusive TAZ. The TAZ had become a primary image for the movement of movements. Yet even Bey was aware of its limitations. "As soon as the TAZ is named (represented, mediated), it must vanish, it will vanish, leaving behind it an empty husk, only to spring up again somewhere else, once again invisible because indefinable in terms of the Spectacle," he explained in his seminal text (1991, p. 101).

Even during the peak years of the Global Justice Movement, actors were keenly aware of the limitations of organizing around the carnival metaphor. Jason Grote, who participated in and organized many RTS actions, explained: "I think the limitations are that, obviously, it's a micro-revolution. It's over and it's over." For others, the party-as-protest model often seemed to allow the political message to become obfuscated within the dancing. For many, there was nothing transformative about dancing in the streets anyway. The notion of dancing in the streets started to wear thin. Many wanted more.

As time wore on, what felt exciting after the Seattle protests in 1999 started to feel like a scripted ceremony. As Solnit explained, "A lot of our demonstrations are like hollow church services where there's no guts or meaning to it and you just go through the routine. We're not conscious and on our toes." There had to be more than street parties, marches, rallies, and fights with police. The authentic play element of the street actions could only remain intact if the actions remained fresh. "It's an ongoing thing," Joe Tuba explained: "We learned a lot from doing that. But then train parties started happening. And that kind of ran its course . . . There is this continuum going on, learning stuff along the way."

Others worried the movement was speaking to itself. "I think the tendency among a lot of cultural activists is just to do cultural stuff and Reclaim the Streets–type stuff," David Solnit mused. "We have people who are not engaged in community struggles. It's good to have parties, but if you are not trying to win something for your community then you do not have the pressure of trying to really communicate things."

"Whenever I meet someone who is doing theater who says that their activism is through their work on stage," Jason Grote groaned, "I always know they are full of shit." He explained:

> I think right now we are sort of witnessing a lot of the limitations to play. There was an article about Burning Man from the point of view of power. You have this amazing thing in the desert and you have all these creative misfits go out and expend energy on this thing. And it's a tricky thing because you don't want to have a movement that's all dedicated to a sort of rank-and-file discipline. But at the same time, it's a real temptation that play is cut loose from traditional activism.

When play gestures merely serve as a pressure release, they tend to lose their vitality. Here they become forms of repressive desublimation (Marcuse, 1955).

Joe Tuba encountered a few of these shortfalls as far back as his punk days before he joined the Hungry March Band: "The problem with that, and this is the problem that punk rock has always had, that it is kind of exclusive. There is a limit to how much it can grow." Yet, the movement continued to evolve. "Like this RTS and post-RTS community is very into spreading itself out. And involving as many people as it can."

EXPERIMENTS IN THEATER

Despite its limitations, RTS New York continued to experiment with different forms of street protest. Throughout the years from 2000 to 2004, RTS NYC would increasingly experiment with theatrical tools to help bring energy and messaging into actual campaigns on the ground.

After Bush's ascension into power, RTS New York planned another trip to Washington, DC, for street theater during the inauguration. This round included a foray into political absurdity. Mocking the baby boomer obsession with the SDS of the 1960s, the group sought to lampoon the right-wingers who had supported Bush's ascendance to power; hence, the Students for an Undemocratic Society (SUDS). Rather than bemoaning the depressing, undemocratic means through which the forty-third president was appointed by the Supreme Court, the group brought a dose of "better to laugh than cry" satire to the inauguration. The press release for the action introduced the group:

WHO ARE STUDENTS FOR AN UNDEMOCRATIC SOCIETY?

We are the children of the political, military, and business elites of America. We have worked for years to undermine democracy worldwide, and seek to celebrate the fact that—with the installation of presidents Cheney and Bush—even the pretense of American democracy has at last been cast aside. We march in support of the property-owning, white heterosexual male who rules by violence.

NO, WHO ARE YOU REALLY?

We're artists, actors, and activists using satire to point out the absurd, massive injustices inherent in a Bush-Cheney administration, and to question how democratic this country ever really was to begin with.

SO WHAT'S THE JOKE?

We're going to be dressing up as "banana republic" dictators and marching around DC on J20, maybe antagonizing some real-life right-wingers, and generally doing media and street performance stunts to illustrate our point(s).

Jason Grote (2002, p. 254), whose fingerprints were all over the press release, described the day:

Something strange happened on January 20, 2001. I don't mean George W. Bush, although that was weird too. There was a fleeting moment when I (and about 50 other people dressed like me) stood bellowing at a National Organization for Women rally. Behind them was a barricade, then Pennsylvania Avenue, then another barricade, then Republicans, and behind them the Capitol Building, its bland white concrete blending into the great gray sky above us all. And while I screamed "John Ashcroft doesn't dance!" in my fake British accent, boogieing spastically like some amalgam of Charlie Chaplin and a member of Devo, the hard brick ground seemed to turn into the boards of a stage. The Capitol seemed like nothing more than pricey set dressing. Everyone, from the NOW protesters to the fur-clad Bushites to the forced-to-be-avuncular Secret Service agents, was transformed, simultaneously, into actors and audience. It wasn't as if DC had been suddenly transmogrified into a theater: it's always a theater. It had, temporarily at least, been transformed from a bad play into a good one.

By the end if the day, the SUDS counter narrative on the lack of legitimacy of the Bush administration became part of the official story of the inauguration. Pictures of the SUDS action, including signs declaring, "Kneel before Bush," "Ignorance is Strength," "Kneel before Cheney," and "OBEY" before a picture of the president's smiling face, could be found over a caption from an article in the *New York Times* national edition. "Anti-Bush protestors outside the Supreme Court before the Inauguration. Many demonstrators complained about the election process" (quoted in Rosenbaum, 2001). "Arguments about the legitimacy of the Texas governor's victory have persisted even as the country accepted the fact that he had won," wrote R.W. Apple (2001) for the *Times*. "Thousands of the doubtful and disenchanted took to the streets of Washington today in angry protest."

For RTS New York, street theater was the next step in the evolution of a protest repertoire. Much of this approach built on traditions of performance art. Here, regular people bring "to life" questions and disruptions of social "conventions" and routines (Goldberg, 1988, p.7). Within this tradition, live art, pranks, street theater, rave, punk, and parties all function as aesthetic tools (ibid.). By 2000, this disposition intersected with the extreme costume ball mix of street theater, carnival, and spectacle seen in the streets of Seattle and in protests around the world (Boyd, 2002; Pranksters, 1987). Here, the street served as a public theater, a commons for debate, participatory performance, and democratic engagement. In this way, activism connected "the realm of play and pleasure" with a street protest tradition bound by few traditional confines (Goldberg,1988, p. 9). "For me, a key inspiration was Dada, the Surrealism, and the Situationists," John Jordan explained. "I was beginning to read up on this. And thinking about ways to make the art invisible." For Jordan, the excitement of RTS was blurring lines between theater and everyday life. Many, such as Jordan, the Billionaire's Andrew Boyd, and William Etundi delighted in watching art intersect with the street activism. Each reveled in the extreme creativity of the movements in which they participated.

BUY NOTHING

On Friday November 24, 2000—Buy Nothing Day—William Etundi planned to stage the first street action for a new project he called Complacent. The previous year, Etundi had been arrested during the RTS Buy Nothing Day action that clogged Times Square. After two years of sitting on tripods in the streets, dancing at world trade meetings, and doing outrageous things Etundi felt like people were still caught up in the spectacle

Guy Debord (1967) bemoaned, caught up in 'complacency.' Playing on this sentiment, Etundi envisioned a stunt to reinvent the Yippie Wall Street prank (reviewed in Chapter 1). He aimed to "create an experience that would make an impression . . . One of those rare spontaneous provocative moments that stick in the folds of memory. . . . that spurs conversation . . . that might make a person think in a way they hadn't before" (Complacent, 2000). The propaganda for the action was vague, even coy. "A novelty? Yes. A risk? Definitely. Something of beauty? We hope so. A world-changing political action. Definitely not" (ibid.). Etundi explained:

> The idea behind Complacent Nation was absolutely about not focus-ing on the politics stuff or creating change. It was about focusing on exciting people. It was about engaging people on the fringes to come more into political movement, and hopefully from there they will learn about progressive politics. And there are a lot of explicit ways I've been trying to create that bridge. But the inaugural actions was all about creating something that was abrupt, exciting, completely insane, and something that was undeniably attention grabbing. You couldn't help but see it if you were there. You couldn't help but be struck hearing about it even a day, a week, or a year later. And so we had a huge party the week before and raised a few thousand dollars in one-dollar bills. Everyone coming to the party had to come with one-dollar bills. Each of those bills was stamped with the word "SATISFIED?" in big red let-ters. And it was stuffed into a bag. I'd donned a suit, a mask—a com-placent mask—hopped onto a telephone booth with a few people and cameras, and tossed these one-dollar bills, in fistfuls, to the shopping masses on the day after Thanksgiving, which is the biggest shopping day of the year in Herald Square, which is the biggest shopping area in New York City. It just happened to be around the corner from the fur-is-murder people, across the street from Macy's. And that wasn't by accident. But what I really wanted to show was just really shaking the crowds of people. The idea was as these fistfuls of dollars bills were wafting around, people were going nuts grabbing it, a few dollars in the air; they'd grab it and it said "Satisfied?" on it. They'd see this complete mayhem, which is what it turned into almost immediately. And see that they were getting crazy over this few dollars, just like flailing in the air.

The action was sure to stir the crowd, a behavior long recognized as poten-tially unruly (Le Bon, 1896). Much of street performance—from Commedia dell' Arte zanies to Punch and Judy slapstick routines—stimulate emotions, from anger to envy to greed or delight (Grantham, 2001). And this was cer-tainly the case on Buy Nothing Day in 2000. A group of us met in the morn-ing in Foley Square, a film crew in tow. From there, Etundi walked to the corner of Broadway, with his not quite smiley face mask and suit, climbed

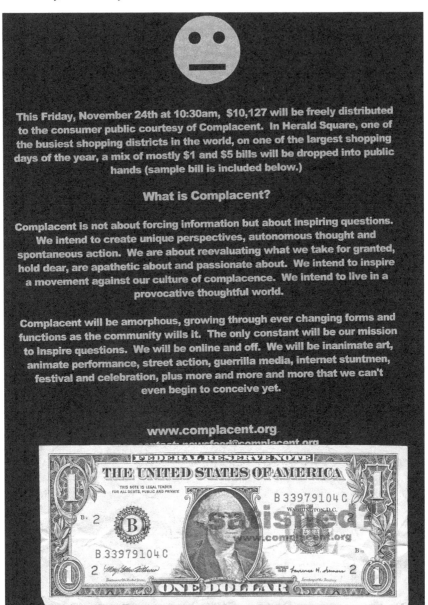

Figure 6.2 Complacent "Satisfied" one-dollar bill. Designed by William Etundi.

up onto a streetlight, looked around for a few seconds, paused and emptied a bag of one-dollar bills he'd earned from one of his parties, pouring out over a thousand bills with the word *Satisfied* emblazoned on them. And sure enough, the shoppers noticed the money floating through the air. Many desperately lunged for the dollar bills. The scene became more and more agitated. One person became furious and screamed at Etundi, saying, "Are you fucking crazy? My kid, I lost my kid." A creepy image of a frenzied mob, took hold in the public theater Etundi helped stir. And Etundi never tried to elude the scene. He stood watching, noting the woman found her child. "The entire time I had no illusion that I wasn't going to get arrested. I was surprised that my charges were just disorderly conduct." Later that night, I met Etundi at central booking and we went out for a beer. Sitting down, we talked about the action, a quiet moment after an eventful day.

"This act was not a direct judgment of consumerism. Not protest to shut down the capitalist structure. Not a world-changing event" (Complacent, 2000). Rather the action was designed to create a situation which inspired people to ask questions, "to step away from what they are used to. To stop on the way to Macy's and grasp at falling dollars and be asked, are you satisfied?" (ibid.).

LIVE ART

Throughout these years, Andrew Boyd (2000) helped theorize about the meanings of the "extreme costume ball" which took expression within the movement of movements. In an interview for this project, he described his thinking about the relationship between theater and activism:

> [W]hen we talk about the uses of play, the way I talk about it is using artistic strategies, which has an overlapping sense with play, thinking like an artist about doing political action. Abbie Hoffman says that all protest, you can extend that to political action, is theater. So protest events that do not consciously think of themselves as theater are often really bad theater. Not always, sometimes there's an organic element. But we're all actors in a way. Sometimes there's an organically beautiful theater to movement, like the kid in front of the tank in Tiananmen Square. His friends had just been killed. He was willing to die. He was caught up in this whole cathartic existential insane moment. He wasn't thinking about theater. He didn't know anyone was filming him. It was an incredible thing.

Boyd, of course, was by no means alone in bringing this perspective to movement work.

"My background was very much performance art, or what is essentially called live art here," Jordan explained. Much of his work has borrowed from an anti-art impulse described by Herbert Marcuse (1969) in his *Essay on Liberation*. Here, Marcuse looked to the transformative possibilities of art to help people feel and see and think about the world and social reality in different ways. The Surrealists, of whom Marcuse was a big fan, worked from a similar vantage point (Rosemont and Radcliffe, 2005). By pushing art out of the galleries into the streets, they helped connect it with daily life. And for this, they were considered revolutionaries (Marcuse, 1969).

John Jordan, who helped infuse a highly aesthetic, even Surrealist sensibility within the movement of movements, brought a similar disposition to this endeavor.

> I was doing stuff that was provocative. One of the key things is the invisibility of art and an understanding that an audience has so many expectations about what art actually is . . . We wanted to create different experiences of art for people who assumed, "I know what art is—art's in a gallery, art's in a museum." And still people would bring enormous expectations to it. So I wanted to bring a set of works where the dimension of art was invisible. Where instead of there being funding or expectations, they would interact with it without even knowing it was art.

In the years to follow, Jordan would observe countless forms of extreme creativity through his participation with the anti-roads movement and RTS. And he was not alone.

Some, such as pagan witch Starhawk, brought elements of public ritual to almost every action in which she involved herself. Starhawk recalled a moment at the G8 protests in Calgary in June 2002:

> We had done several days of actions. And the last day, nobody had planned anything, so the pagans decided we would throw an action that was a ritual. There's a park in the center of Calgary. We mixed up all this clay and water and made mud. And the people took off all their clothes and became mud people. If you are a mud person, you can't talk normally or walk normally. So the mud people went writhing through the streets of Calgary. And we had a prophesy, saying when power meets greed, the fortress falls and the ancient people rise. We'd stop and we'd proclaim the prophesy and then we went to all the oil companies and we danced and we had mimes and planting seeds and then leaving a mark of mud on the oil companies' windows or walls and moving on. Calgary had never really seen anything like this. It started off with sixty or eighty people, by the time we got through the downtown, we had hundreds of people just following us, just mesmerized. At one of the drug companies, I saw this businessman taking off his shirt standing there with this totally tranced out look on his face with a scab of mud on his forehead. I went over and said, "Are you okay?" And he said, "There's a lot of energy here." [*laughs*] "I can't leave. I'm supposed to go back to work, but I can't leave." He went all the way down with us. And finally at the end, we did a spiral dance in this open area and there was a big market by a river. Then finally everyone went into the river and washed off. It was beautiful. It was really one of the top actions and top rituals.

Differentiating between ceremony and ritual, Starhawk suggested, "I think that one was obviously transformative. It was not reinforcing any status quo."

One ritual Starhawk's group often uses is called a spiral dance. "It starts with a circle and then it spirals in and people get close and it teaches people to see each other. And then you spiral back out and in and build the excitement and the energy," she explained. "It's a way of raising power and raising energy which usually turns into a chant or an ooom." The More Gardens! coalition often ends its fundraisers with spiral dances, which help everyone to connect. When done publicly, such as in the middle of a mass protest, the spiral dance creates a highly participatory ritual space.

Throughout such demonstrations, the struggle becomes one of rearranging ways to use public space. Andrew Boyd explained:

> You are constructing these moments. And again, it's artistic strategies. You think about the symbolism, you think about the staging, you think about the character, about composition, concepts of art from set design, from photography, from portraiture. . . . It's a whole resource kit that is often not made use of by political people. And it's powerful. If you look at any of these events, the Democratic convention, [Bush's] landing on the aircraft carrier, it's all Madison Avenue.

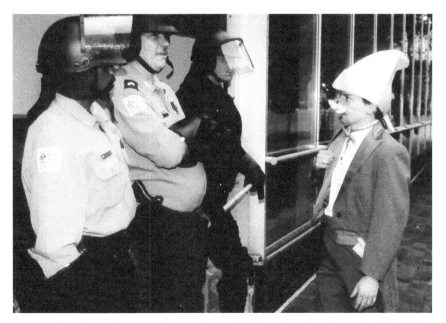

Figure 6.3   One of the many incarnations of Andrew Boyd, as loan shark in Washington at IMF action 2000. Photo by Caroline Shepard.

From his work with United for a Fair Economy to the Billionaires for Bush, Boyd has made a career of borrowing from popular educational and theatrical forms (see Boyd and Duncombe, 2004) to highlight the issue of income inequality and the corrupting influence of money on electoral campaigns (Boyd, 1999, 2000, 2002). He has also made use of irony. When he was in college at University of Michigan, Boyd found out the school was conducting military research on campus. So, instead of staging protest as others had, Boyd and company formed a group called the Nuclear Saints, who called for more military research, not less (Barto, 1983). A press release from November 14, 1983, established the rationale for the action.

> On Monday, November 14, 12 members of the student organization, the Nuclear Saints of America, entered the laboratory of Professor Thomas B.A. Senior, demanding an increase in military research on campus. Professor Senior's lab was chosen as the sight of the action because of NSA's fervent support for the Professor's work on electromagnetic pulse shielding.
>
> The action is intended to demonstrate the organization's commitment to national defense. By volunteering to aid Senior, the NSA are working to ensure the reliable functioning of America's first strike capability. The NSA have come to do military research, and they will not leave until they get some done.

It included a rib at conventional campus activists.

> The NSA have also realized the necessity of purifying the laboratory after its defilement last week at the hands of a band of brutal leftist thugs. At 3:00 pm, the NSA will commence a religious ceremony to cleanse the lab of the evil spirit left by the agents of darkness.

Boyd would recall the ironic Nuclear Saints stunt as a key moment in the mythology of the Billionaires for Bush. It was also a useful example of the efficacy of play-based organizing. "When you've got a super-serious target, it's one way to take away the aura of authority," explained Boyd some two decades later. "Like what we did with this guy in the military research lab." Clever, silly and none too earnest, many of the gestures, including the mockery of the earnest Left, the world would see with the Billionaires could be witnessed in the absurdist Nuclear Saints prank.

One of Boyd's favorite pranks with United for a Fair Economy (UFE) was a mid-1990s Boston Tea Party Action. The goals for the action were twofold:

1. to counter Republican claims that the flat tax is good for working families
2. to reach the broad public with this message

He described the prank:

So this Tea Party thing was doubly interesting because they were staging an event and we restaged it by intervening. These were two guys, two Republican congressman, Dick Armey and Nick Townsend. One's from Texas and one's from Louisiana. They'd been campaigning for what they call a "tax reform," which was a flat tax or a national sales tax. They were pushing to get rid of the entire tax code and institute this very regressive tax system. It seems fair because it was simple and was treating everyone the same way regardless of whether they had eighty billion dollars or negative assets and seven kids. So it was a flat tax versus a sales tax. So they were promoting that and they came to Boston and threw a cask of tea overboard from the Boston Tea Party ship, the historic one where it all happened back in 1773 or whenever it was, symbolizing their liberation from the IRS tax code. So we called up pretending to be Young Republicans and found out what their basic plan was. We read the stuff they were talking about doing in the *Wall Street Journal.* And so we kind of thought how to restage this in a way that sort of brought out the truth of what they were actually advocating. You know, you can give a press conference afterward and say how they were wrong, or you can get in there and mix it up. So we got in there and mixed it up. We got there before they did, set up our people in a way that they wouldn't notice them. And then [the Republicans] were about to throw their tea overboard and at just the right moment, we had this little dinghy which had been hiding in the Boston Harbor on the other side of the [tea party] boat, sort of padding furiously underneath where they were about to throw [the tea]. And the dinghy boat had two people on it. One had a construction hat and the other woman had a kerchief and they held up a sign that said "Working families life raft." And they started saying, "Don't sink us with your flat tax. Don't flatten us with your flat tax." "We're the working family life raft; this tax will be terrible for middle-class taxpayers." And then [the Republicans] were sort of caught dead in their tracks 'cause the photograph caught these guys [in the boat]. They are about to throw this thing overboard, but then not doing it, because our story line was that would be a bad thing. And then we had all these sort of rich people on a boat. They started saying, "We're the Rich People's Liberation Front. We want this tax plan. We want this tax plan."

Boyd's boat tipped over at the exact same time that Dick Armey's group dropped their cask of tea overboard. "They threw it overboard and we capsized at just that moment," Boyd explained:

People ended up in the water. This is the Boston Harbor, mind you, so it's not cleaned up like the Hudson. So it was a huge thing. The photos were in the *Boston Globe* and it was looped on CNN. It was Tax Day.

But if you see the picture, you'll see basically how we restaged it. That's the point. We're staging something and we understood how they

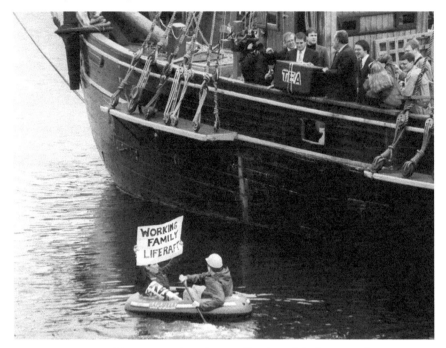

Figure 6.4 Boston Tea Party action. From collection of Andrew Boyd.

were staging and what the various things meant that they were trying to invest with meaning. And we invested them with different meanings, sort of creating a stage around their stage. Not disrupting them and not stopping them, but restaging them.

Through the action, Boyd and company offered a compelling counternarrative to the shrill politics of Republican tax cuts. "[A]ll politics happens in a very mediated way, it's all about spectacle," explained Boyd. "It's all about symbolic communication with an audience. It's all about storytelling and mythology and using and repurposing symbols and stuff like that they were doing. But we did it the same way." Instead of screaming about what was wrong, their performance challenged the story line. "It may be play," Boyd mused. Here, part of the play of social movements is changing the rules of the game. For Boyd and company, their disruptive performance also served as a more inclusive production in democratic worldmaking. As Boyd noted:

> We're not storming the boat. We're telling them to do their thing. And here's what it means for all of us. Again, you're respecting the symbol system that they've set up. But you are reinterpreting it. You're restaging it. And in a sense you are hijacking their power, their prestige, their

star status that turned out all the media. If we were going to stage something on our own, who would come? But no, we hijacked all the media and the spotlight. They already had a stage. And they had a stage because they were powerful.

The prank gained media coverage on CNN and around the world (Ellis, 1998). A student of organizing, Boyd recognized what the action incorporated: "good research, symbolic engagement, surprise and stealth, timing and discipline, upstaging, straight/satirical combination, appropriate tech, 'media wrenching,' media spinning, and control of the confrontation." In terms of things which did not work so well, Boyd conceded the action "didn't hold the field, didn't stay in character, and didn't document ourselves." Still, the prank sent Boyd on a trajectory from Boston's UFE to RTS New York and the Billionaires for Bush (or Gore). Along the way, he articulated his ideas about artful activism, conceptualizing the movement actions he participated within as an "extreme costume ball" (Boyd, 1999, 2000, 2002).

Part of Boyd's work was articulating a set of ideas about activism as a meme for others to emulate. Good artists borrow; great artists steal. William Etundi described this viral dimension of the politics of play:

> I think the biggest assets to the politics of play are, to borrow some words from marketing, the viral aspects of public display. Like we create an interesting action, it's five people. And fifty people see it. Of those fifty, ten people are into it. And those ten people go out and create an interesting action that a hundred people see. And of those hundred, twenty people go out and they are inspired and they do something exciting. And you start getting this exponentially increasing thing. And I think that's the biggest strength of the politics of play.

New York activist Kate Crane concurred. Mindful of how many people got involved with activism through their experiences with the Billionaires, she noted:

> They were able to plug so many people in who otherwise would not have gotten involved. Like the main PR person for the Billionaires, she's an ad executive who has no activism experience. She just knocked herself in full force and ran with it. There was a lot of it that people could plug into; they could feel it, they could identify. Here in New York because New Yorkers are sarcastic, elsewhere because it was fun. And also they were able to take their template and replicate it over and over again.

Throughout the decade, a movement of ludic groups seduced countless new bodies into political engagement and participation. Yet the process of getting people out was far from simple. New York party promoter Abby Ehmann, who organized parties and used those ties to rally protesters against New York's Giuliani Era XXX zoning law, adds: "I have to say, it has become more easy, because more people are pissed off. And also, a lot of the protesting has become more fun." Through groups such as the Billionaires, Ehmann suggested the new activism "saw that the way to get people out was to do it via nightlife. Like the Billionaires for Bush and the people who are making politics more palatable." Citing examples such as Critical Mass, she suggested it is a way of expanding a political arena. And from there, people got involved in many different kinds of campaigns. Etundi explained:

> You see that in More Gardens! and Critical Mass and especially in RTS. If you look at those early RTS meetings, that was my first experience with political organizing. You know, Mark Read, Beka, Andrew Boyd, so many people gelled there and went on to do just faaabulous things. And it really spawned a whole lot of stuff. The Billionaires were inspired by that. Complacent came directly out of RTS. A lot of other projects have. And then these separate projects have spawned people to doing separate projects.

Here each project moves tactics forward. When they failed to do so, the groups lost their vitality or worse, fell prey to perhaps the most searing critique such a group can endure. "You know, the Billionaires got on my nerves; it got boring," Kate Crane noted.

One of the largest criticisms of the politics of play is it lacks gravitas. To counter this charge, many have used research to substantiate group claims. Some have done it to better effect than others. For much of the 2000 election cycle, the Billionaires for Bush (or Gore) argued that there was no difference between candidates George Bush or Al Gore. Corporations had bought both of them. They argued the economic policies of Clinton/Gore would be no different than what Bush's would be. To support their claim, the Billionaires noted inequality had grown substantially under Clinton/Gore, as a by-product of a neoliberal economic program which dominated both conservative and liberal governments around the world (see Harvey, 2005). This was a fair and accurate claim. Yet, the group failed to account for the findings that poverty went down among almost every group of US citizens from 1993 to 2000, something that did not happen with Reagan or Bush. Under Clinton/Gore, poverty in the United States actually declined in ways not seen since the Great Society years of the 1960s or afterward (Blank, 2000). When I brought up this point during the first Billionaires for Bush (or Gore) meeting held at Judson Church in New York City in the summer of 2000, I was shouted down. Play loses its utility in a campaign when provocation and defiant sarcasm becomes an abiding practice,a substitute for ideas connected with coherent claims or substantiated with comprehensive research. Part of how ACT UP or Science for the People supported their causes, however unpopular, was to highlight the ways research substantiated their claims (see Epstein, 1998; Moore, 2008). It is vitally important for activist groups to back up their arguments with coherent research. Otherwise, ludic protest becomes bluster, rather than a compliment to a well-coordinated campaign. As for the Billionaires, as the years progressed, the group's critique felt more and more prophetic: billionaires actually were running things.

THE TWENTY-THREE-STORY TOWER

While Andrew Boyd, William Etundi, and Brook Lehman followed RTS New York by forming new groups—the Billionaires, Complacent, and the New York City DAN—the remaining members of RTS continued the group's work. In December 2000, the group held a permitless parade through the East Village and the three Starbucks (known as "the Bermuda Triangle") at Astor Place, followed by the SUDS actions in Washington, DC. Upon returning from the inauguration protests in the winter of 2001 RTS turned back to the politics of neighborhood life on the Lower East Side of Manhattan. The aim was to do an action a month for as long as possible.

The group's first action of this period would be a street carnival/circus in opposition to a proposed thirteen-story tower which would loom over Houston Street. The action was to coincide with a community board meeting in which the board was scheduled to vote on the building. Working with a large anti-displacement coalition, which included members of the old Lower East Side Collective. Jason Grote drafted a flyer announcing a Friday night "Anti-Displacement Street Circus!" Its advertisement of the carnival as a burlesque show drew the attention of a graduate student named Larry Bogad who was completing his PhD dissertation in Performance Studies on "electoral guerrilla theater." At the time, Bogad had been wanting to draw his theater friends into this form of political engagement, but with little success. He explained:

> [I]n New York in 2001 when I met you, I was very much wanting to do this kind of thing. But my theater friends were theater friends. And my activist friends were organizers. They weren't doing theater. And that's in the streets and I always had that separation, whereas I was in the middle. So getting to know Reclaim the Streets people in the city was a great moment. I was very much looking for that. And finding that affinity group was a big thing for me.

In terms of his first experience of RTS in New York City, Bogad recalled:

> Well, it was an event where there were a lot of RTS people involved, but it might not have been an RTS event. But it was about preventing something that has now gone forth, which is a big building on Houston

Street, where there was a parking garage. There was Reverend Billy doing his thing. What brought me to the event was the great creative flyer
that talked about a radical circus in the streets and a human pyramid
that was going to be built.

The flyer, advertising a circus in the street, was posted throughout the
city and on the Internet. The e-mail announcement for the event began with
the subject line: "March 23: JOIN THE ANTI-DISPLACEMENT CIRKUS
OF THE STREETS!" (quoted in Moshenberg, 2001). It continued:

> WHO: Reclaim the Streets NYC, Reverend Billy and the Church of Stop
> Shopping, CHARAS/El Bohio, the Lower East Side Anti-Displacement
> Coalition, 23 or more random street performers, and maybe YOU!
>
> 23–23–23
>
> WHAT: An ANTI-DISPLACEMENT STREET CIRKUS featuring
> performers, jugglers, fire-eaters, hellraisers and LIVE NUDE HU-
> MANS and possibly NON-HUMANS! And maybe YOU! Note: this is
> a NON-ARREST ACTION! We are NOT PLANNING on BREAK-
> ING ANY LAWS! Also, there will be a 23-PERSON PYRAMID!
>
> 23–23–23
>
> WHEN: Friday, March 23, assembling at 5:30–6pm, then parade to
> LUDLOW and HOUSTON, the site of a proposed 23-story luxury
> tower (ugh!), then CIRKUS at like 7pm we guess but WHO KNOWS
> really!
>
> 23–23–23-
>
> WHY: To fight the forces of displacement and gentrification the only
> way we know how, which turns out to be doing cirkus acts and stuff
> like that. . . . Ludlow and Houston is the side of a proposed 23-story
> luxury tower that would drive up rents and chase the poor residents—
> mostly Latino and Asian—out of the Lower East Side.
>
> 23–23–23
>
> HOW: I DON'T KNOW!

"That was the great teaser, almost Mark Twain-y," Bogad observed.
"And that brought me in. I was the demographic. Here I was, being mar-
keted to by the movement." He continued his story:

> I saw the flyer and said, "I gotta go." And I couldn't get any of my more
> conventional activist friends to go. I went, there was a bunch of people
> doing great stuff, people flying around in wings in a big formation, like a
> bunch of birds following each other, this wonderful little Utopian creative

gesture, brush stroke in the street. And there's Reverend Billy. And it wasn't even the most radical costume ball type of event. It was quite modest by RTS terms, but just to add those few touches to it were wonderful.

And in between the birds and the anti-displacement sermon from the Reverend Billy, the group did actually put together the small human pyramid, maybe not twenty-three stories, but still. After the action, most of us went over to a friend's apartment in Chinatown, where we ate dinner, drank, and listened to Brad Will regale everyone with his off-tune, absurd radical folk tunes.

PLAY AS A STEPPING-STONE IN POLITICS

Stephen Duncombe (2002A,B,) had long suggested there was an actual method to this brand of ludic politics. Each prank built on ingredients for a carnival of activism. The bits and pieces of community theater and culture provided a focal point around which to build collegiality and connection. Yet, more than this, they functioned as an easy entry point or gateway into political activity. As actors supported each other and gained new tools, other engagements in more formal political work become feasible. Throughout the years RTS New York served as a "stepping-stone" to more formal politics. From 1999 to 2004, the group involved itself in successful campaigns to save community gardens, win back pay for immigrant workers, and preserve civil liberties after 9/11 (Ness, 2002; Shepard, 2004). And along the way, players discovered new repertoires—collective action forms—of political action.

Such a politics is at its most vital as a bridge between individual, group, and community needs. For William Etundi, this included two competing dimensions: nightlife and neighborhood activism. "I was going to raves when I was like sixteen years old." And, his mother brought him to demonstrations in the Bay Area. "That was when I was coming of age, eleven or twelve years old. It helped me lay the foundation for sex and politics, which is of course a lifelong process." Once in New York, the play of RTS served as just the sort of stepping-stone into New York City politics and organizing that Duncombe described. "With RTS, I got really enticed with the New York City political scene," he explained. "From there, I got to learn more and more about other spheres of organizing in the city, a lot of the community-based organizing, which is incredibly strong here. And it slowly but surely became my entire life." And politics overlapped with party culture. "It's drawing from a lot of different bits and pieces, from a whole lot of different experiences, trying to bring them together to create something that is rooted to do real work and create progressive social change." Incorporating "elements of graffiti, of party culture, of hip-hop culture so we can make the stuff more interesting," Etundi reasoned. "We can make it enticing for other people to bring their voices in and create a real exponential, physical growth."

Throughout our conversations, Etundi identified a challenge that has vexed the movement: that is, translating the movements' political wanderlust into neighborhood struggles across race and class lines. "The real challenge to creating a creative movement has been to move creative energy into specific policy change out of the Lower East Side into the South Bronx and into neighborhoods of color, where the issues are more urgent." In such spaces, there may not be as much "financial or cultural room to go dance in the street." For Etundi, this is the greatest "challenge to this movement of the politics of play."

In the second chapter of this book, Panama Alba pointed out that play takes place and is understood in wildly specific cultural contexts. For it to serve as a viable model Andrew Boyd suggested activists should be aware of what it can achieve and what it cannot:

> I don't know if it's good at lowering utility rates in poor zip codes. It's more of a kind of swarming pattern. It doesn't have a sustained, kind of meticulous 'eyes on the prize' kind of a thing. That requires more of paid organizers. People on the ground who are fighting for their own rights, in combination with the Alinsky model. There are critiques of the Alinsky model. I don't mean that exclusively. I just mean that kind of thing, which is much more brass tacks.

The challenge remains how such a politics can influence or compliment neighborhood-based campaigns for change.

DIRECT ACTION AND POLITICAL PERFORMANCE FROM CHICAGO TO CHIAPAS

With activists moving through RTS, the More Gardens! coalition, and the Billionaires, those in the movement of movements increasingly recognized that all direct action could and should be understood as a form of performance, which communicated movement goals. "Martin Luther King understood the power of theater," noted Andrew Boyd. "But it was not necessarily true that everybody who was getting hosed down in Selma understood theater." Yet, there those who viewed the street as a space for dramatic interaction and performance (Goffman, 1959; McAdam, 1996). From this perspective, the police perform a theatrics of power with uniforms, badges, batons, wagons for arrests, and high-tech gadgets, while activists hope to stage a more liberatory drama. The police tend to be more interested in the theater of fear, which contains crowds and supports the status quo. The aim of activist theater is to shake up the plotlines so other stories find expression.

One of the most dramatic forms of political theatre is non-violent civil disobedience, often described as direct action. Civil disobedience challenges the legitimacy of authority while creating an alternate set of solutions with one's own actions; in this way, it serves as a form of theater that works to advance narratives of social change and renewal. "Direct action introduces the concept of play into the straight predictably grey world of politics," argued John Jordan (1998, p. 113). To make his case, Jordan borrowed from Victor Turner's (1969) view of play as both unserious and a liberatory force with total disregard for social mores. "The playfulness of direct action proposes an alternate reality but it also makes play real; it takes it out of Western frameworks of childhood make believe—and throws it in the face of politicians" (Jordan, 1998, p. 133). Such forms of direct action are difficult to reconcile with other more serious forms of political engagement. "The state never knows where this type of playing ends or begins," Jordan noted (p. 134). "Its unsteadiness, slipperiness, porosity and riskiness erode the authority of those in power."

In many cases, play overlaps with a form of political theater which invites audiences to join in a joyous performance of social renewal and abundance. Such street theater is intended to seduce audiences into participation in a social change drama (Ornstein, 1998). "You just get a real response," Tim Becker explained in describing the response to the theater used to highlight the plight of the community gardens. "People seemed to love it. It helped them feel good about the gardens and feel good about being politically active, without feeling they were part of something really radical or they would get in trouble in the office."

As Andrew Boyd's story of the Tea Party Action highlights, by the mid-1990s, activism took an artful performative upswing. A few words on this moment are useful as they establish the groundwork for what would become the movement of movements. In his interview, San Francisco activist David Solnit suggested this shift began somewhere between the Zapatista Uprising in 1994 and the actions at the Democratic National Convention in Chicago in 1996. He recalled:

> [At] the 1996 Democratic Convention in Chicago, there was an anarchist, radical gathering called Active Resistance. One of the areas that I worked on was called 'Art, Theater, and Culture.' We organized a muralist from the San Francisco Mission District, some puppeteers, a mask maker from Chicago, a wide range of artists and musicians and dancers, and we spent a week together making art and theater. We ended up organizing the demonstrations for Active Resistance. What was so incredible about that was that for one of the first times, we had a demonstration where the art and theater wasn't sort of icing on the cake or a decoration. The entire logic of the protest was organized as a street theater pageant. We took over the main six-way intersections in Chicago.

I attended the Chicago Democratic National Convention protests Solnit refers to. And certainly there was an absurd defiance to the whole thing. This is not to suggest it made much sense at the time. It did not. Field notes from the days included an appreciation for all that felt wonderful and flawed about the street demonstrations. While coherence seemed to be lacking within the cacophony of puppets and signs, the overall message of the demonstration was a street level critique of business as usual. The "Stop the Racist Imprisonment Binge" stickers that activists passed out seemed to embody a raw, authentic rage against the three-strikes laws being passed across the country. Participants carried puppets in a procession accompanied by a marching band, activists, bystanders, and "everybody in the community" recalled L.J. Wood, who was also in attendance.

"We had a theater pageant and a twenty-foot corporate power tower dragged along by voters, consumers, and taxpayers in all these different costumes. People walked out of their stores, door, and kitchens, and the kids smiled and waved," noted Solnit. "It just had such a different quality and when the police started cracking down on it they just looked very outrageous. They were in unfamiliar territory. They were dealing with a giant puppet and theater pageant with eight hundred people."

"It was a little problematic in that we didn't realize how intense the police pressure was going to be at that point," explained Wood. Yet, the art helped the demonstration feel vital. "To have art and culture at the center of it, moving artists from being the decorators to actually being in the center," mused Solnit. "And that was actually the catalyst for forming Art & Revolution." It was not a traditional protest. Instead it felt like one of the 'extreme costume ball' like street carnival protests seen over the next decade (Boyd, 2000).

Despite the innovative qualities of the street demonstrations, many in Chicago seemed fixated with the history of Chicago 1968. Much of the city yearned to rekindle something of a progressive tradition of action and power. But few could put their fingers on how. David Dellinger, one of the Chicago Eight, was an enduring presence throughout the week. While he attempted to get arrested, the Chicago police refused to be provoked or give the world another image of Chicago police wielding batons. He was not arrested until the last day of the convention. "He had to work at it," Wood concurred. Over the next few political conventions, police would become increasingly sophisticated about not participating in the activist story lines.

Four years later, the police raided the convergence space where puppets and props were being made before the 2000 Republican National Convention in Philadelphia, confiscating the props before a single rally. And the space for play was reduced. "That's obviously no accident," noted Larry Bogad, who lived in Philadelphia while attending college. "They had plainclothes police or what have you inside the space already. And they arrested everybody, I forget, but I think it was sixty-four people, puppetistas, destroyed all the puppets." This, Bogad noted, is common practice in Philadelphia. If materials are disposed of, they cannot be used as evidence in court. "So they destroyed all the puppets. They claimed all the paint thinner was flammable for making a bomb. They said [the activists] were making a slingshot, but it was a stick to hold up a puppet arm."

"There had been a series of crackdowns, particularly on art and culture," explained Solnit. "It's a little hard to articulate, but I think that the police understand that when you control visual space, giant puppets can actually hold a street much better than a black bloc ready to fight." Yet there was more to it. "The other part is that whether its street theater or clowning, we're developing skills to confront power that they are unskilled with, that put them in very unfamiliar territory," Solnit explained. "They are better skilled at violence and physical confrontation. Yet humor and silliness and art and theater, they just don't know how to relate to it." Here, play serves as a different way of confronting power. It aims to disarm, breaking down social controls. In the streets of Chicago, "a combination of theater and playfulness shifted the terrain with the police. It wasn't that we just make art, we were also self-organized. When the cops started rushing in, we all grabbed [the art] so the police couldn't get it," Solnit explained. And activists used it as part of street tactics to hold the space. "But I think what was different was that we had something proactive and positive. That we had a theater and a celebration and a festival going on made it so it did not matter whether the police showed up." Competing protest narratives intermingled throughout the actions as ghosts of Chicago's antiwar past intersected with the style, tactics, and aesthetics of the Global Justice Movement coming into being. While Dellinger looked backward, the group that would become Art & Revolution built on the collective intelligence of Food Not Bombs and the poetry of Zapatismo.

Throughout this period, the movement of movements borrowed from the multiplicity of narratives flowing from the Zapatista "one no and a thousand yeses"—no to neoliberalism and yes to humanity, culture, and difference. "And right after the uprising in 1994, Marcos was called the Subcomandante of Performance Art," Solnit mused. Instead of another left-wing movement aiming to take power, the Zapatistas played with power; they told stories with it, yet they did not try to hold it in any traditional sense. And, gradually, a qualitative shift took place in the way movements conceived of their struggle. Art and culture became a means to engage in an anti-systemic critique which connected multiple issues and sources of oppression. Yet the challenge remained: how to link this critique with a winning political strategy that led to shifts in people's lives? This was the question the Global Justice Movement would face in the years to come.

SUPERBARRIO MAN AND THE STRUGGLE TO BRIDGE A PRAXIS DIVIDE

In the spring of 2001, members of RTS found a very practical way to bridge the praxis divide between the political wanderlust of the movement of movements and core economic issues about wages, salaries, and work, and then acted on these local manifestations of larger global problems. Recognizing the global dimensions of trade policies—such as the North American Free Trade Agreement (NAFTA)—groups such as the LESC and RTS worked together to address the local dimensions of such transnational problems. During spring 2001, RTS collaborated with the Lower East Side Community Labor Coalition (CLC) greengrocer campaign.

That spring, members of RTS New York, many of whom had spent years on the picket lines with the CLC, tapped into their network to support the campaign. The group held a brainstorming session. By the end of the meeting, the group had come up with a plan to stage a theatrical action, in which SuperBarrio Man, a Mexican pop culture hero, wrestled "union busters large and small," on May Day, the international worker's solidarity day. The point of the performance was to highlight some of the themes of the long, drawn out campaign. The group put out calls to various supporters to take part in the performance. Andrew Boyd, of the Billionaires, would serve as the referee for the action. When Bill Talen, aka Reverend Billy of the Church of Stop Shopping, dropped out as the emcee, the group recruited former dramaturge Ricardo Dominguez, a cofounder of the Electronic Disturbance Theater (EDT), a group that developed the "virtual sit-in" in 1998 in solidarity with the Zapatistas. Dominguez, who was in Rome meeting with the Italian direct action group Ya Basta, was recruited through a series of phone calls and e-mails to participate two weeks before the action was to take place. "[N]ot up to speed on this SuperBarrio performance," he responded in an e-mail (2001) to the RTS mailing list. "[W]here and when is it?. . . if I can . . . I would be more than happy to play!" Many would be. Jerry Dominguez, the lead organizer with UNITE, which was helping organize the greengrocers, would play SuperBarrio Man. Jason Grote and Matthew Roth would play union busters, and RTS newcomer Larry Bogad played the "Objective Press," constantly denouncing SuperBarrio as a cheater and extolling the virtues of the bad guys. Steve Duncombe played one of the union-busting henchmen and helped recruit organizer Jerry Dominguez to play the lead. I would play one of the "ring bimbos" who announced the rounds of the match.

Jason Grote (2001) was not actually at the meeting in which he was drafted to participate. "Well, I picked up the latest issue of *Variety* and they tell me that I'm still on tap to play BarrioMan this May Day." He was later informed he was actually slated to play a union buster. Still, he wrote, "As per my usual contract with RTS, I've got a few requirements." These included a copy of the video footage of BarrioMan. In addition, "Like before, I will be needing the tractor trailer with the full-service gym inside." And finally, "for the last time, can someone tell the catering people that I want the crusts cut OFF of my fucking sandwiches?" That was followed by the caveat, "OK, OK, number one is for real. Does anyone have any BarrioMan footage?" This rambunctiousness was a constant part of the group process when RTS New York was functioning on all cylinders.

By mid-April, rehearsals were scheduled and a call for participants in the action went out over the RTS e-mail list:

MAYDAY 2001 WRESTLING MADNESS
SUPER BARRIO MAN VS. MULTI-NEFARIOUS BOSSES

The odds may be stacked against us
The money may all be in the BossMan's Hands
But come Mayday we will collectively smack THE MAN down to the MAT until he cries UNCLE

As the first Mayday of the new millennium approaches, propaganda-ad copy ballyhooing the miracle of the "new economy" is as relentless as ever, despite the obvious emptiness of the rhetoric. For many workers there's nothing new about any of it. Greengrocer employees are locked in a fierce two-year-old struggle to gain the basic right to organize. Sweatshop garment workers toil invisibly in the middle of Manhattan. Immigration officers threaten them all with deportation while the Bosses pick their pockets and starve their families

OUR RESPONSE: Reclaim the Streets, in coalition with the Community Labor Coalition, will march with thousands of immigrant workers to demand their rights. . . . the requisite pack of rabble- rousers will be stopping by greedy Greengrocer stores and garment sweatshops, staging wrestling matches between SUPER BARRIO MAN, people's champion, and various offenders of common decency . . .

WHAT YOU CAN DO: Join the March for the Rights of Immigrant Workers!!

L.M. Bogad, whose first RTS action was during the twenty-three-story tower campaign, became active with the group after reading the call for SuperBarrio participants on the e-mail list. Like Grote, Bogad had training in theater. He described becoming involved: "We met to rehearse and I was the new guy. So this guy, Ben Shepard, was very cool about that. He said, 'Are you Larry from the e-mail?' which was great 'cause it's hard to be the new guy." As an outsider to the group Bogad appreciated the gesture. "Sure, be COINTELPRO all the time and get an ulcer, but while you are doing that try to be friendly to the new guy, he might not be an FBI agent." The RTS strategy for dealing with agents provocateurs was always to put them to work for the group (if possible). Bogad talked about the SuperBarrio Man action:

What I liked about it is that it's savvy interculturalism. I thought it was really apropos and smart as well as being festive. To take a real folk hero of Mexican wrestling for working-class kids and audiences, to take that SuperBarrio character, who is a real performer, obviously, in Mexico and say, "Let's take his costume. Let's do a knockoff version of that." 'Cause we have Latino workers; we have UNITE and the Community Labor Coalition, and a lot of workers who could enjoy the symbolism of this person. Let's make our own SuperBarrio Mayday wrestling madness in the street against the thugs, the union busters, the Billionaires, the Money Devil, and all these cats. The Money Devil was Garret, who got arrested for wearing his mask. He was El Diablo del Dinero, the money devil. All the creative characters doing cool stuff. And I knew a little bit about stage fighting, that little bit of theater background. I said, hey, you can pretend you are pulling someone by their hair this way. And it looks like you're really doing it. The union organizer who played SuperBarrio man was great because he knew martial arts. He was graceful and could move around and pretend to fight. So it's skill sharing. The labor organizer who was willing to wear the funny costume, maybe not too worried about his conventionally defined masculinity. He was totally into it. The fact that we had a couple who played accordions together as the sound track for our live show, again, it's this do-it-yourself stone soup kind of aesthetic. It's like if they both played tubas we'd say "great." Make that work. And it's funny. It adds to the humor, it's like, who are these accordion guys?

Matthew Roth, who was also involved with the action, described the scenario:

> The idea was bringing the people's hero, SuperBarrio Man, who wrestles the corrupt politicians and businesspersons and mob bosses. And who is almost defeated every time, almost unmasked every time so that they may get his real identity. But with the power of the people, the crowd's cheering, he gains strength from that and is able to defeat the corrupt, evil overlords. And so we had our own SuperBarrio in New York. And I was Phil the Dark Knight with my cadre of Fashion Whores, who bound SuperBarrio Man with the power of credit. Merely flashing their cards stunned him. And enabled me to sweep in and nearly win. That wily bastard. He somehow escaped. The crowd is cheering and all these people are going crazy. *La gente unita. . . .* I was overwhelmed and of course he won as usual.

Bogad elaborated:

> It started being a piece of street theater. It was mobile. So it went along the permitted march route of UNITE for this march for immigrant workers demonstration, which started in Union Square, appropriately enough. So we first performed in this rally context. And then the rally, of course, turned into a march. And we marched all the

way around the city, passed some sweatshop bodega kind of places that we were protesting, stopping there, and we were going all the way to the IMF building, which again was something that was cool about UNITE being a progressive union that draws a bigger picture, connecting the local to the global. And RTS too being down with that, having an international perspective, work local, think about global issues and how this all tied together. The show, of course, was a blast. It was a professional wrestling type of outrageous fight, which of course, being SuperBarrio Man, the bad guys are going to try to take his mask off, which is the greatest defeat for a Mexican wrestler to have your secret identity revealed. Which becomes ironic. Everyone winces, "he's going to lose his mask, oh my God" and then cheers when he gets his power back, even though the Billionaires are all ganging up and bludgeoning him three to one. And our ref is looking the other way all the time, you know. So we had a lot of fun shtick like that.

Roth played a spoof of Phil Knight, who at the time was the CEO of the Nike company, which had made a habit of supporting sweatshop labor. "I had on those Lycra supertight, flex black spandex pants things that runners wear and a bright yellow shirt," he recalled. "I had a nice cape with a 'swoosh' on it and it said 'Dark Knight' on the back. And some funky bluish, purplish runner's shorts, kinda hiked way too high up. I looked actually quite ravishing."

Throughout the afternoon, the roving performances took place in front of greengrocer shops that paid workers substandard wages. "We pulled out the ropes and had the full-on mock wrestling match on the street in the name of SuperBarrio Man," explained Roth. A later performance would take place in front of a former Donna Karan subsidiary sweatshop in the garment district on Fashion Avenue. By the time it reached Seventh Avenue, the procession passed the headquarters of Human Rights Watch, where Bob Kohler stood outside monitoring who was getting housing from the Human Resources Administration. For much of that spring, the Global Justice Movement of movements overlapped with campaigns juxtaposing local and global issues. The streets were alive with a cross-section of local struggles that mirrored global issues related to poverty: housing, wages, human rights. Here, historic conflicts between anarchist and reform-minded thinking, between radicals and liberals, seemed to resolve themselves within activist practice and creative direct action.

With each successive round of the SuperBarrio performance, the tension and temperature seemed to rise. Each performance highlighted the struggle of workers to find a different way to work in the world. Audiences included fellow activists, the greengrocers underpaying the workers, media, and by extension decision makers, as well as the public. Matthew Roth outlined the show's multiple audiences. "The first is the

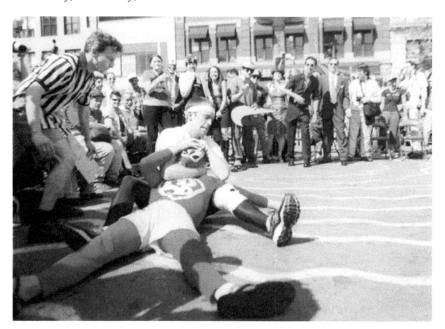

Figure 6.5   Matthew Roth wrestling SuperBarrio Man. Photo by Caroline Shepard.

sort of radical engagement with the unknowing public around you. The group occupied a lane of traffic on the street." Yet, gradually the scene stirred up a frenzy. Roth continued:

> So on one level it's engaging the public. And we saw it very clearly. Within minutes of the action, there was an enormous crowd around us. The police were trying to separate the crowd from traffic. So we're right there in the middle of a thoroughfare that's not intended for people. And we didn't have a permit for the performance. The march part was permitted, but what we were doing wasn't. We weren't asking permission to be on a roadway that's not intended for pedestrians and certainly not intended for pseudo–mock wrestling matches.

SuperBarrio Man was able to prevail in round one at Union Square, after which the march set off to the site of the most infamous antiunion greengrocer, East Natural on Thirteenth Street and Fifth Avenue, for round two. Bogad recalled:

> What ends up happening is we're surrounded by a massive police presence. I think there were as many police as there were demonstrators. And they are doing what I call their own little theater of domination,

where they are criminalizing things, passersby might be thinking we must be psychotic if there are hundreds of cops surrounding us. We must be really dangerous. So I think it has that effect on passersby. It's obviously a little intimidating to us, especially if you are not just a regular RTS member but one of these immigrant workers out there to express your feelings on this issue. But whatever it is, you're a little intimidated by being surrounded by police. And if your papers are not together, all the more so. Certainly. If you're 'sans papiers' or even if you're up here from El Salvador, you're having flashbacks, you're uncomfortable. It's not a good feeling. So it affects the people.

Not long into the match, the legal observers began to whisper that the police were planning to arrest a number of activists when the wrestling matches ended. The interaction between police, activists, and the audience—which included many undocumented workers—produced competing stories and performances, as a joyous theater of social and economic liberation intersected with a display of raw power and control by the police. "It's really a performance and counter-performance, 'cause why are we doing this?" Bogad explained. "We're doing it 'cause it's fun. We're also doing it because it creates a bit of a carnival spirit, where it's like, 'Wow, I went to that demonstration and it was a damn good time while still dealing with our issues.'" Yet that performance clashed into a wildly different kind of theater. Just as the Radical Cheerleaders began to perform outside of East Natural, the

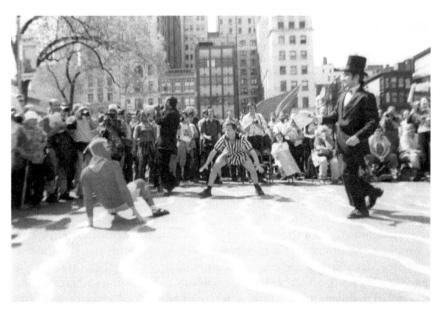

Figure 6.6   SuperBarrio Man street theater with Andrew Boyd as referee. Photo by Caroline Shepard.

police arrested one of the Billionaires who'd been wrestling; his charge: "masquerading in public." The crowd began to chant, "Shame!" "Let Him Go!" "No More Police State," and the ubiquitous "Big Sticks, Small Pricks!!" "Now, being surrounded by police," Bogad ruminated. "That's the opposite kind of energy, that's trying to cancel it out, where it's like, 'I went to that demonstration and it was a drag and I felt intimidated. I'm not gonna go next time.'" Word spread the police were looking for anyone who'd worn a wrestling mask. So those in masks scattered. And, the police moved straight into the crowd with billy clubs swinging. One of the Radical Cheerleaders who had been performing was arrested (see Anderson, 2001). Bill Talen, aka Reverend Billy, who was teaching a class on political performance at the New School, had taken his kids out to watch the show. They stood across the street. As the melee broke out, one of Talen's students was arrested. By this point, the SuperBarrio performance was supplanted by a theater of domination. Bogad watched it take shape.

> [T]hey end up arresting Garrett, the Money Devil; they don't arrest the real money devils in the IMF Building, they arrest the fake one, amusingly enough, for wearing his mask. There is the mask law. And the irony being, of course, SuperBarrio Man doesn't want to lose his mask in the wrestling match, and the super-villains are trying to take off his mask. That's the fictional story line. Of course, the police will make you take off your mask. So Garrett got arrested, as you know. Thirty-six hours in jail, months of court, and charges are eventually thrown out because it's completely ridiculous. The judge deems the case "facially insufficient," which is funny legal terminology—after all, they arrested him because his face was insufficiently exposed due to the mask. They used this 1845 mask law that has nothing to do with your freedom of speech. But of course, it's being selectively applied to activists. And what that's about, on one level, is just raising the social cost of participating—the financial, personal, emotional costs and labor of participating in a democracy. It's a chilling effect.

It was clear to everyone that the police intimidation and arrests were designed to turn people away, chilling interest in future protests and their political content (see Bogad, 2003).

As the other cases in this study suggest, authentic, unregulated play often functions as a threat to business as usual. Much of the action's vitality stemmed from the subversive, unpermitted performance, linking a very specific grievance, stating what was wrong with the situation in an ironic, dramaturgical fashion. Bogad elaborated on the point: "We're not standing up there screaming at them, but we're doing something that does satirize them and show them for the bad cartoon characters in our cartoon." The group performed at the scene of the crime—in front of the shops where workers were paid two and a half dollars an hour. "Or they're not getting paid," noted Bogad. "It's just outrageous. So that's a little more confrontational, but still in a playful way." With SuperBarrio Man, theatrical confrontation was remarkably effective at communicating a message about economic injustice. The day after the protests, New York Attorney General Elliot Spitzer filed claims against East Natural, Abigail's, and Hudson Market (all owned by the same family) for back wages due to employees, who were paid an average of $2.60 an hour (Ness, 2002). Joyfully speaking in character, Stephen Duncombe—one of the primary organizers—questioned whether Spitzer would have acted without all of the protests and pickets. "It sends a clear and loud message to other greengrocers about what happens to those who underpay their workers, block organizing, and hire thugs. Is it mere coincidence that these charges were filed a day after the appearance of SuperBarrio Man, Champion of the People?"

The theatricality of the May Day action combined with the communication to the attorney general and other stakeholders, including the local city councilwoman, as part of a multipronged approach. "You put a little bit of creative effort into making a certain kind of a visual and you can get more play than you might have thought," Bogad explains.

Yet, none of this could prevent an effort by police to shut down the action. "The police are as out of control as I have seen in my lifetime," John Mage, a radical lawyer and longtime observer of police misconduct, observed after the event. For many, the police seemed to be trying to shut down the space for play and performance which accompanied the unsanctioned guerilla theater. "Again, it's bringing down the carnival," noted Bogad. "We're saying we're trying to build up something of a carnival, a play space."

A vital ingredient of the carnival is that everyone is welcomed to join in the action. Such forms of political performance function like improvisational jazz, never performed in quite the same way. Those involved find new connections between themselves and their communities. The mix cannot take place without the interplay between audience and musician, storyteller and listener. Here, the full-participation carnival becomes "a play space to imagine other worlds and to liberate ourselves" explains Bogad. With no distinction between leader and follower, performer and audience member; everyone is a leader.

For Matthew Roth, the connection to such a politics was transformative. "It wasn't until after I discovered that form of expression and that form of performance that I realized exactly why I could never go back to doing the traditional marches." Rather than walk passively through the stations of protest, he vowed he would to take a proactive stance: "That way . . . I'm creating in my own right." When the state seeks to shut down the carnival, it is shutting down free-flowing experience of community and possibility. This connection between self and others helps participants experience a feeling of authentic democratic living.

Yet, when this form of authentic community take shape, it is often followed by restrictions. Herein, a regulatory politics of fear, mass arrests, and selective enforcement of policies inhibits political participation. "Now you can't have a mask and we're going to take your puppet away," Bogad explains. "And you can't have this, and you can't have a banner that's too big."

Despite these efforts, by the end of May Day 2001 dispatches reported mass protests in Zurich, Taiwan, and South Korea, where a crowd of twenty thousand clashed with fifteen thousand police. Economic security, jobs, and the right to organize were the focus of mass mobilizations across the globe. New York City was no different. SuperBarrio Man serves as a best-practice example of the use of play in a larger campaign. LESC's Community Labor Coalition (CLC) had worked on the greengrocer campaign for years. Many RTS members had been in the meetings and the picket lines. When the campaign needed a dose of energy, the group added a jigger of play to the campaign. Yet, this ingredient was never disconnected from the larger organizing effort.

COMMUNITY BUILDING FROM DIABLO CANYON TO THE LOWER EAST SIDE

Much of the vitality of the politics of play finds its foundation in the process of radical renewal, which took place between the birth of Gay Liberation and the "emerging wisdom" of the Zapatistas (Marcos, 2004). For David Solnit, this process dovetailed with the antinuke activism of the 1970s and 1980s. Renowned campaigns targeted the Lawrence Livermore National Laboratory in Livermore, California, and PG&E's Diablo Canyon energy plant near San Luis Obispo, California (see Epstein, 1991). Both Solnit and Starhawk were active within these campaigns. Prefigurative community building accompanied the direct action of these campaigns. Members of Lower East Side organizing groups such as the queer CIRKUS AMOK as well as RTS New York build on this impulse to play and organize. From Diablo Canyon to the Lower East Side, an impulse to paint a canvas with an image of a more colorful and caring democracy inspired a new generation to engage and act.

"In '82, I got involved with the Livermore Action Group, which was sort of the direct action wing of the antinuclear weapons movement," David Solnit explains.

> It was a chapter in the threat of nuclear war and people chose disarmament, with the distribution of resources from the military to human needs. There was a campaign in the Bay Area focused on the Livermore nuclear weapons lab. And so people were lobbying for de-escalating the nuclear arms race. So people did a mass direct action campaign in 1982 and '83 with well over one thousand people getting arrested. And it

included spending a couple of weeks in jail. That was an incredible hub of networking and creative ideas and innovation. So there was a lot of creativity in the protest and the demonstrations themselves were very participatory and horizontal. A lot of people had costumes. It was a departure from walking down the street or listening to speakers at a rally.

While the Livermore group built on the ideas of A.J. Muste's pacifism, it also found room for the queer aesthetics and the creative DIY culture of punk and prefigurative politics which has long been a central part of anarchist organizing. The actions also built on the consensus-based decision-making models of the Quakers. "It was incredible," Solnit mused. "The thing about decentralized or horizontal organizing is you create frameworks that create these wide-open spaces where people are very diverse and work together." Over the years, waves of protests overwhelmed the Livermore weapons lab as the case for nuclear disarmament found expression in countless different forms through the blockade.

Here, a respect for a diversity of tactics allowed a range of direct action approaches to flourish. "There'd be an area for the religious people, a creative theater area, an anything goes tactically area. It allows huge amounts of different cultures to flourish," explained Solnit. The result was a sharp departure from more linear models of protest. The entry level to be part of the action was extremely low; conversely, participation was high. And creativity flourished. This diversity allowed a wide range of groups, rooted in a range of protest traditions, to coordinate. "There were Christians who were praying, and pagans doing spiral dances, and punks doing street theater, and all kind of crazy old radicals doing all sorts of political things," explained Solnit. The effect was a powerful display of opposition. "The real theater of it all was people blockading cars with their bodies."

A social eros took shape within the mix of direct action, respect between the participants, the space they shared, and the community this created. Starhawk described this feeling during the campaign to shut down the Diablo Canyon nuclear energy plant:

> I think I felt that really way back in Diablo Canyon in the very first nonviolent direct action, being encamped with people. Really, I think I was down there for about three weeks, where decisions were made by consensus; where there was this tremendous amount of care and good vibes from people. It's really transformative. Some of the people who had been at the G8 [protests in 2005] were saying they'd been at the [antinuclear protest] in Avion and there had been a camp there and the process had been so inspiring to them that they came back inspired to create something like that.

Larry Bogad, who also participated in the G8 actions Starhawk mentions, described how this community-building impulse propelled his work with RTS New York. "I think it was great to see, when you started working with a group, the personal connections, being part of the whole affinity group building, how different issues called for different techniques and tactics." The human dimension included many of the most basic of human struggles. "You know, within the affinity group, who's busy, who's not. Who's having a kid and who's not. Who's overwhelmed with work or who leaves town or whatever." For a period between 2001 and 2004, Bogad found that RTS New York offered a useful space in which to utilize elements of creativity, play, direct action, and performance in his organizing. It was also a sort of laboratory for the politics of play.

As it organized the affinity group followed a series of stages from banter in meetings, through rehearsal, and eventually performance. "The play came out in several modes. Play came out in our rehearsals and in our performances, and those are two very different things," Bogad explained. "In the rehearsal, we are in our 'safe space.'" He laughed, in homage to the new waves of Bush era domestic spying. "It makes me feel special to know I have an audience," Bogad mused. "And it's nice. But there we are playing together . . . making our costumes together, which we often did. That's an act of creativity together too." Thus, even the most routine activist engagement becomes an opportunity for expression. "Rehearsing and playing around, trying different shticks and different scenarios. That's fun and that's in a totally more free space, 'cause it's like our space, that we're making it warm with our own creativity."

From the rehearsals to the day of the scheduled protest, the dynamic shifts, as Bogad explained:

> Now in the moment of play in the actual action, of course, there's a different dynamic at play, because now we're directly engaged with others that are not in our affinity group. Then it's passersby and it's the state and other activists that are not into what we do and other activists that are into what we do. The media, passersby—that's the difference between rehearsal and performance. And the stakes go up. You don't do over. You can do over on the next city block, but whatever you do, that's what you did. . . . But when you have your first interaction with a policeman and you have this clown character and he says this, what do I say to him? Now, it's the time. You're on. Lights up. And you tweak it and you have a doubling. There's you and there's your character, together in the moment.

For RTS, as with many creative troupes, play helped support a creative, interactive group process. Bogad described the third level of play within the group:

> The third part of play which actually permeates all of this is the play within our affinity group of banter. Of making the room warm, when

we're all at the Life Café drinking and eating something and hanging out and talking and playing around, I think that's part of the play, 'cause we build our own interpersonal culture of playfulness, of irony, that has different tones to it. I think that's part of building the trust and the affection. And that's not about sewing the costumes. I'm saying when we're just hanging out and not getting down to business, right? So when you have an RTS meeting and there's schmoozing for a lot of it, that's part of what's happening.

Here, play involved multiple levels of participation. There is the spirit of frivolity, and then there's the performance itself. The play's the thing Hamlet used to catch the conscience of the king. "In Hamlet, the king blanches and goes white and calls the whole show off," noted Bogad. Yet he is also realistic about which publics one is addressing. While the performance may not function to shift the terms of engagement with the state, there are many things it can achieve. "We're about building a movement culture that can spread and more people can join the movement and get into it," Bogad explained. "And get those people in the middle to join us . . . to get excited and active and engaged." Thus, play is about creating a different kind of democracy.

For the members of RTS New York, play involved both creating a supportive culture of resistance and community as well as serving as a catalyst for personal freedom. "That all of this boils down to, perhaps, liberating ourselves I guess is an obvious point," said Bogad. "Modeling our version of citizenship—which means to be playful and participatory as citizens. And giving that model of how to behave as citizens, not just as consumers." Thus, for Bogad and others, "To be a citizen means to be a voter, to be a citizen means to be a consumer, to be a worker, a producer. All of those things, of course, you are doing every day." Yet there is also the flip side of the play dynamic. "But for us, it's also about being a trickster," he explained, alluding to the mercurial, disruptive side of the human imagination (Hyde, 1998; Wilson, 1990).

Through engagement in these less than linear confines, one encounters a struggle to find a place for different perspectives on social life, political participation, and authentic democratic experience. It is a way to cultivate a participatory theater of living in which everyone is invited to be part of the drama of social change (see Boal, 1990).

SUMMER 2001: FBI MEMOS AND A MASQUERADE PROJECT

By the summer of 2001, the movement of movements was churning forward at full steam. The protests over the Free Trade Area of the Americas (FTAA) in Quebec City in April produced some of the most intense confrontations yet seen with the young movement. Many would describe the confrontations between the protestors and police over the wall surrounding the old city as hair-raising, thrilling, and a bit ominous (Graeber, 2002; Herbst, 2002; Kauffman, 2004). The FTAA protests in April successfully challenged the validity of the global trade system, and RTS worked with the CLC to win back wages for workers in May. Throughout the summer, a living wage campaign at Harvard University captured the attention of the country, as workers' conditions became a topic of debate, political deliberation, and action.

By this point, play had become a part of the movement's very discourse. When activists catapulted teddy bears over the wall erected to separate protesters from the trade summit, most thought of this prank as an ironic gesture of ludic opposition to the tear gas wielded by the summit trade security forces. Yet, the police found no humor in the gesture. And activist Jaggi Singh was charged with possession of a weapon—the 7.6-meter catapult used to hurl the teddy bears. The defense charged that the catapult was a theater prop (Rabble Staff, 2001). When Singh was held in jail for some seventeen days, another group came forward to take responsibility. They specifically distanced Jaggi from the prank in a tongue-in-cheek press release from April 25, 2001:

> Prominent perma-protester Jaggi Singh has been nabbed and charged with possession of our catapult.
>
> Jaggi is not a member of our group, and has never been a member of our group. Nor will we ever let him become a member of our group. Nor will we ever let him become a member of our group, as his sense of humor does not meet our rigorous standards . . . Jaggi was not involved with any aspect of the project's planning, not with catapult construction and deployment. Nor does Jaggi have the chutzpa necessary to smuggle a 25x10 foot catapult into the most heavily fortified city in Canadian history.
>
> Furthermore, we admonish him for managing to steal credit for our catapult. While it may be his fault that the police were stupid enough to charge him for its possession, he should have known better than to take a look at it during the protest. It is no wonder fellow activists call him Braggi Smith.
>
> The catapult was deployed by members of the medieval bloc (they wore pots on their heads, and shields made of pot lids). (Deconstructive Institute for Surreal Topology, 2001)

Singh was eventually freed, yet not after enduring a long ordeal. Still, those involved tried to keep their sense of humor.

Many considered the Quebec protests a thrilling success (Graeber, 2009). Yet, with most every success, increases in control cultures followed. And panic followed. The political marginalization of anarchists—"the terrorist or anarchist black bloc hysteria," as Jason Grote describes it—was gaining steam. Long before September 11, the powers-that-be sought to delegitimize activists. A common tactic was to brand them terrorists or anarchists. On May 10, FBI director Louis Freeh testified before a Senate committee hearing: "Anarchists and extreme socialist groups—such as . . . Reclaim the Streets . . . —have an international presence and, at times, also represent a potential threat in the United States." (see FBI, 2001).

First Ron Hayduk and then L.A. Kauffman (2001) posted the text of the FBI report to the RTS e-mail list. The memo listed several categories of left-wing groups, including:

> Anarchists and extremist socialist groups—many of which, such as the Workers' World Party, Reclaim the Streets, and Carnival Against Capitalism—have an international presence and, at times, also represent a potential threat in the United States. For example, anarchists, operating individually and in groups, caused much of the damage during the 1999 World Trade Organization ministerial meeting in Seattle (FBI, 2001).

Conspicuously absent from the list were those training to fly jets without an interest in learning to land, or those with specific plans to attack the United States who Richard Clarke (2004), the chair of the US Counterterrorism Security Group, had tried to warn the government about throughout 2001. Instead, the FBI director set his eyes on the organizers who wielded teddy bears and organized street parties.

In the days after activists became aware of Freeh's testimony, members of RTS reveled in the absurdity of the moment. While some found it horrifying; others thought it was a reason to have a party. Still, the FBI test presented what many understood as a very real threat. RTS was on the radar of the US government.

In 1994, RTS London had faced a similar crisis. John Jordan recalled:

> The Criminal Justice Act, which was an attempt to pretty much kill all counterculture in the UK . . . It was targeting ravers, targeting direct action people, travelers, so there was all this very resourceful DIY culture that was already there, very involved in partying, all that stuff. So there was already a kind of everyday creativity, a rave community, that was one of the bodies involved in this campaign. There was all that influence coming in. There was a one-hundred-foot tower built entirely from stolen scaffolding with a sound system on top. It was all that party protest stuff already happening. And that was the beginning of when it took off.

RTS London actually gained strength by organizing against this law. "It was one of those wonderful moments where the government tried to pass the act, yet it was an example of a law that created a movement," explained Jordan. "It doesn't happen very often. It really brought together all these different constituencies." And instead of cowering, activists responded creatively. "There was art and there were these traditional forms of direct action," Jordan explained. "The law called all forms of direct action criminal. On the day itself that the law came in, we actually occupied one of the building sites." Not only a street party, "it was also a direct action itself because it was a criminalization of the body itself. All forms of direct action had become criminal." Hundreds converged to flaunt the new rule. "That day, the day that the Queen signed the law, we went on-site. We'd produced just hundreds and hundreds of signs which said 'criminal' that people just wore over their necks." The group used every tool they could to respond to the police campaign to kill the group and the movement it represented. Still the group continued.

Through all of this ongoing repression and struggle, Jordan became ever more aware that play could effectively counter such social controls. And he brought this experience to Quebec. When things got hot with the cops during the FTAA protests in 2001, Jordan (2003) reveled in the profoundly silly response to the police: "Witnessing a large medieval catapult firing teddy bears and soft toys over the fence erected around the summit of the Free Trade of the Americas in Quebec . . . Pulling the fence down and dancing on its back as it bends." Here, play was part of a smarter, more thoughtful response to the opposition. "Seeing the clouds of tear gas rise above the city, fired at the rate of one per minute for three days and nights, laughing as someone expertly hits the gas canisters back towards the police with an ice hockey stick" (ibid.). The point was to play with power rather than fight it.

For Jordan, this rambunctious engagement helped transform the world of protest turning the streets into a living work of art. "It felt real to me," wrote Jordan, "more absurd, more adventurous and often more dramatic than any theatre" (Jordan, 2003). It was also fun. "[P]laying was always in the tactics," Jordan explained in our interview, especially his post-RTS projects, which emphasized the seductive "irresistible" qualities of activism. "The rebellion has to be pleasurable," Jordan insisted.

The teddy bears notwithstanding, many observers were troubled by the almost militaristic iconography of the Quebec protests. L.A. Kauffman, who was at the action, explained:

> I had a big problem with the aesthetics of the Quebec City protest, and with the aesthetic drift of the Global Justice Movement more generally. Our side was becoming more and more militaristic. All those people— mainly, but not exclusively, young men—dressed in black, looking all menacing and ominous, getting off on confrontations. They had unwittingly become almost a mirror image of the repressive forces that they were up against. And the spirit of carnival that had been so striking in Seattle, that sense of a carnival of resistance, was getting lost. (Kauffman, 2004, p. 380)

In response to the increasingly macho tone of the protests, L.A. Kauffman, Mark Leger, and David Crane spent the summer of 2001 organizing
a new project group, the Masquerade Project, which aimed to provide an
aesthetic intervention for a Global Justice Movement that was increasingly
characterized by images of quasi-militaristic black bloc types. "[I]nstead of
'BOMB-WIELDING ANARCHISTS DUELING WITH THE UPHOLD-
ERS OF LAW AND ORDER,'" the news about the Masquerade would
show a far more ambiguous "slippery image—one of queer bodies in carnival together in contradiction to these strange and oppressive police officers
. . . They would present an image of how people in the New World dressed,
behaved and cared for one another" (Herbst, 2002).

Similarly, RTS New York started thinking about ways to organize a
different kind of bloc, with a less militaristic presence at the next convergence action in Washington, DC, scheduled to coincide with the IMF/
World Bank meetings in mid-September. Under the heading "Big Meeting! Traveling Carnival!" an e-mail announced a meeting at the Charas/El
Bohio Community Center to organize a carnival block:

> Calling all RTSers, Anarchist Clowns, Radical Cheerleaders,
> YaBas, Marching Bands, Puppeteers, Masqueraders and other
> kindred anti-corporate globalization protesting freaks.

The call noted RTS NYC was hosting an open meeting on Wednesday September 5 at Charas/El Bohio Community Services Center to plan for a
traveling carnival block to go down to Washington, DC, on September
29 and 30 to protest the IMF/World Bank meetings. "Who better than
a bunch of clowns to make the point that the humanitarian claims of
the IMF and World Bank are a fucking joke?" wrote Steve Duncombe
(2001). "So please come with your ideas, your friends, your sense of
humor, and most of all: yourself. See you there, XOXO RTS/NYC" (quoted
in Duncombe, 2001).

That day, September 5, a crowd of nearly one hundred activists filled
a room at Charas/El Bohio where we had met to organize so many other
actions. I facilitated the meeting to discuss plans for the IMF convergence. Kauffman announced plans for the Masquerade Project. She
explained the point was to decorate gas masks with sequins to bring a
more colorful flair to the actions (Herbst, 2002). Others followed with
a proposal to have a clown bloc at the action. "One of the most popular
sites on the web is the 'Kill Clown,'" one observer noted. "People actually like seeing cops beat up clowns." So they decided not to do a clown
army, but instead would put out a call for a "Silly Bloc" with a time and
a place to meet up in Washington. Most walked out feeling like it had
been a productive get-together. A work session was scheduled for the
Masquerade Project the following week. The time for play in a social
movement action seemed to have truly arrived.

A PLOT SHIFT

What happened the following Tuesday, September 11, is now history. As many recall, it was a startlingly beautiful autumn morning. I was trying to get to Hunter College that morning for classes in the doctoral program at the School of Social Work. As I left my house in Brooklyn, someone ran up to me and screamed, "Someone flew a plane into the Twin Towers!" And I thought they were crazy for acting so hysterical. Yet the subway was not working well. And by the time I reached Union Square during rush hour, I was forced to take the bus up to the school on the Upper East Side. Smoke teemed through the air.

Angry that the city could not handle an accident that sounded like a little air traffic confusion, I took the nearest bus up to school. As more passengers got on the bus, it became one of those communal New York moments. Different passengers brought different bits and pieces of information as they entered the bus. When a man walked up and proclaimed, "They also hit the Pentagon," I stopped thinking it was an air traffic accident. "Now I'm starting to get scared," said another rider, echoing what many felt. "Now I just want to go home." I felt the same way looking behind me at the smoke rising from downtown. One woman on the bus was convinced Osama Bin Laden did it. I scolded her for rushing to judgment. There would be a lot of rushes to judgment in the days and years ahead. Within the duration of the bus ride, both of the towers would collapse.

All at once, the movement of movements faced the end of play. Kauffman (2001) wrote a dispatch for her e-mail column stating that "everything has changed" and the Masquerade Project was scrapped. And Kauffman gave the gas masks to the relief workers digging through the wreckage downtown. "It's now official: In the wake of the September 11 disaster, the IMF and World Bank have indefinitely postponed their planned late-September meetings, and the raucous street protests that were to greet them have effectively been canceled."

That September 12 at about noon in Union Square, the day after the attacks, we all sat in the park. A group meeting was called for many who had been involved in the actions. Some RTS people arrived; Jason Grote and L.A. Kauffman were there; Andrew Boyd, Priya Warcry, a few ACT UP folks, and some others who met in the grass at Union Square. There was a huge cloud of smoke coming up behind us. Everybody was shell-shocked. Kauffman had buttons she'd made which pled, "Our Grief is Not a Cry for War!" We talked about the need not to blame Islam. Some talked about ways to get downtown to help, even if they were not wanted. Others called for direct action. A group from C Squad planned to go downtown. And Kauffman declared, "The Global Justice Movement has got to become a global peace and justice movement." It was the first time I'd thought of, wow, I guess this is where we are going to have to take this thing. "That was such a haunting meeting," Kauffman (2004, p. 382) recalled in an interview a few years later. "The smoke from Ground Zero got closer and closer until that horrible stench surrounded us and we had to flee. We went and reconverged in the back of the New York City Independent Media Center because you couldn't breathe."

A second meeting was scheduled for later on that night at Charas. I stayed home and had dinner in Brooklyn. Jason Grote attended the second meeting. By that evening, many were aware that things had changed. Grote and I talked about the end of that spirit of rambunctious possibility: "I think that everybody was traumatized . . . I saw you that day (September 12) and people were meeting in Union Square and the smell was in the air. And the thing is, too, that the hair shirt Left never really went away."

There were always those who were hostile to more flexible or pragmatic approaches to organizing. This antagonism dated years before September 11. Yet, after the bombings, dourness came roaring back with a vengeance. It was particularly on display at the September 12 meeting at Charas/El Bohio. Grote recalled:

> But part of what happened in the meeting that day, at the earlier meet-ing at Union Square, there was a mass shrine. Someone had put a flag of the earth in George Washington's arms. And there was a very active and vibrant peace movement happening there that was really holding the mourning, the grieving that was going on. Even there was debate there. There were American flags there. But it wasn't hostile. It was divided. It was very civil. People were talking. Some people were taking photos and I understand paranoia, but it was a weird activist hostility. And I was thinking, here are people having a really constructive not hateful response, and these are the people who are supposed to be the Left. And they are full of anger. The day that it happened I was feeling ambivalence too. Here we are fighting global capital, the WTO, etc. . . . At the time I had a really hard time figuring out my own feelings and fantasies of 'smash the WTO' with this. It wasn't rational. It was a gut thing. John, who was involved with RTS, was asking people how they were feeling and he wrote to the [e-mail] list saying, "let's not forget that we got into this because we wanted to alleviate suffering." And I needed to hear that . . . And the next day, there was a meeting about a people's response to this at Charas . . . There was a lot of talk about what we could do in the face of a lot of helplessness and futility . . . The strategy of play didn't seem to fit with this . . . That sort of humorless hair shirt Left came roaring back.

Grote would drop out of organizing after the Charas meeting.

The week after September 11, Kauffman (2004) busied herself with a frenzy of organizing. All the while, Union Square was becoming a space for peaceful remembering with art and stories and pictures on the sidewalk to accompany the often poignant "missing" signs all over the city seeking information about lost loved ones who were probably not going to be found. Kauffman (2004) recalled how that feeling was translated onto the street:

> There was an extraordinary protest shortly after September 11 that got virtually no media coverage. I think it was on the Friday night after the Tuesday attacks. It was a nearly spontaneous march that went from a candlelight vigil in Union Square up to Times Square. It was very emotional, and very non-ideological. It wasn't about the intricacies of interventions and imperialism, it was just all these people who did not want to see mass slaughter committed in our name as revenge for the mass slaughter that had just happened in our city. (p. 282)

Before long, though, the street actions stopped feeling as useful. "[E]ach succeeding protest became less interesting and compelling. It felt like all the nuance and emotion was drained out . . . and all that remained were the sorts of groups that have ideological certainty no matter the circumstances," Kauffman (2004, p. 382) recalled. "Money for Jobs, Not for War" signs started appearing at all the demos. "I always paraphrase that one as 'Money for Soul-Draining Wage Slavery, Not for War'—with fewer and fewer homemade or heartfelt signs" (ibid.). October 7, 2001, the day the bombing of Afghanistan began—many of us participated in an anti-war march that went from Union Square to Times Square. I ran into Kauffman and she said, "I'm getting really bored with this knee-jerk anti-imperialist politics." Then she just walked off. "I was disgusted," she explained (Kauffman, 2004, p. 283). The world had changed and so had the feeling on the streets. The carnival of activism was over.

7 From Play to Panic
Ludic Organizing in Absurd Times

> It's such a bizarre and weird time in the world. . . . This presiden-
> tial race has become the biggest dick contest in history. "Your dick
> started an unnecessary war!" . . . "Your dick is soft on terrorism!"
> Has this kind of dick waggling happened before outside of a pro-
> wrestling context?. . .
>
> Then there is the Bush administration trying to keep us in a state
> of panic all the time, like raising the Terror Alert so that we're not
> at ease but always on edge. And it's always the most ridiculous stuff
> like, "An ATM was targeted in Midtown Manhattan."
>
> But I'm so used to raised terror alerts, I'm unaffected. I'm like,
> "It's orange. Does that mean I have to take off my shoes?" Mean-
> while, clog sales have gone through the roof. People think that it's
> Halliburton that's benefiting from all this; no it's Birkenstock. It's a
> huge clog/mule cartel conspiring. Slip-on shoes are the future.
>
> Comedian Margaret Cho (2004)

The early 2000s were an absurd time. And it was the comedians who
seemed to understand this better than anyone. In the days after the bombings of 2001, retired generals dusted off their uniforms for TV appearances as a corporate, military, involuntary entertainment, prison-industrial
complex churned into high gear; war coverage began a twenty-four-hour
news rotation. Funding for the military, policing, and security structures
skyrocketed, at the expense of everything else. Repression increased and
immigrants were detained. "[T]hey're scaring Americans into supporting
their power grabs by essentially yelling 'They're coming to kill us!'" jour-
nalist Maureen Dowd (2006) put it. Much of it felt like a crass attempt to
panic the public into support for an aggressively conservative social and
economic agenda (Harvey, 2005).

While the story of activism from ACT UP to Seattle involved robust
forms of direct action, the playing field was radically altered in 2001. The
US Patriot Act, passed in a panic-like atmosphere, shifted the context for
activism (with the Clinton era 1996 anti-terror law increasingly being
applied to activist groups). While the powers-that-be had long sought to
redefine protest groups—such as Earth First! and RTS—as terrorists, discourses linking protesters as national security threats gained credence in
the fall of 2001 as fear became a driving force of national politics.

And play was eclipsed. "Now," explained Jason Grote during our 2005
interview, "there is a lot of fear of play." This is anything but new. Barbara Ehrenreich (2007A,B) reminds us the Romans strove to suppress the

ecstatic Dionysus cults because of their capacity to subvert the status quo. Conservatives tend to harbor similar fears (Reich, 1970). And the Bush era was no different. Bush's Attorney General John Ashcroft went as far as to cover the female breast on the "Spirit of Justice" statue at the Justice Department. The gesture was an emblem of an antisex, anti-play cultural apparatus of the period. Still activism continued. This chapter considers the ways activism and play shifted and evolved with the terror alerts and panics of the era.

RECLAIM THE MOVEMENT

Throughout the fall of 2001, RTS and other New York activist groups reeled and debated ways to move forward. William Etundi and Andrew Boyd organized a candlelight vigil downtown. Members of RTS New York, who had been meeting for several weeks while trying to get a grip on things, decided to put together a broadside about what had happened to the movement since the terrorist bombings. Members of the group brought copies of the broadsheet, penned by Steve Duncombe, to the vigil. "Reclaim the Streets says . . . Reclaim the Movement," it declared. Since 9/11, many of us had been mourning those lost to the attacks, the US escalation, the eroding of civil liberties and the Global Justice Movement created over the previous years. "We built a Peace Movement," the paper read. Yet, this movement was "different than the movement we had before. For all its faults—and there were many—the Global Justice Movement was flexible, anti-authoritarian, creative, fun, increasingly popular and thus effective—not qualities one could use to describe the often alienating Peace Movement."

The day before the action, members of RTS organized a prop-making party at Charas. It would be our final meeting at Charas, which lost its request for a stay of eviction on December 18. A space for the enemies of neoliberalism to conspire and comingle—that made it a target. We would have to look for another meeting space without it, and soon. Things were about to heat up again. A new convergence action was already scheduled for New York City around the meetings of the World Economic Forum (WEF).

THE WORLD ECONOMIC FORUM, NEW YORK CITY

On January 15, 2002, the *New York Daily News* published an editorial targeted specifically to activists. "Confab Welcome, Crazies Not," it declared. "New Yorkers have suffered enough of late . . . You have a right to free speech, but try to disrupt this town, and you'll get your anti-globalization butts kicked. Capish?" It was the latest in a long series of cases of "protest panic" dating back to the days after November 1999 when the WTO meetings were disrupted in Seattle (see FAIR, 2003;

Graeber, 2004; Shepard, 2005). Since then, the potential appearance of masked anarchists had inspired fear, trepidation, and expensive security details in towns where world leaders converged for meetings of the G8, IMF, WTO, and now the WEF. Despite the demonization, an action was in the works.

"Bad Capitalist, No Martini!"—a spoof on the old bumper sticker, "Bad Cop, No Donut"—to mock rogue policemen, that would be the RTS slogan for the protests of the WEF meetings, chock-full of fat cats, who deserved similar mockery. It was also a push to bring bodies back into the streets. The slogan was generated at a convergence space in a warehouse off the West Side Highway in midtown. A plainclothes police officer sat inside the car just outside the entrance of the space, in a not too subtle

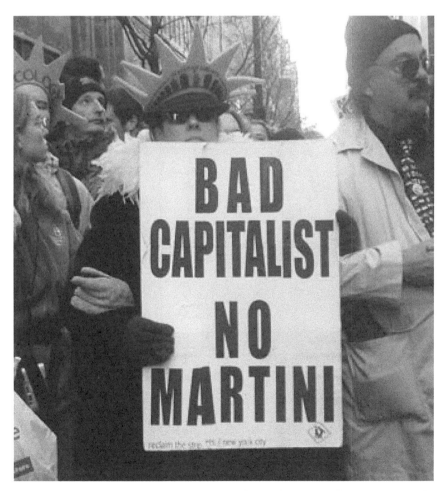

Figure 7.1 "Bad Capitalist, No Martini" photo of L.A. Kauffman at the World Economic Forum, NYC 2002. Photo by Jim Glaser.

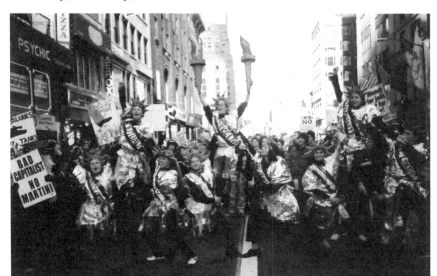

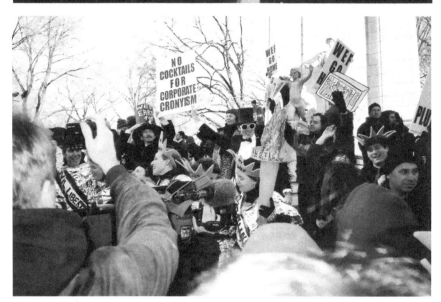

Figure 7.2   World Economic Forum carnival block. Photo by Caroline Shepard.

message to those inside. Still the action planning continued, with activists from Spain and California dropping in nightly to help make puppets and prepare for the action. "[D]ance on the ruins of the world!" the RTS press release proclaimed in solidarity with Argentina, whose economy had crashed. "Tango and Samba to Protest the WEF . . . Come one, come all! On Saturday, 2nd February, at 11:30 a.m. in Columbus Circle, Reclaim the

Streets will tango. And samba. And make a Considerable Din." So, "RTS invites everyone—musicians, dancers, artists, flappers. . .—hell, even the NYPD. Cops tango too, right? Anyhow, RTS invites the masses to come and shake their booty in solidarity with all those who get screwed by the McDonaldization of the globe." It concluded, "People Before Profits! Public Space for the Public!" With these words, the group proclaimed the movement was ready to reengage.

When most every "liberal" interest group, the unions, and NGOs bowed out of participating in the protests, a group of anarchists risked arrest to lead a buoyant march attended by well over ten thousand people. A phalanx of police squeezed almost everyone who arrived. Still a makeshift drum corps maintained a festive opposition, complete with a street samba band reclaiming beats and urban possibilities. While the people called for increased expression, the police called for repression. Faced with a police force that had betrayed every guarantee it had made in negotiations prior to the action, the crowd began to sing, "We all live in a Military State, a Military State, a Military State," to the tune of the Beatles anthem "Yellow Submarine." Music and dance would be a way to cope with increased social controls. "I think that music and dance are ways of keeping cohesion, keeping your courage up when you are in a tense situation, of linking together," Starhawk, who was at the head of the march, explained. "The civil rights movement was brilliant at using those tools." The Global Justice Movement was still learning to cope with this challenge.

So, it was not surprising when police tried to coordinate, control, and stifle the spontaneity out of the WEF actions. I was planning to drum with the samba band during the march. But once I got to Columbus Circle, a policeman snatched my drumsticks out of my hands. "So what do you have to hit the drum with then—your hand," Larry Bogad observed with a laugh when I related this story to him. "Amazing, 'cause you could stick somebody in the eye with that," he noted, reveling in the absurdity of the moment. "What about umbrellas? They have to take your shoes too. They could take your shoes 'cause in theory you could take them off and throw them at someone. You could show up naked but then you'd get arrested for walking around naked." Only after the Republican National Convention in 2004 would I find out that confiscating drumsticks was official police policy. Under the subheading "Carrying Signs or Objects," the legal guidelines for the Republican National Convention, dubbed "Operation Overlord II," acknowledged that people do have a right to participate in First Amendment–protected activities:

> However, where it can be shown that the object carried, i.e., a wooden pole with a sign attached or a bat, has the potential for being used as a weapon, the police may prohibit the carrying of the object during a demonstration. Persons who insist on carrying objects that are

potential weapons should be directed to put the object down or to leave
the area of the demonstration. If they refuse to do so and continue to
congregate with others in the demonstration, they may be arrested for
Disorderly Conduct. (Doepfner and Sweet, 2004, p. 5)

Under such a glare, most anything could be viewed as a "potential . . .
weapon."

Despite the increased policing at the WEF, there were those who found
ways to cope with the increased police controls. Starhawk called it one of
her favorite actions:

> After the big march, which was very frustrating because the police
> totally controlled the space, we all ended up in Grand Central Station.
> We were all eating in the food court. Some people said we want to do
> something; we want to do a spiral dance. We ran upstairs and started
> to circle in this big dome. Of course, police are so uptight there. They
> were wanting to arrest everybody. And immediately a security guard
> came over and said, "you can't do this performance here." And we kept
> spiraling and drumming. We said, "it's not a performance, it's a reli-
> gious ceremony." He went to get backup. We kept spiraling. I looked up
> at one point and noticed we had a perfect circle of riot cops.

The festive gesture helped break down the hyper-control of public space.
Starhawk explained:

> That really worked with the spiral. We had the riot cops around us
> and we had an audience around all these stores and galleries and we
> had a great circle. So I think they were hesitant to really move in. But
> finally a cop walked up to us and said, "Enough." I took that as our
> cue to do what we call waving a cone of power where we all throw our
> arms up in the air and ooooom. So we did that and I guess evidently
> our cone of power was strong enough that they did not move in on us.
> And then we moved down and someone sang "Amazing Grace." They
> couldn't really move in on a whole group of people singing "Amazing
> Grace." By the time that was over, I was pretty sure they weren't going
> to arrest us.

Throughout the weekend the police seized and arrested those they felt
looked like "obviously potential rioters." And activists around the city
spent the weekend in jail. Years after the action, the police admitted in
court to using undercover officers to infiltrate group meetings and protests, while sending "undercover officers to distribute misinformation
within the crowds." This tactic, of course, had been rejected a generation earlier after the abuses by the police against antiwar and civil rights
groups (Dwyer, 2006c).

By far, the most troubling piece of news from the police testimony was the reported thirty "proactive" arrests of activists with "pipes and masks" said to present "an obvious threat" (Dwyer, 2006c). Activists had brought shields to protect themselves. Reflecting on the experience, New York activist Eric Laursen (2006) noted the NYPD will "continue to peddle these lies even after they're discredited in court." Hence, "As the Miami cops like to say, 'You can beat the rap, but you still got to take the ride.' And in the memory hole of history, they'll keep 'arresting' you, over and over again" (Laursen, 2006).

9/11, THE ANTIWAR MOVEMENT, AND THE STRUGGLE AGAINST THE BLUE MEANIES

In this context, much of the vitality of the Global Justice Movement ebbed after the 9/11 attacks. Less people came to meetings. Yet, activism continued in multiple circles, albeit in different forms. Countless interviewees expressed frustration with the dour tenor of protest after the attacks. Not that all protest needed to be fun or entertaining, but many still hoped for it to feel powerful and democratic, not rigid or stale. Many had come into global justice organizing out of old left groups such as the International Socialist Organization (ISO) and the various Trotskyite sects, which operate with an entirely different ethos. "I don't think play came up," mused global justice activist Marina Sitrin, who got her start in organizing with the Young Socialist Organization. "They were more interested in ways to take state power."

"They organize authoritarian little protests, wave their uniform homogenous signs, and get their permits and make friends with the police," observed Kate Crane, reflecting on the organizational approach of the sectarian group International ANSWER. "I don't want some creepy hierarchical structure where the grand leader tells me what to do."

Musician Joe Tuba experienced a similar dynamic when he was in college in 1997. "I was kind of desperate to get involved with something. And the only thing that was on my campus was the ISO, which is a pretty personality-draining, very boring and stilted and archaic kind of group." He described the group's routine: "They'll go out every Sunday [with their newspapers] and even if you try to write something for the paper. I wrote something for the paper and I never heard anything about it. It just disappeared." It is a very top-down model. "[T]hey are just really centralized and controlled," Joe explained. "All they really want to do is read a lot of books and decide what is the exact right thing to say. And push it on everybody. There is no interaction and there is no collaboration."

In contrast, Matthew Roth argued: "I think a big part of it in politics and play is to engage someone without prescriptions, to engage them by inspiring them, to engage through narrative." He likens the experience to enjoying being carried away by a great story. For Roth, play benefits organizing by not being pedantic. "You are not sitting someone down and scolding them. None of this paternalistic 'you need to do this because.' It's not the negativity." Here participation invites, rather than lectures; it lulls and entices people to take part in a dialogue. For Roth, this is "anarchism in its true spirit." Instead of a monologue, "consensus" finds expression in a "politics of play. . . from the streets." Such organizing creates new forms of collective power and mutual aid (Newman, 2004).

By 1999 Joe Tuba had found the Hungry March Band. Here, an abundant cacophony of participants were invited to perform and contribute in any way they could. Joe Tuba described his first encounters with this open participatory model:

> I was really desperate to get away from that kind of ISO paradigm. And I ran into some anarchist kind of people—like the gardens movement and Reclaim the Streets. And they both were a really good fit. I wasn't looking for anything specific. But they both really worked out because you were directly doing exactly what you wanted to do—making a garden or taking over a garden or taking a street. You were physically, actually directly doing what you wanted to do and making it attractive to people—as opposed to selling a funny newspaper that's really kind of blatantly propagandistic and badly written.

Tuba recoiled at the paternalistic model he had seen with the ISO. "They basically want to assault you on the street and go, 'You need this. You really need this.' They are like Christian evangelists," he explained. "'We know what we're talking about. We've studied. You need to take this home and take it to heart and join us.'"

"They always had the answer," reflected Marina Sitrin. "It was a hierarchical relationship." And that, of course, is the antithesis of democratic organizing. "[I]t's totally a top-down approach," Tuba concluded. "It's a totally patronizing and infantilizing thing. It's this whole vanguard mentality."

By far the greatest critique global justice activists have of this sectarian organizational model is the repetition of the same techniques over and over. "Here we have the signs that all say the same thing. And we're all chanting the old plug-in chants, it makes you fade into the background already 'cause you're a walking cliché. Your eyes skip over clichés on the printed page," explained Larry Bogad. "If someone says he smelled as good as a rose then readers don't even really read that 'cause it's a terrible cliché," Bogad elaborated. "And I honestly feel it's the same thing with protest. If you're doing a cliché or acting like a cliché, people just skip over it, like yeah, yeah."

For activist artists, such as Bogad, the goal is to build on a genealogy of aesthetic intervention to help make authentic contribution to current social movements.

We're aware of our predecessors from the early 1970s, late 1960s. We're aware of their influences from the Wobblies, doing some fun outrageous stuff. We have this genealogy that we're trying to bring up because it gives us a sense of continuity in the counterculture even . . . We're part of a culture that crosses, hopefully, boundaries of identity and boundaries of race, class, gender, but also boundaries of generation.

A DIFFERENT MODEL

With the Global Justice Movement, activism took a step in a new direction. Sitrin remembers things changing in 1999. And much of this came with a recognition of joy and beauty in action. "Seattle was both powerful resistance and a celebration of life . . . I saw beautiful protest. I also saw people organize where they were all listening to each other. It was a huge break. Joy and power in one moment."

In Seattle, the politics of play found its full expression as a creative direct action, hip-hop, and dance which complimented an expansive blockade. In the years which followed, many aspired to build on this win by supporting a movement culture in which laughter was honored and pleasure valued. Here, what the community activists hoped to create was embodied in their organizing. "Community is very much part of it," explained Starhawk, who was also in Seattle. "I'm trying to organize in a model of decentralized direct democracy, make decisions that way, plan our actions that way, and incorporate as much of a vision of art and play and culture as you can."

The community element feels like it is front and center for these struggles. "[You have to] be able to confront the system and have the community that can confront that system," L.J. Wood elaborated. "I always think of the revolution as something that's already happening, so I try to build the world we want to have into the organizing we're doing today. But at the same time, if you look at what we're doing, you have to confront the system."

"I think there really is a contrast," Jordan explained, adding:

I think play engenders enormous creativity. I think you can develop enormous community. On that level it is absolutely essential. It is way more attractive than other forms. It's compatible. It's the ability to create warm convivial spaces. If there was more play within those traditional models, they would benefit from it. It's always radical groups that are about creating space, that offer that unknown and unexpected. As a thing that opens up possibilities. It's much more exciting.

Jordan's entry into such a politics began when he inadvertently witnessed a street rally turn into something entirely unexpected. "[T]he A to B march turning to riots, that was my first experience of playful protest, the space being completely turned on its head." He saw that "there are other ways of protesting." Here, ludic activity opened spaces for something completely different. "How do you engage people?" The answer was with actions that felt desirable, with modes of interaction that inspired questions, that used "tools of the system to engage the system with *détourné* and situations," Jordan mused, referring to the old Situationist lexicon. "I would feel a high that was so wonderful."

"The traditional protest groups like to play by the traditional rules, meaning that they want the barricades. They want everything legal," concurred New York antiwar activist Ben Mauers. "But being in protest there has to be a little danger." Without this, a movement is easily ignored and contained. "It has to be creative. It can't be the usual stuff anymore. It's out. We have to do different things for the media to listen to us. To get people involved," Mauers continued. "Play can be very important in protest, just to get to the creative part of the brain. How was Abbie Hoffman able to lure people—by doing creative types of stuff. We need to bring that element back in." Rather than repeating the routine, "we have to get people to think."

By 2002, "politics felt very cold," L.A. Kauffman (2004, p. 383) mused. "And it made me sick . . . to think that the movement that I was part of was merely showcasing the shrill and the simplistic, was dominated by people with cold and creepy politics." So, she started a new antiwar group in the fall of 2002 with members of Lower East Side Collective and the New York RTS group.

AN ABSURD RESPONSE TO AN ABSURD WAR

Matthew Roth described his experience with this antiwar affinity group:

> The most fun I ever had in a single event was Absurd Response to an Absurd War, which you were in, my friend. I remember that beautiful perm you had with the perms for perma-war during the fall antiwar march in Washington, DC. We're leading up to the assault on Iraq and the drumming up of the weapons of mass destruction and the yellow cake power, whatever, everyone saying how Iraq is the worst terrorist threat there has ever been. Al Qaeda/Iraq. Al Qaeda/Iraq. All this stuff, if we didn't know, we felt was absolutely wrong and totally beyond logic. It was absurd.

Absurd Response was the name for Kauffman's new LESC-style antiwar affinity group. Faced with the post-9/11 drive to war in Iraq, it attempted to mirror the absurdity, thereby amplifying the image of this lunacy.

At the time, philosopher Slavoj Žižek suggested there was a rationale for such thinking. "The only way to signal you are serious is, at the level of form, is to make fun of yourself," he explained. This is where the circus-like carnivalesque finds appeal. "This pseudo-Heideggerian jargon, we live in fateful times, the destiny of humanity is threatened blah, blah, blah—I think you cannot talk like that," Žižek elaborated (quoted in Clover, 2005). So one has to find different ways to engage the serious, especially when the country is looking at starting a war.

For most involved with Absurd Response, the feeling remained that the world was witnessing an absurd situation—a "war on terrorism" a sitting vice president predicted could last fifty years—that required an absurd response (see Shepard, 2003). The job of activists was to spotlight the flawed logic of the nation's shift toward perma-war. For many, the best way to do this was with guerilla theater. There had been absurd wars before, but, unlike the Gulf War of the early 1990s, the Second Gulf War began with a mobilized movement already on the ground and running. As the Global Justice Movement flirted with becoming an antiwar movement, questions about aesthetics had everything to do with political strategy and movement building. Here a politics of authenticity had to contend with the defiant joy of the Seattle era protest model. Confrontation with police would translate into almost certain political repression. So instead of righteous indignation, many turned to a colorful, festive theater, full of joy, intelligence, and humor. Here, direct action intersected with a topsy-turvy carnival (Bakhtin, 1981, 1984). The point of this model was to create a festive energy that dismantled social hierarchies. We've all laughed along with a great joke. Everybody wants to be at a party where everyone is free to have a good time. The point is to punch holes in social pretensions. After an entire year of post-9/11 mind-numbing seriousness, the possibility of a joke's capacity for catharsis was considerable. The first 9/11 anniversary marked this. And activists celebrated at a Reverend Billy show with Kurt Vonnegut at St. Mark's Church in the Bowery. Roaring and laughter filled the space. Somewhere within our public life, some of the sentiment of the "better to laugh than cry" satire, the spoofs of late-night TV, had to be unleashed.

The point of such protest would be to relink protest with optimism and a feeling of possibility or rejuvenation. The festive atmosphere of a great action could be bridged with the transformative aspirations of the carnival. The aim of an absurd response would be to create a brand of protest that merged the joyous ecstatic spirit of exhilarating entertainment with a political agenda of progressive political change. Within this festive revolutionary theater, progressive elements of political change would be linked with notions of social renewal, moving spectators to join the fun, to become part of the concrete action of social change (Ornstein, 1998).

The thinking was that the group could create a less righteous, even ironic response—an alternative to the wing-nut or sectarian responses. Our first meeting produced a simple commitment to organize a festive feeder march to join the larger antiwar march taking place in October 2002 in Washington, DC.

Of course, the group had been to DC before. In the days after Bush succeeded with his Supreme Court 5–4 election shuffle, RTS New York had formed SUDS, a satirical play on the 1960s group SDS. Dressed as campus preppies wearing "W" hats, members drove down to Washington for the inauguration on January 20, 2001. "Tell Us What to Think—Obey!" would be the group's slogan. The group's chants served to lampoon old left slogans and comment on the new plutocratic regime: "Whose Street?! Wall Street?!" "No Justice, No Problem," and the crowd-pleaser "What do we want—fur coats? How do we want them—full length!!!" When a counterprotestor chanted at SUDS, the group would counter or agree with them. When a group of actual collegiate right-wing preppies sang "nah nah nah nah, hey hey hey good-bye" to President Clinton, SUDS interjected with "democracy."

This time, however, instead of campus preppies, the October 26, 2002, action would highlight a group of patriotic ladies with bouffant permanent hairdos who supported the war. "Perms for perma-war" would be the slogan. The group carried signs with themes from Orwell's *1984*: "War Is

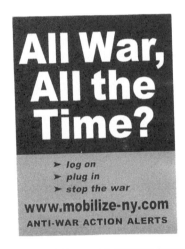

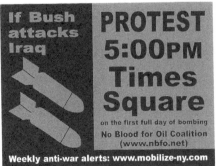

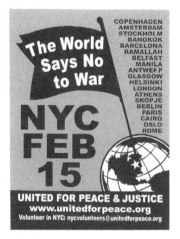

Figure 7.3 Absurd Response stickers—"All War All the Time," "The World Says No to War," "If Bush attacks Iraq, Protest 5:00 PM Times Square," by L.A. Kauffman. These stickers could be found around New York in 2002 and 2003. Courtesy of L.A. Kauffman.

Globalization" and "Ignorance Is Strength." The slogan "OBEY" embodied much of what the group felt was being demanded by the current administration. The point was to offend the banal.

The morning of October 26, 2002, members of the group arrived late, threw on oversized wigs (each with a different letter spelling P-E-R-M-A W-A-R), and met up with other activists at the Washington Monument. Some bowed to the giant phallus with Reverend Billy; a few put on the "Dickheads for Cheney" gear, which included rubber dildos.

But just getting everyone together to pull off the Absurd Response was a challenge. Matthew Roth recalled the scene:

> That day I was a "Dickhead for Dick," a dildo for Dick Cheney. I was actually kind of concerned when we first arrived. There were, like, four people there. And an hour later more showed up. But there were only maybe ten of us or twelve of us. And I was like, this is a really small thing to carry this concept out. And we had a couple of placards and this absolutely gorgeous banner, which said, "An Absurd Response to an Absurd War" in sparkly sequins, like bright. Then the wigs came out and people got made up. And then someone snapped a dildo on my head. Then the Reverend Billy showed up. And then I was like, these twelve, fifteen people, however many, it was a pretty small group, it suddenly had more energy and more excitement and vibe than anything I'd seen before. And okay, all right. I can go and march the march and feel good about this . . . it's satire.

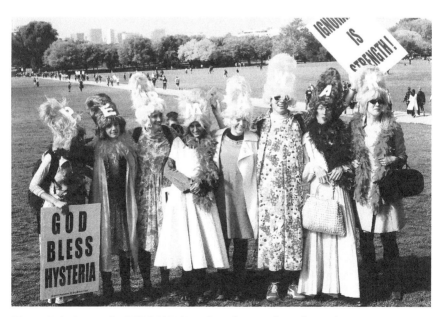

Figure 7.4 Perms for PERMAWAR. Photo by Caroline Shepard

Others passed out palm cards to explain the point of the theater: "Are you ready for Perma-War?" the literature asked. "Iraq is only the beginning. The Bush Administration is drawing the United States and the world ever closer to a state of permanent military engagement. So what do we do?" The back of the card answered: "Throw a party!!! Activism doesn't have to mean droning speeches, dull chants, and tired slogans. To sustain the growing movement over the long haul, we need humor, theater, music, flamboyance, irony, and fun."

The Perms were carrying hairspray cans with perma-war product sprayed on them. The point was to compare one product line—hair spray—with another—perma-war. As Bogad explained: "We think there could be a big future for Perma-war Inc. Keep that hair up. My hair is standing up already."

Joined by Reverend Billy and the Church of Stop Bombing Choir and a group calling themselves the Spirit of 1976 Gone Wrong, a group of anarchist clowns, jugglers, fire-eaters, strippers, puppeteers, drag kings, and missile dicks marched from the Washington Monument to the Vietnam Memorial to feed into the larger march of disgruntled citizens. Two clowns dressed in red, white, and blue cheered and danced spastically to the call for war, screaming "tee hee," bouncing to and fro, calling for the crowd to join them. "War makes me happy!!!" Larry Bogad recalled them screaming. "'Peace is stupid.' They were just really berserk, insane, absolutely sociopathic clowns."

Confronted with counterprotestors, the group switched gears from exaggerated pro-war chants, "We need oil, we need gas, watch out world we'll kick your ass," to the deconstructive chants, "March march, chant chant, rhetoric rhetoric, rant rant."

In other cases, the clowns joined the other side and started yelling at the group. For most of the day, this was an effective ploy for disarming counterprotests and the media coverage of them, yet not everyone appreciated the irony. Early on in the day, the group stumbled upon a group of counterprotesting pro-war Iraqis. This group actually charged the Absurd Response feeder march. The clowns' overture incited not a playful theatrical scene, but an agitated screaming and shoving match which could have turned violent. A couple members of the Absurd Response had to pull one of our friends out of the fight. Having had its fun, the group marched backward, onward, and away for another joke.

"Are you guys right-wing drag queens?" one confused observer asked me as we walked away.

Amidst the cacophony, the group functioned on the brink of total confusion and miscoordination. "When you do the opening space thing or whatever you want to call it, a lot of this is improv theater, folks," noted Bogad. "It's like, you know, we have a costume; we have a concept; we think about it. But things happen. And also we're interacting with reality. I'd say that we're riffing on reality."

Amidst hoards of earnest protestors, many with earnest "How Many Iraqi Children Will Die?" signs, Absurd Response spontaneously declared:

"We love bush, we love dick, all you peaceniks make us sick" or sang, "We Shall Overbomb" and "All We Are Saying Is Give War a Chance."

Faced with mind-numbing reified protest clichés, the Absurd Response directly lampooned the slogan "The people united will never be defeated" with "The people who chant this will never be creative. The people, bad slogans, will always be defeated." "Bad slogans, repeated, insure that we're defeated." "Power to power." Or members chanted "All war, all the time, perma-war is peace," while the perms for perma-war formed a Rockettes-esque perma-war kick-line.

"The things we're saying are so absurd, they are as absurd as the motif we're organized under, that I can't stop but laughing the whole time," mused Matthew Roth, who grew up in and out of a commune. Thinking about this crowd, he speculated, "Like they grow their beard in order to do this. Like the rings of the tree, they can say this hair started in 1968 when . . . anyway." While Roth supports a left politics, he argues there are better ways to communicate a message than this. "The delivery and the methodology are so stale. It burns me, it squelches me. It makes my heart hurt."

As the rally and march wore on, irony percolated throughout the crowd, as different march participants were drawn into an absurdist political moment. Roth described the aha moment which takes place during such events.

> It's when you first saw that rabid Republican who you are standing next to and they heard what you are chanting, breathe in and realize, "wait a minute, they're not with us." It's this 'aha.' It's that humorous moment. That to me was taking performance and the politics of play to a different level. It was completely within the structure of a protest and yet the content was completely different. And we were still delivering a message that people still got and totally felt. It was this liberal crowd of antiwar protestors. They totally got it at the end. But it took a second and it was in that taking a second that they had to think for a second. It's like that moment when there's an answer that your teacher is trying to get you to get and if your teacher just tells it to you, you don't get it. If your teacher shows you and leads you to the answer, you're of course like, "So that's how long division works." I think it has a similar effect in the mind when you use satire, when a person has to do a double take and think, "wait a minute."

For Roth, this approach shifted the story lines away from the conventional antiwar narrative:

> I remember this classic scene when we were marching around the El-lipse within a group of normal protestors and of course it's infectious and they're picking up on it. We're coming up to this federal building

on the left and this long-haired dude is up on top of this pillar over-looking this crowd of people and he's chanting antiwar slogans and they are all chanting back. And then we come up. And he hears this, "What do we want?" And we say, "War" and "Always." And from a distance, he just recognized the cadence of the chant. And he chants it. And then we get close enough that he stops to hear what we're say-ing with his fist raised up in the air and I'm looking up. It's just this classic iconography, this moment, if this were 1970, this would be an anti–Vietnam War [protest], this would be this radical movement here and we're him and he's us. And this second, his face just turned black, he was so pissed off, like, "what are they saying?!" And then he cracked up. And he went through so many emotions—whoosh! And then he was just laughing and chanting our cheer. And his fist was up in the air again. And everyone around him is doing it. And they got it. They were completely engaged. They were pulled in by this form of storytelling.

Throughout the day, more and more people sang along and applauded to renditions of "We Shall Overbomb," joining us for the chorus, "Deep in our hearts, we do believe, we shall live in war forever." The "'W' Stands for WIMP" chant calling for the war to begin ASAP also proved to be a crowd-pleaser. "War is good for children, it builds strong bones," followed by "Bomb Iraq, start the war, we don't need no peace no more." With the crowd swelling, Absurd Response was joined by a group of George Wash-ington University students and members of RTS Washington who led the crowd in a rendition of the perma-war hokeypokey. "You put the money in, you put the money out, you put the sanctions in, and you shake it all about," as everyone danced. "What do we want—perma-war! Why do we want it?—for higher ratings!" Drums improvised along with variations of the jazzlike call-and-response.

"I'd have to say my favorite chant was, 'Three Word Chant,'" Roth remembered fondly. "'Three word chant, three word chant!!!' And then 'Four words are more! Four words are more!'"

The point of the Absurd Response carnival was to open a space for dif-ferent kinds of participation as well as to puncture the righteousness of the often pious activist scene. As Bogad explained: "Anybody could show up. So we had a guy show up in a caveman kind of costume, with a club, doing the Neanderthal thing, banging his club and saying 'Bush! Bang! Boom!' A Neanderthal who likes bombs was his thing."

"Everyone's in drag, wearing these huge perms with dresses, just delight-ful. We start chanting and everyone is just electrified," Roth recalled. "They loved it. They start taking up the chants. There's this magnetic experience of, 'All right, I can be completely irreverent and say these satiric things' and it makes perfect sense. Everybody gets it. It's the aha."

Much of ludic quality of the action was aimed at amplifying the lunacy of the rush to war of the Bush administration, creating a funhouse mirror image of the extreme Right. Bogad explained:

> The funhouse mirror is just this idea, I'm not just going to duplicate you because I'm not just going to just reinscribe your position, 'cause that's a waste of my energy. But I will [mirror it]. And it's not just going to be a simple inversion or a simple exaggeration. But it's going to be a cartoon of the positions we find reactionary and destructive. And so again, the Bombshells again are these glamorous upper-class women who just send these kids off to die for their fortunes. And they just dig it. So there they are.

"[W]e turned back to that carnival model," L.A. Kauffman (2004, p. 384) explained: "People loved it and responded really well to reintroducing satire, humor, color, dance, music into the movement. It helped that some of the satire was directed *toward* the movement."

By the end of the day, the Absurd Response got ten- to thirty-second news coverage on most of the networks, a predictably sarcastic story in the *New York Times*, and a cover story in the *Washington Post*. It declared "100,000 Rally, March against War in Iraq" with the "Party for Perma War" on the front cover (Reel and Fernandez, 2002). The question remains though, is it a good thing if this ironic theatrical protest is the image of the antiwar movement the public sees?

Despite the controversy of the action, Kate Crane still felt the absurd response was an appropriate one for that moment in history:

> When we were doing Absurd Response before the war actually started, that felt incredibly appropriate. We all knew back then that the reasons for going to Iraq were a lie. We knew that it was a sack of bullshit why we were going to war, that it was absurd. It was like, "Are you kidding me?" To use that idea was a better way for people to hear that it was bullshit.

Mostly importantly, the message was getting out. In the week after the protest in Washington, more positive coverage of the antiwar movement followed. The *New York Times* changed their tune and followed the *Washington Post* line that the October event was perhaps the largest antiwar protest since the Vietnam era. "Rally in Washington Is Said to Invigorate the Antiwar Movement," read the *Times* headline of October 30, 2002 (Zernike, 2002).

Later in the week, the group took the perma-war message to the West Village Halloween parade, where the antiwar humor engendered widespread support. The Absurd Response effectively communicated a range of ideas that many were feeling. Some of the most serious of participants in New York's political culture were engaged by the Absurd Response's playful politics. "I remember at that Halloween parade one of my dour ex-girlfriends was like, 'you guys are the hottest thing in New York City activism,'" Crane boasted. "Sometimes it's that you can have the same idea and convey it three different ways. When you convey it in a way that can make people think, that can make them laugh, you can hold their attention."

For many in the group, the feeling was that humor was the greatest response to this strange convergence of events. The group put together a small website highlighting our antics and calling for new members to join our weekly antiwar events e-mail list. Here, the public was invited to continue to challenge the elite-engineered hysteria. Whether this shifted the power dynamics of the push to war is another question. But throughout the fall of 2002 and early 2003, Absurd Response brought a bit of lightheartedness back to the theater of protest. The core message was that fun and freedom are essential tools for activists working to create a better world.

Back in 1965, in the face of threats of violence from the Hells Angels, Allen Ginsberg (1965/2000, pp. 9–10) wrote a pre-action treatise on how to handle such potentially disruptive situations. In his surprisingly still contemporary tract, he offered a mind–body view of keeping cool and creating a theater of protest. His little essay serves as an outline for the transformative potential that protest offers when we are critical of ourselves and joyful at the same time:

> If imaginative, pragmatic, fun, gay, happy, secure propaganda is issued to mass media in advance . . . the parade can be made into an exemplary of spectacle on how to handle situations of anxiety and fear/threat to manifest by concrete example, namely the parade itself, how to change war psychology and surpass, go over, the habit image reaction of fear/violence . . . This is, the parade can embody an example of peaceable health which is the reverse of fighting back blindly. (pp. 9–10)

Perhaps that was just it: the parade can be an example of another way of being right with others and ourselves. Attacks from the Hells Angels need not bring out the worst in us.

"BETTER TO LAUGH THAN CRY"

The months of activism from October 2002 to March 2003 when the Iraq Invasion began were some of the most exhilarating, depressing, riveting, and charged I can remember. If a mood became too intense—another bombing or shift in the public's jittery nerves—it shifted the emotional political climate. Still, many felt relieved to laugh. "War is so 20th Century," a sign at one of the rallies read. "Somewhere in Texas, there is a village missing an idiot," another sign proclaimed. Activists chained themselves together in Hillary Clinton's office the day she voted to approve the war in 2002.

    Despite the unsettling premonition that war was going to happen regardless of whether voters wanted it or not, whether they cried or not, activists planned a final push against the invasion. In doing so, they often faced formidable obstacles. A new antiwar group, United for Peace and Justice (UFPJ), fought a fruitless legal battle for a permit for an antiwar march in New York City on February 15, 2003, only to see its request dismissed as a security threat. Born in Porto Alegre, Brazil, cities around the world responded to the World Social Forum call to "Say No to War." Rallies were planned for some 180 cities around the world.

    Members of the RTS/Absurd Response team called for a Fat Saturday festive party for a WORLD WITHOUT WAR! to meet at the steps of the New York Public Library. "Why—BECAUSE WAR IS SO LAST Millennium," the call declared. "A festively ironic, theatrical carnival-like feeder march to join up with the large anti-war rally/march on Saturday, 15 February, at 11:30 a.m. at the Lions/Public Library. Celebrate Mardi Gras, Reclaim the Streets says 'Give Up War for Lent.' And Dance." The call was open to everyone: "musicians, dancers, tap dancers, artists, sinners, wingnuts, even the NYPD. Anyhow, RTS invites the masses to come and shake their booties in solidarity with everyone . . . a majority of Americans who thinks this is dumb." After all, it concluded: "Invading IRAQ is just so ten years ago!!!"

    The RTS/Absurd group would be part of the "red" bloc of activists, whose actions absolutely presented a risk of arrest. Others from religious or labor groups tried to participate in safer actions, but no one was going to have an easy time of it on February 15, 2003. Members of the Absurd Response team wore feather boas and Marge Simpson wigs and carried noisemakers. Signs included the ubiquitous "All War All the Time?" and "God Bless Hysteria" in homage to the rainbow colors of the alerts police swarmed through the streets. Remnants of the roving samba band from the WEF protests the year before also planned to meet at the carnival bloc. Once there, sounds boomed from both the band and a mobile version of the RTS sound system in a grocery cart. A queer bloc also met at the space, as did countless photographers and journalists. Crowded beyond measure, all bets for keeping the bloc together would be for naught. The street was clogged with bodies for as far as anyone could see. Police and photographers clogged the steps with activists, with everyone braving the freezing weather. The plan had been to follow the marching band, but the streets were so clogged it was hard to follow anything.

    As soon as the group left the library steps, many of us were separated within the sea of people. In the name of crowd control, police separated everyone, arbitrarily placing blockades wherever they could. Some Absurd Response members passed the time organizing rounds of the antiwar hokey-pokey, while others fought through police barricades. This seemed to last hours. In the meantime, the police pounced on protesters, actually pushing activists into 42nd Street and crushing others into dead ends. Even my father, a retired reverend, had to fight his way out of protest pens, working with a group of octogenarians to break through the police lines. The police sent horses to break up feeder marches heading to the main rally at Central Park, separating the crowds into smaller groups, while pushing marchers off sidewalks with batons. In the end, they arrested nearly three hundred people (Dunn et al., 2004). And miraculously, RTS/Absurd Response reconverged with the folks with a working sound system. The group zigged and zagged through the side streets, avoiding police or being pinned into pens, before making our way through the police to get a bite. Eating at Howard Johnson's in Times Square we watched what looked like a riot outside, as police pushed people to and fro. It was the apex of the Absurd Response.

Two days later, a *New York Times* editorial compared the weekend's mobilization with the Czechoslovakian Velvet Revolution of 1989 and the Revolutions of 1848. "The fracturing of the Western alliance over Iraq and the huge antiwar demonstrations around the world this weekend are reminders that there may still be two superpowers on the planet: the United States and world public opinion . . . millions of people who flooded the streets of New York and dozens of other world cities." Bush would suggest the actions were like a giant "focus group" that he could safely ignore.

Still February 15 was recognized as the largest day of protest in world history. And with it, activists succeeded in communicating to the world and history that much of the world was against this war from the very beginning (Cortright, 2005).

By the time then Secretary of State Colin Powell made the case for war before the United Nations a few days later, he knew the information he was about to present was not entirely accurate. A heady cold winter wind blew through the streets of New York as Powell headed to his vaulted stage at the UN where he claimed, "Saddam Hussein is determined to get his hands on a nuclear bomb. He is so determined that he has made repeated covert attempts to acquire high-specification aluminum tubes from 11 different countries" (quoted in Media Matters, 2005).

Over time, history would prove the protestors to be right. "I participated in a hoax on the American people, the international community, and the United Nations Security Council," Lawrence Wilkerson, Powell's chief of staff who drafted the UN address, confessed after he left office (quoted in Media Matters, 2005).

"If Bush attacks Iraq, Protest 5:00 PM Times Square," read the pink and black Absurd Response stickers designed by L.A. Kauffman. On March 20, we received Kauffman's ominous e-mail: "The war has begun; it's time to get out in the streets! However you choose to express your feelings on this sad and ominous day—through solemn vigils, loud marches, or nonviolent direct action—we urge you to take immediate and visible action." That dark afternoon, the skies poured with rain and we felt completely futile. The protests in Times Square made for film noir-ish sights of activists scuffling with police in the rain, as the ANSWER sound system, permitted by the police, droned on into the night. News throughout the evening followed reports of demonstrations across the country. It detailed the rise of a new kind of antiwar activism, stories on Bush's failed diplomacy, a demonstration in Times Square, the Dixie Chicks against the war, in San Francisco over one thousand people got arrested for actually shutting down the city's financial district.

Once the war started, many felt compelled to communicate to the rest of the world that there were Americans against the war. On March 22, just two days after the start of the bombing of Iraq, UFPJ had already scheduled yet another citywide rally for "Peace and Democracy." Once again, stickers for the event could be found around the city. Yet unlike on February 15, this rally had been awarded a permit. I showed up that Saturday expecting a bit of a funeral march. In the week before the rally, few in the normally festive RTS/Mobilize New York affinity group were feeling very festive. It's hard to be ironic when people are really dying in the streets. We put out a call for a funeral bloc at the rally, asking people to come as pallbearers and hysterical mourners: "Bring your prayer beads and talismans. Wear Black. Grieve with Righteous Anger. And get ready to march for our ailing democracy . . . Reclaim the Streets Says: Mourn with Militance."

Strangely, that Saturday turned out to be buoyant. Two nights before the rally, a call went out from a renegade RTSer calling for a "baguette bloc" to protest the anti-French tide taking hold across the country, while thanking the French for their hard line against the war: "A wildly militant march of folks celebrating everything French, wearing berets, blue and white striped shirts, smoking Gauloises, and pumping their baguette-clenched fists up and down in the air, shouting 'Tous ensemble! Tous ensemble! Oui! Oui! Oui!'" (a French anarcho-syndicalist chant for "All together! All together! Yes! Yes! Yes!"). And sure enough, that day most were wearing berets and moustaches, eating Brie, faking bad French accents, singing "The Marseillaise," etc. While I was not as ready to be silly, there was a certain ring to the "French Kiss for Peace" and "Eat the Props" chants lead by Andrew Boyd and Ricardo Dominguez as we munched on baguettes. The exuberance of the day was undeniable. The Tranny Brigade chanted "We're queer! We're cute! We're antiwar to boot!!!" Reverend Billy made peace with authentic protestors. The Glamericans wore their feather boas and carried signs proclaiming: "War is Tacky, Darling" and "Peace is the New Black." The Frenchies spoke for all our "nausea." ACT UP members screamed "War is so heteronormative." And so on.

The action was striking. There are times when I do this that I feel like we actually are coming so close to imagining and actually even creating a far more caring world. I was in awe. I just couldn't believe how many people were out dressed to the nines to speak out against the war. Despite police arresting activists for standing in a park, a quarter of a million people marched against the war that Saturday. And, certainly, many of us felt that energy, despite the destruction happening in the world.

Yet the joyous resistance did not necessarily work for everyone involved with the ever-morphing RTS/Absurd Response team. "We were going to do a funeral bloc. I felt like that was appropriate," Kate Crane recalled:

> Our friends wanted to do a baguette bloc, with the pinstripes for peace. And it was fun, but I was like, I don't feel it. I know that in this other part of the world I probably will never see, people are getting blown to bits and their houses are getting destroyed and their villages are being leveled and the government's lying to us. And I don't feel like being joyful. I feel like it's flippant. I feel like it's disrespectful to the devastation that's happening.

The baguette bloc would be the last action of the Absurd Response team.

THE CARNIVAL WEARS THIN

Andrew Boyd, who helped organize the baguette bloc, reflected on the use of carnival in the age of the War on Terror:

> When you talk about the carnival thing, it was a great tactic. But then after 9/11 we couldn't use it. Partly our particular segment of the movement took a long time to recover and figure out with enough time passed that you could have a fierce joyous street carnival kind of thing, especially in this city. It was hard, it was really hard. And we, the movement, had become closely wedded to that energy and that tactic and that kind of display. It was hard to find a compelling, inviting, mass, organically shared sort of open architecture, easy to engage in kind of thing that wasn't based on play and carnival and celebratory kind of stuff when things were not celebratory.

Carnival notwithstanding, many were becoming weary of the large-scale actions organized by antiwar coalition groups. Longtime activist Michael Shenker, for one, missed a space where individual input could have an influence:

> People want to be on a creative journey of self-discovery . . . No one is being forced by anyone, except maybe by circumstances. People have different personal needs. Realization and utilization of individual potential. And then the joy of working collectively with other people so that that is recognized by other humans and esteemed by others and appreciated by the collective. And that in essence is nonhieratical. This is why I have problems with groups such as ANSWER and UFPJ. Seattle was an incredible inspiration for me. It appeared we were moving in a direction of popular brilliance of small collectives. And all of a

sudden, when things get really serious . . . We have this war in Iraq, let's just turn things over to x, y, and z. You go to one of those marches, you feel like a cog. You feel like cattle.

"We haven't stopped the war in Iraq," Starhawk mused in our 2006 interview. Yet she spoke for many when she noted, "at least I can look myself in the mirror and say I'm looking at a woman who has done her damnedest." For many, the stage everyone was performing on was as much for memory, and even history, as it was the streets around the world; the audience was as much the international community as it was the Bush administration. The waves of history are never easy to predict, and they should not be quickly demarcated. "The administration's deceit in justifying the war set the context for the political problems the White House began to face afterward," scholar David Cortright (2005) wrote. "The ways in which social movements influence policy are not always readily apparent. They often emerge in unanticipated form, or in future impacts." He suggested: "While the antiwar movement did not succeed in preventing the invasion of Iraq, it helped to set the terms of the debate and exerted considerable influence on public opinion. The Bush administration rammed through its war policy, but it lost the more important struggle for hearts and minds" (2005, p. 96).

In the weeks after the war started, activists continued on a small scale of direct action. San Francisco set the standard for the country, becoming a national epicenter for antiwar activism, with loosely coordinated affinity groups facilitating the goal of shutting down the city's financial district and even a few highways. New Yorkers from the direct action communities of ACT UP, and the more radical types within UFPJ, formed an ad hoc coalition to plan a massive nonviolent civil disobedience. The city was buzzing with action. On March 26, a group covered themselves in fake blood and chained themselves down across Fifth Avenue. That night, stories of their action spread around the world (M26, n.d.).

Decentralized, autonomous actions were scheduled to begin at 8 a.m. the following day, Thursday, March 27. The target of the action was the media–government collusion promoting the war for corporate interests. The goal was to stop business as usual. The Rockefeller Center area was chosen as the target since many media companies and other corporations have offices there or nearby. The plan for the day was for a massive die-in on Fifth Avenue at Rockefeller Center, with coordinated actions planned by affinity groups throughout the city. I arrived that Thursday morning with about thirty minutes before I had to get to work. The sidewalks from Fifth Avenue to Rockefeller Center were clogged. Police had already set up police pens, where activists milled about and chanted. Eight a.m., the time for the action to start, came and went. The police, who had blocked the entrance to Rockefeller Center, stood not knowing what to think. Suddenly, a horn went off and activists pushed over the police pen, stepping onto the streets and lying down for a 'die-in.' Crowds of protestors roared as chaos took hold. Traffic stopped. The police struggled to reestablish control. Cameras, journalists, and police were everywhere. I mugged for several of the cameras as I cheered the activists, only to realize the paparazzi I was oozing for had no press credentials. They were police, recently legally released to photograph activists (Powell, 2002). Subsequent actions would continue under auspices of this anti-war coalition dubbed M27 after the date of the die-in.

The week following M27, the amalgam of antiwar groups which organized the civil disobedience actions continued to meet. The coalition was bound by three central points: calls for additional massive nonviolent civil disobedience during the national day of action; respect for decentralized, autonomous direct action affinity groups; and a corresponding legal protest to stop business in New York while people die in this war. On April 7, the M27 coalition planned to target the Carlyle Group. If ever there was a time when I felt like I was onto the right target, April 7 was it.

RTS planned to work with the Glamericans and Circus Amok, a queer performance art/free circus. The Glamericans organized a call for protest just the week before. At our one joint meeting, we all agreed that no one wanted to get arrested. After brainstorming protesting the war-profiteering Carlyle Group, we decided to go as mock billionaires. After all, the Carlyle investment fund was making billions on the war, with a defense contract whose stocks continued to escalate as the war continued. The group was run by a group that included the forty-first president, George Bush, with his secretary of state James Baker as their counsel, and former Tory leader John Major, Bush's main ally during the First Gulf War. Some have even noted that the Bin Laden family was part of the group. The Carlyle Group had done nicely with their connections to the Bushes and the Saudi royal family. The scenario was simple enough. The protestors would converge at the Carlyle Group offices on Madison Avenue between 58th and 59th as the emblem of the warmongering profiteers.

The Glamericans made the signs and wrote up the call, which was sent out everywhere, including to the New York Billionaires, who forwarded it to their lists. "Looks like RTS is also joining in as Billionaires," one of their e-mail posts noted. "Join Glamericans, Reclaim the Streets, Circus Amok, and other fabulous protesters in our mock pro-war stance. We're talking over the top and we need you to help make it over-the-topper," the call declared. "[C]ome in corporate drag—business suits or fancy dress. SLOGANS: 'MORE LIVES TO THE GALLON' 'WAR IS GOOD FOR YOUR PORTFOLIO.'"

The demonstration was supposed to start at 8 a.m. Monday morning on April 7th, 2003, I was running late. It took a while to find the top hat I'd used the last time I dressed as a billionaire during the WEF protests the previous winter. Running down from the F train at 63rd, I'd lost the exact address of the protest. So I just followed the roars of the crowd and the riot cops I noticed running through the streets. The police led me straight to the fabulous, decadent-looking billionaires, dressed in gothic vampire makeup most appropriate for sucking the blood out of local economies. There the mock vampires were busy celebrating the war profiteering taking place at the Carlyle.

"We started off about 8:15. We all had some nice banners," mock vampire Ben Mauers recalled, noting that things were going just fine. Around 8:35, the police, who had surrounded the entire group, started squeezing in. "They're going to arrest us," a few people started saying. "Nah, I'll go talk to them," I responded. "Can I go to class? I have class at nine and would love to leave," I told one cop. No comment. A few of us busily called in to work or to cancel appointments as we watched the police arresting the protesters. I grabbed the one other RTSer nearby; we stayed close. The group was never told to disperse. Slowly, the police then began arresting random people standing on the sidewalk. "I got there at ten of eight with my donut and my coffee," recalled Tim Becker. "And it was, like, no time at all [*laughs*]." He had not even finished his donut and coffee before the cuffs were around his wrists. All in all, some 94 people were arrested.

The arrestees were taken down to 1 Police Plaza, where the activists commiserated and conspired. A short history of New York activism could be read in the stickers throughout the cells; fading "Mayday is Jay Day" from the Million Marijuana March of 1999 and Spanish "Silencio = Muerte: ACT UP Wall Street" stickers were on the benches. The cells even had a few old RTS stickers for the June 18, 1999, protest. Of all the protests we've done outside of corporate targets, few of us had ever seen the police move in so fast. For the Carlyle Group, there was little interest in a protest about the profits the first Bush is making on the war, which his son who was president stood to inherit.

Throughout the day, activists were interrogated about their political associations. Later in the week, the *New York Times* reported that the NYPD said they had ceased using the "demonstration debriefing form" (Rashbaum, 2003a, 2003b). This was not the experience of those inside the jail, who were questioned for much of the day. I was out of jail by 6 p.m.; others were in way after 11 p.m. Our charges were disorderly conduct and failing to disperse. After the demonstration, Stephen Duncombe, who was also arrested, recalled, "I've been going to legal protests in New York City for more than a decade and I've never seen anything like this. They arrested us for peacefully standing on the sidewalk and with no warning."

The Carlyle Group protest was another one of those occasions when activists ran into the limitations of the play model. We went there intending to play billionaire vampires in support of the Carlyle Group. Yet as Tim Becker points out: "They [the police] made you wear that makeup all afternoon long." I did not even have time to take off my billionaire top hat before we were swept up. Yet this might signal that the group had actually hit a real pressure point. "I don't think the theater made any difference that day. That was just an extra point," Becker pondered. "But there is no real way of knowing. There is all conjecture. That's like seeing yourself in history. And how much are you really cooking up."

The dramatic confrontation still communicated a powerful message about the Carlyle group, argued Ben Mauers. "The most important thing is that we are getting the message out to people," he noted. "When we did the Carlyle protest, we had mainstream TV actually cover what the Carlyle Group is." Before the action, knowledge of the Carlyle Group was limited to conspiracy literature (Briody, 2003). After the April 7 action and similar protests in other cities, the Carlyle Group's role in the war became a central point of contention for even the most mainstream critics of the Bush administration's policies. *New York Times* columnist Maureen Dowd (2006) echoed the group's arguments in a later story, noting: "The creepy John Grisham–style Washington firm called the Carlyle Group, suffused with Arab connections and money, and seeded with Saudi money (including bin Laden family until after 9/11), even gave some thought to investing in the ports." In the following months, A7's counter-public critique jumped from the counterculture into the public sphere of national debate. "It's about getting the information out there," Mauers explained. "I think that the theatrical forms of protest are one of the last legitimate forms of journalism in many ways."

After the arrests, activists fought back, suing the city. "The Carlyle arrests are part of a pattern of NYPD harassment in which lawful demonstrators are arrested and jailed with the short-term goal of clearing them off the streets and the long-term goal of deterring them and other New Yorkers from participating in future demonstrations," said the Center for Constitutional Rights's Nancy Chang in announcing the lawsuit against the City of New York for the Carlyle arrests. After all, the charges against all the plaintiffs involved in the Carlyle case were dismissed. One plaintiff, Sarah Kunstler, was held for twelve hours and charged with two counts of disorderly conduct. "It was frightening to learn how easy it is to be arrested without warning and hauled away for peacefully exercising your free speech rights," she said.

I have often wondered what drove us to reject a politics of authenticity in favor of a brash, absurd response during the antiwar mobilizations. "Camp and tragedy are antithesis," Susan Sontag (1964/2001, p. 63) explained in "Notes on Camp." "The whole point of camp is to dethrone the serious. Camp is playfully anti-serious." Instead of frothing with anger, such engagement allows organizers to maintain a "more complex relation to the serious." To a degree that's what we were trying to do. And we were not the only ones doing so. Actions were planned for the entire year.

CANCUN, MIAMI, AND CONTROL OF PROTEST

In September 2003, the WTO meetings were to be held in Cancun, Mexico. Like much of the activism during this period, the days were filled with the inevitable highs and lows of direct action, negotiations, and street performance on a tragicomic stage. Throughout the week of protests, activists succeeded in propelling their message, even as they were forced to contend with some very difficult news during the negotiations. Early in the week, a South Korean farmer activist committed suicide in protest of unfair trade policies. "Well, it was very heavy when Kun Hai Lee killed himself," recalled Starhawk, who was at the action. "But when you are in actions like that, each day feels like a year." In that time, the activists convened a memorial. "The day before, we had marched up to the barricades and pulled the fences down, which was also fun, and then we sat down and had a memorial for him," she remembered. Later in the week seven activists left the streets but not their message behind, as they reconvened on the beach, with their fists in the air, to deliver a defiant message, painted in red on their highly toned backsides: "We Are Winning."

For Starhawk, the display of direct actions ranging from playful gestures to serious street actions reflected a breadth of responses. Yet, in the end the talks failed to produce a deal. "I think in some ways, it's just a way we can sustain doing it," Starhawk mused on the play element within the movement. "I think that we are seeing that around things like the WTO and G8, that although they are still wielding enormous power and they are still winning,

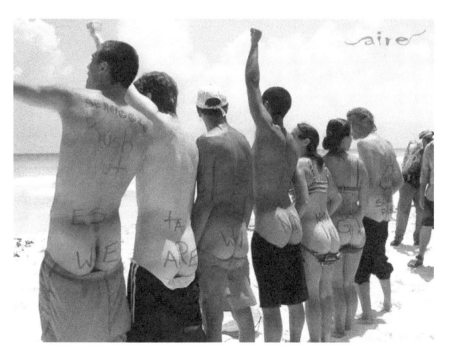

Figure 7.5 We Are Winning Butts Accion Informative en Resistencia. Photo by Mike McGuire.

they don't have the kind of assumed legitimacy that they had before." After all, "The WTO talks collapsed at Cancun." And the movement's critique continued to enjoy a great deal of support (see Reich, 2006).

The success in Cancun was not repeated during the protests at the FTAA meetings in Miami later that fall. Police prevented most any movement or form of protest. For New York activist Beka Economopolis (2003), who attended the action, the implication of the police actions was simple: activists would be arrested and removed from the streets regardless of whether they were innocent or not. While the illegal arrests and bogus charges could be easily beaten, these police practices were able to discourage participation. "This chilling effect remains: civil liberties are trampled, lives are disrupted, and a deterrent is delivered," she wrote after returning. This aggressive policing approach has since come to be known as the Miami Model. The Miami episode cast an ominous shadow over the protests planned to coincide with the Democratic and Republican National Conventions the following summer. It was all part of the era of the Patriot Act.

PATRIOTS AGAINST THE PATRIOT ACT

"WE ARE SO FUCKED!" was the RTS slogan in the days after 9/11; one of the group's countless bratty "better to laugh than cry" screams as it held on for dear life as the 9/11 attacks were played as justification for more killing. RTS had used absurd responses to the situation as long as it could. Soon we started to wonder, "Where do we go after irony ceases to be effective?" What were the most effective activist responses to the use and abuse of the narratives of the War on Terror? Facing the limits of camp, the affinity group struggled to fight the ideological uses of the Patriot Act by actively backing the campaigns for Patriot Act Free Zones taking place all over the country. The city was sponsoring Resolution 909 to oppose the Patriot Act. So the group decided to support the resolution.

As summer turned to fall, Resolution 909 gained considerable momentum. Support from the City Council increased and hearings were scheduled. The hearings presented a telling challenge for RTS. By the time Resolution 909 came along, the group was faced with the question: what do you do after postmodernism? You can't live on irony alone; there is too little to show for it. Irony recedes in relevance when political situations become too dire, when there is an urgent need to engage in dialogue with the political mainstream and new approaches become necessary. What was the best way to move? "Carnival is supposed to be a liberatory action, which means that we shouldn't be chained to it," argued Larry Bogad. It is not always appropriate or useful. "The use of irony is situationally determined. Depending on the context, irony can be either a post-hip cop-out or a challenging, effective way of engaging publics. Irony always includes the risk of a misfire in communication," concluded Bogad.

RTS organizer Steve Duncombe argued that in terms of pure politics, for many activists Bush and the Patriot Act appeared so absurd that parody came perilously close to reality. Further, while the Absurd Response was a great way to make politics fun, the political terrain was shifting. Irony works best as an inside joke to mobilize and appeal to a subculture. Yet it is limited in its ability to demonstrate what kind of world we really want to create. If we are going to suggest that another world is possible, we'd better be able to suggest that this world is more than simply ridiculous. So the affinity group used its e-mail list, sponsored street parties, even a rant in support of a culture of resistance to the Patriot Act (see Shepard, 2004).

The City Council finally passed the resolution by winter of 2004. Udi Ofer and Glenn C. Devitt of the New York City Bill of Rights Defense Campaign noted: "Given that the Council convened to deliberate on the resolution only a few blocks from Ground Zero, it was hard not to appreciate the historical significance of the vote. It's largely in the name of the New Yorkers who perished on 9/11 that the federal government continues to push through anti-terrorism policies which needlessly sacrifice our most fundamental rights and freedoms."

Riding home one night through the snow after one of our biweekly drunken RTS "meetings" and "planning sessions" in the midst of the campaign, a friend explained that even if the world she lived in was going completely to hell on a macro level, she still had to do something at home. Taking care of her own community was the only thing she could see doing. Few answers to bigger questions emerged. Irony and play would still be necessary and fun parts of the strategy to be used when they seemed tactically appropriate, and when coordinated with extensive research and political savvy. For now, street aesthetics had successfully complemented a legislative campaign to make one city and the United States as a whole a little more free. New York City just became a Patriot Act Free Zone, or so we hoped. As we'd learn with the Republican Convention, this was barely the case.

WHERE THE FUN STOPS—REPUBLICAN NATIONAL CONVENTION NEW YORK CITY

Much of the city's approach to the RNC was regulate, control, or shut down unsanctioned expression, direct action, or play. The NYPD legal guidelines for "Operation Overlord II" specifically listed "Swarming/ Critical Mass" and "Marching Bands" as targets (Doepfner and Sweet, 2004, pp. 13, 17). Police were warned that "Lacking supplies, protestors have resorted to the use of paving stones, bricks, mailboxes and road debris. Protesters may utilize devices such as wrist rockets, slingshots, large rubber bands, paint ball guns, lacrosse sticks to launch projectiles" (p. 17). Cognizant of the Jaggi Singh incident that occurred at the

Quebec City FTAA protests in 2001, the police went as far as to note: "Catapults have been constructed to hurl objects, such as stuffed animals, bricks and bottles over security lines and at police officers" (ibid.). The teddy bear launch in Quebec was an absurd gesture. But the police did not seem to appreciate the playful aesthetics of the flying teddy bears. "Our style of festival is their style of disorderly conduct," members of RTS wrote on a flyer years earlier. Much of the RNC would involve just such an interplay, between a Kafkaesque administrative approach toward crowd control and an impulse toward freedom.

Throughout the days and months leading up to the RNC, members of RTS felt there was not enough defiant rambunctiousness and play in the actions and cultural response to the RNC. So RTS/Absurd Response formed a new spin-off: the Clandestine Insurgent Rebel Clown Army (CIRCA). As the groups had done many times in the past when we ran out of new ideas, we again turned to the creative work of RTS London (Jordan, 1998). When RTS London planned a guerilla gardening action for May Day 2000, we followed suit, organizing our own gardening action the same day (Duncombe, 2000). The group would pull together pieces of the Billionaires, SUDS, and Absurd Response for its performances as clowns at the RNC (see Shepard, 2005).

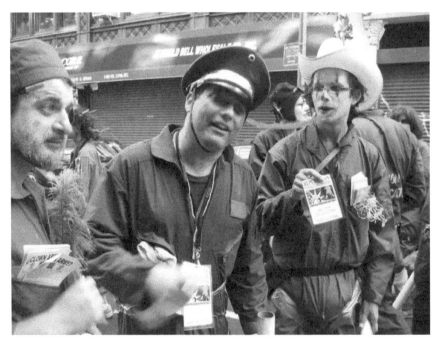

Figure 7.6   NYC CIRCA photo—Jason Grote, L.M. Bogad, and Steve Duncombe with bulge. Photo by CIRCA NYC. From the collection of the author.

New York's CIRCA drew rave reviews. "Acts of creative street the-ater stole the show, with creative expressions suggesting that America's activist movement may have come of age," one reporter noted (Wheeler, 2004). "Running helter-skelter down side streets perpendicular to the protest thoroughfare, the Clandestine Insurgent Rebel Clown Army played a virtual game of freeze tag with journalists and photographers before suddenly retreating in chaotic fashion," observed this writer dur-ing the massive rally on Sunday August 29, 2004: "They wore dirty green army fatigues, fake passes identifying them as Republican del-egates to the convention, and ridiculous clown paint on their faces." The reporter interviewed one of the clowns. "Our hero, Dubya, is in town for the Republican National Clown Convention, so we've got our credentials," Larry Bogad explained. "We're the Big Top delegation, from right between Kansas and Missouri. We're ready. We're just as big clowns as they are" (quoted in Wheeler, 2004). Here play found its way into the mix.

But for the most part, there was not too much room for clowning dur-ing the RNC. The police cracked down on the massive Critical Mass ride the Friday before the actions began (see Shepard and Smithsimon, 2011). August 31, 2004, A31, was the day planned for direct action. While activ-ists saw the day as a space for expression, the police saw demonstrations without permits as threats to public safety. Throughout the day, activists were arrested merely for being associated with the protests. A street-party bloc was planned for Union Square. "The only time that instruments got smashed was with the Rude Mechanical Orchestra last year," recalled Joe Tuba, who planned to perform. He described the scene at Union Square. "I showed up just in time to see the Rude Mechanical Orchestra play-ing in Union Square and take off into the street . . . The Infernal Noise Brigade right behind them and they went a block away and got penned in and everybody got arrested." The police were acting on specific orders to slow down the band. "Marching bands and amplified music may be used to interfere with the police radio communications and to signal dif-ferent messages to protesters," stated the police protest manual for the RNC, adding: "increases in beat are used to indicate an attack, while decreases are a signal to withdraw." Therefore, "Persons marching or parading within the city without a permit may be subject to arrest under Penal Law, Section 240.29 Disorderly Conduct" (quoted in Doepfner and Sweet, 2004, p. 17).

That day, acts of political freedom—public performances, bike rides, and old-school civil disobedience—were targeted and restricted. Random acts of spontaneous expression were targeted and restricted. While the theme of the convergence was "Let the Fun Out," it might as well have been "Go to Jail Fast." Nearly three hundred bikers were arrested at the Friday night Critical Mass bike ride and by Tuesday, A31, over one thousand people were arrested in the largest number of mass arrests in the history of US political conventions. This writer was arrested by plainclothes officers and held before it all began. When lawyers tried to track me down in the system, they were notified that the city could hold me for twenty-four hours without charges or information about my whereabouts under the Patriot Act (Shepard, 2005).

Fear ran wild. "Far too many New Yorkers were far too quiet," civil liberties advocate Norman Siegel proclaimed after fighting for the release of activists held for over seventy hours during the convention. "Our freedoms are not taken overnight, they disappear gradually."

"In the history of political conventions, there have never been so many people demonstrating opposition to their government," former Chicago Seven member and California state senator Tom Hayden told demonstrators on September 1, 2004—even as many remained confined on Pier 57, the dirty makeshift holding space for arrestees used by the city. Hayden noted that the 1968 generation never saw the kind of preemptive arrests, control culture, and repression which had become common features of recent protests (Slackman and Cardwell, 2004).

In the months after the convention, some 90 percent of the charges against RNC activists were dropped, as police were generally unable to substantiate their claims. In many cases, the police were found to have lied, omitted information, and misrepresented evidence (Dwyer, 2005).

FIGHTING AND PLAYING ON

Despite the crackdown, many stayed involved, even when things seemed really desperate. "I spend a good 40 percent of my life and work fighting depression. If you don't bring some light and goodness to this, for me, I'd never get out of bed," explained Kate Crane. "I don't know if things can change," she confessed. Yet, "sometimes it's just putting the right energy out there. The choice is to sit at home and be depressed or go have a circus party with your friends and in that act, to be embodying the world you want."

Over the next few years activists continued to stay engaged and build models of a better world within their activism, sometimes with play or direct action; often with both. "We are not blocking traffic. We are traffic" is the motto of Critical Mass. Cars make up traffic, and so do bikes. Few people expect car drivers to ask for permission to clog the streets. Bicyclists were claiming the same space for themselves. The arrests of hundreds of bicyclists during RNC protests were only the beginning of a long legal fight between bikers and the police over the definition of a "procession." Yet, the ride and the battle over the police tactics toward it would remain a source of controversy (Shepard and Smithsimon, 2011).

In February 2006, New York State Supreme Court judge Michael D. Stallman ruled against the city's injunction against Critical Mass (Dwyer, 2006b; Stallman, 2006).

"The City's attempt to stop the Critical Mass bicycle rides was soundly rejected by Justice Michael D. Stallman of the New York Supreme Court," noted attorney Norman Siegel. "We are, of course, pleased by the decision. Hopefully, New Yorkers will be able to continue to ride their bicycles in the streets free of arrests, harassment, and hostility in ways that guarantee public safety for all New Yorkers." While the fight continues, it appears the unpermitted authentic community ritual has withstood the city's assault. Despite the pattern of repression, gestures of freedom often prevail when activists do their homework, fight, stand up for themselves, play, and stay focused on the task at hand.

IN THE END

Narratives linking protest with terror accompany new forms of thought control. As capital intersects with state power, the system appears more than capable of absorbing disruptions. Yet, the need to speak out and offer alternatives remains imperative. And when done effectively—with disciplined research, a clear target, a well-communicated message, and a winning strategy—it still remains effective. In the age of terror, the capacity of civil disobedience to disrupt the everyday mechanisms of power appears vastly restricted. For this reason, prefigurative community-building protest remains a vital source of inspiration and organization. If anything, activists suggest they need this kind of activism to live, to feel pleasure, and to carry their work forward. In the tragicomic theater of contemporary urban life, playful responses inspire continued creativity, advocacy, the occasional frustration, and risk. Yet, as the Critical Mass battle suggests, when combined with direct action, research, mobilization, and a clear legal strategy, then play helps sustain and move campaigns forward. Between street parties and bike rides, advocacy and fun, the possibilities of play in public space—and by extension democracy itself—remain both paradoxical and compelling.

8 The Limits of Play
Radical Clowning vs. Tomato Picking

"Let's be unafraid. That's what they taught us. Let's be fools. Let's be ridiculous. Let's rise up. Let's rise up and change this world. Somebody give me a Yes-Men-allulia here!" . . . Once we understand we are controlled by clowns, you can be a clown yourself. Once it's clowns versus clowns then maybe the best idea might win. And the best idea is compassion.

> —Reverend Billy, 2009, in front of an
> immigrant detention center in New York City

To be sure, the quality of clownishness and childishness easily appears to adhere to authentic acts of protest in situations where the radical opposition is isolated and outrageously weak while the Enemy is almost everywhere and outrageously strong. "Maturity"—by definition—rests with the Establishment, with that which is, and the other wisdom then is that of the clown or the child.

> —Herbert Marcuse (1972, p. 51)

"White Power!" the Nazis shouted. "White Powder!" the Clowns shouted back running in circles throwing white flower in the air and raising separate letters which spelt "White Power!"

"White Power!" the Nazis shouted once more, "White Flowers!" the clowns cheered and throw white flowers into the air and danced about merrily."

> —Alex in Pictures, 2007, at a KKK Rally in
> Knoxville, Tennessee in which White supremacists
> were foiled by a group of clowns

Throughout the years, social actors the world over have explored different approaches to performance and protest. Questioning the accustomed boring rallies, the bursts of action, and the frustrated tears, in the mid-2000s a new cohort of actors experimented with an innovative form of radical street performance and community building. In so doing, they helped expand an activist's repertoire with a distinct play strategy. And the image of clowns running through the streets found its way into the public consciousness in cities around the world. The Reverend Billy and Alex in Pictures quotes above refer to the ways clowns challenge social mores. Earlier chapters of this volume considered the pranks of clowns including ACT UP's Operation Ridiculous and Wavy Gravy. This chapter considers some of the advantages and limitations of the radical clowning models which took shape in the summer of 2005.

FROM SOUTH CENTRAL TO EDINBURGH

On August 20, 2005, Time's Up! declared August 23 "Bike Lane Liberation Day" in New York City. That Tuesday, a group of bikers wearing clown costumes started a bike ride at St. Mark's Church in the East Village and rode up Second Avenue (for more on this, see Shepard and Smithsimon, 2011). Earlier that summer, clowns zapped the G8 meetings in Edinburgh. A subculture of clowns was featured in David LaChapelle's documentary *Rize*. Here, African American clowns occupy the LA streets where urban life is thought to offer little but a generous dose of grief and oppression. *Rize* details a subculture inspired by Tommy Johnson (aka Tommy the Clown), who started a new dance movement as a response to the Rodney King riots of 1992. It involved a highly physical form of dance which modulates between tribal and contemporary urban hip-hop steps, offering an alternately despairing, angry, and joyous style of clowning. As an alternative to the state-programmed default of gang life, drugs, violence, and prison, those in the subculture formed troupes of friends who paint their faces like warriors, share space, and dance. Here, groups of "clowns" and "krumpers" perform, compete, and build community together. The film never turns its back on the despair of the circumstances that surround the kids; yet it emphasizes emotional outlets created by a cohort of youth who have grown up in a warfare state characterized by mass incarceration, HIV/AIDS, police corruption and brutality, and widespread loss.

WHY CLOWNING?

LaChapelle's South Central is not the only place where people turned to clowning as an answer to the neoliberal police state with its mantra of "There Is No Alternative." Clowns could be seen intermingled among the groupings of "flex, temp, full-time, part-time, casual and contortionist workers, migrants, students, benefit claimers, New Dealers, work refusers, pensioners, dreamers, duckers, and divers" invited to bring "drums, music, banners, imagination" to the actions against the G8 in Edinburgh, Scotland, in July 2005. The point of the carnival was to subvert business as usual, to assert "desires for FULL ENJOYMENT with fun in the city—and begin to make capitalism and wage slavery history."

   In the center ring of this circus of resistance was the Clandestine Insurgent Rebel Clown Army, or CIRCA. Organized by John Jordan of London's RTS, Larry Bogad of the United States, Jennifer Verson of Bristol, and others, CIRCA first emerged to protest Bush's visit to Buckingham Palace in 2003. The following summer, a group in New York City zapped the Republican National Convention.

I asked Bogad why his affinity group of seasoned movement activists had decided to make use of clowning as a technique at the G8 protests. He began with an caveat about the politics of debt relief, the forcible opening of markets, the politics of neoliberalism, the G8 meetings, the anniversary concert for Live Aid, celebrities, and politics. "So what is the role of the trickster within this whole spectacle?" Bogad pondered. "In the face of this, we wanted to articulate a radical analysis, to confront the media power, the euphemization, the celebrity power." Much of the action took place in a highly mediated stage. "As usual, the movement was demonized in much of the press. During the protests, images of a policeman crossing clubs with a black blocker on the front of newspapers. So we wanted to interrupt the flow of this imagery." They did so as a band of silly clowns. Throughout the week of the summit, the world was treated to a range of ridiculous and telling theatrics including the much-publicized gesture of a clown kissing a policeman's riot shield. Here, Bogad suggested:

> We interrupted what I refer to as the *hegemonologue* coming from the media, which relentlessly depicted the protestors as terrorists and Bob Geldof and Bush as heroes. The point was to be disruptive but in a creative, nonviolent way, engaging people, opening up a creative and personally freeing space for ourselves as well. As opposed to just being angry and ulcerating, we were opening up a different, more engaging, playful space, with an energy that is more than sustainable, it's beneficial. It can reach police officers, passersby, put them in a creative/interpretive/nonthreatened space as well. Some may even pause and think: "They're absurd . . . but maybe they are both absurd *and* they have a point." That's the idea of the wise fool. Our press release stating that these debts were fundamentally illegitimate was quoted, even in some right-wing papers, because we were being such buffoons.

CIRCA's "Anti-Official Communiqué #8.86: Operation BROWN-NOSE," written by "Colonel Oftruth and General Confusion, Edinburgh, 30.06.05," addressed the demonstrators at the Make Poverty History march:

> We are so proud of you, so in love with you, we share your compassion and desire to TRULY make poverty history. We admire your realization that the only real way to end poverty, in the global South or in the suburbs of Edinburgh, is to stop the Great Eight's amusingly antisocial habits—their rather nasty slapstick routines—kicking the poorer nations with war, arms sales, and bullying trade policies, manipulating their markets and plundering their resources while dangling the crumbs of 'debt forgiveness.'

With their communiqué, CIRCA aimed to upend the pomp of the G8. Clowns have long taken on such struggles toward disequilibrium. Geoff Hoyle, of San Francisco's Pickle Clowns, has argued that radical clowning involves a "joyful sharing in attempting an insurmountable task" (quoted in Schechter, 2001, p. 20). The Pickle Clowns often refused to leave the stage even when others suggested their time was up. Instead, they stumbled into a circus trunk and bumbled about. "But their movement is rebellious, at least so much as their bodies cannot be completely controlled by them or others" (ibid.). Through the flying and careening of silly bodies, CIRCA's opposition offered a rambunctious critique of the docile bodies and politics thought to be necessary to support neoliberalism.

CIRCA drew inspiration from Walter Benjamin to Abbie Hoffman, RTS to Joseph Beuys. John Jordan recalled the day he wrote the CIRCA communiqué:

> I picked up this old book that I had bought years ago and never read, called *The Death Resurrection Show*, looking at the relationship between shamanism and Western popular culture, the repression of shamanic cultures in the period in the beginning of agriculture in the West. Yet, that culture, the shamanic culture and the dynamics that were within it, continued in clandestine form as popular forms of culture, especially with clowning and later rock and roll . . . Somehow the clown bit of it just hit me. And it felt like just pulling together these many, many interests in my life. Years ago, I had thought of the idea of a clown army . . . But, I kind of let it go. It was one of those weird things; I pick up this book; I go fuck, "I really wanna do this clown army thing again." I meet someone a few evenings later who described an activist dressed as a clown during the RNC actions, I think it was the Philadelphia Clown Block. They picked up a tear gas canister with a large red hankerchief and then blew their nose with it and of course reeled across the street in absurd yet hilarious pain. And I found it extremely funny. An image it just kind of burned into my imagination. I actually went home that night and wrote the first communiqué of CIRCA. Bush was coming to town. And I thought, okay let's give this a go. And I sent it out. And then got Larry (Bogad) and Jennifer, and a couple of the other clowns involved. Clowning could bring everything together. What I had seen with activists, they start to build this activist armor, they stop feeling things . . . clowning stripped that armor down, it opened up vulnerability. Clowns feel everything directly, they have no skin between themselves and the world. It was a bit of a trojan horse, a psychological tactic to get activists to rediscover their spontaneity and their emotions and on the streets it would replace confrontation with confusion . . .

Shortly after this, Larry Bogad entered the group.

The clown army began when I was in England teaching political the-ater . . . And John Jordan, who was a founder of Reclaim the Streets in London, where it first really started, sent out this call for clowns for the Clandestine Insurgent Rebel Clown Army, which didn't yet exist yet but was going to form to muster and storm the palace when Bush came to town, under the premise that we're upset that there's been no court jesters allowed in the palace since 1549. And we were so excited they were inviting another fool, but then we found out it was Bush. It was the wrong kind of fool. And now all these fools that we have marshaled into this basically clown army are going to march on them to show them how real fools should be. So we were going to speak, not truth, but mirth to power, 'cause he was the real abuser. So that was our point. I answered the call, which I got from a mutual RTS friend, and John got back in touch with me. It was an example of a social network integrating into a great action. And so we got down there and met in an old movement resource building, a little place called LARC, the London Action Resource Center. There was a van full of bobbies, of London cops, sitting right outside when I got there, so I knew it was the place.

Not long after the group formed then a note arrived from Chiapas, Mexico. "To the compañeros and compañeras of the Clandestine Insurgent Rebel Clown Army," the note began.

"An army of rebel clowns?" Again I tried to picture it: red noses and machine guns, combat boots and cream pies, military marching and slapstick tumbling—what a ridiculous vision, far too many clashing opposites to make serious sense.

I turned inquisitively to my trusty compañero Durito. His hard black eyes rolled back in their sockets, and if one could hear an insect breath-ing, then a tiny yet deep exasperated sigh would have been audible above the patter of rain on the huts' tin roof. "You're trying much too hard," he whispered, "stop thinking like a guerilla—start thinking like an idiot, it wouldn't be the first time." I took a deep breath, chewed the end of my warm pipe and delicately picked my nose. . . . it hit me, 'The Clandestine Insurgent Rebel Clown Army!' I laughed out loud . . . A fighting force that exists between chaos and order, obedience and disobedience, reason and madness—how perfectly absurd. That the world is absurd, we know. That to change the world requires as much, if not more absurdity, is less well known. 'Serious' politics is often much too knowing to see its own folly whilst 'Frivolous' politics is often ignored until the hindsight of history discovers the prophetic wisdom in its folly. Twenty years ago when we came to the jungle from the city, we had the absurd belief that with our guns and ideas we could convince the campesinos to join the revolution . . .

Fellow clowns, rebels and combatants of CIRCA I wish you the indestructible luck of fools in your many struggles, wobbles, pratfalls and pranks.

I wish you pockets filled with hope that never runs out and hearts filled with musical beats that build a future of life, liberty and dignity. . . .

From the mountains of the Mexican southeast.

The note was signed by Subcomandante Insurgente Marcos. Yet there were those who suspected it may have been penned by one of the rebel clowns.

Bogad, who took part in the early clown actions in London before joining them for the G8, found play in much of the group's work:

First of all, again, in our making costumes together, in our rehearsing. It was absolutely about theater games. And then we kind of made up and riffed on our own theater games as well. So we'd do games of mime or gesture or playing with a deformity. That sounds pretty serious, but it's serious play. One of the things we did was: now imagine you have a deformity, now make it something you are really proud of. Then you are all going around the room as these tragic clowns, these buffoons who are like outcasts. My character had been disemboweled in the war, so he was always holding his guts in but making the best of it.

Activists around the world joined actions planned for the G8 meetings in Scotland in 2005. A veteran of years of street activism, David Solnit immediately recognized that the clowns threw off the police. "Clowning puts them in a different space," he explained. "It dramatically shifted relations with the police. It kind of opened a space in people's imaginations."

Solnit was not the only person to make this observation. "I think it can be a very effective response because it's not what they expect. In Scotland with the G8, just when the clowns showed up the cops started laughing," recalled Starhawk, who was also at the action. "They didn't know quite what to do. A bunch of guys show up with Molotov cocktails and sticks, the cops know what to do. They're primed for that . . . A bunch of clowns show up, now what do we do?" Scampering about, cowering, begging, pleading, and not really leaving, the clowns seemed more than comfortable playing with power, while inviting everyone, including the police, into their game.

"The clown thing involved play, and playing an enormous amount," John Jordan confessed.

And game playing, and politics, but touching each other and not taking ourselves seriously and learning to let go in the process. During the process, one of the old RTS people who is now involved in clowning in Belgium came up to me and said, "Can you imagine what it would have been like to play at RTS meetings? What it would have done and how it would have changed the social relations in that meeting?" And I have seen it. You do enter a space of trust; you enter a space which is more convivial. And for me, the key of any radical politics is trying to create an atmosphere which supports warm, convivial social relations.

Here, the silliness helped open up space to create community. None of this is to suggest there were not arguments or disagreements. But play was sufficiently suffused into the process that few took it too seriously. "It's also a space in which you learn," Jordan reflected. One sees this with children at play. They learn from play experiments with what is real and what is not; here problem solving and active imagination become part of an engaged mind (Wenner, 2009; Piaget, 1962; Winnicott, 1971). As the Surrealists recognized play is a space to walk on the precipice between reality and possibility, between work and leisure; it is a fantastical space in which to explore alternate ways of worldmaking.

And without it, groups can get bogged down in reality principles in which creativity suffers and is stiffled. "Now I look back on RTS, and what an irony that all these experiments with theater and pleasure and play and carnival, and yet in the process itself there wasn't any of that," mused John Jordan.

> Even though we talked about prefigurative politics all the time. And with the clowns, my point was that if clowning was going to be part of the protest tactics, then it had to be part of the process. There was an awareness of how transformative a lot of the clown exercises were. We had transformative moments in the process and not just in the streets . . . A lot of the clowning was very much about breaking down your kind of armor, letting go.

While the limitations were many, CIRCA was profoundly effective in communicating to multiple publics, including media. As John Jordan observed:

> [M]edia really found it impossible to criminalize the clowns. They tried. But it was pretty damned cool. We saw people feeling some kind of empathy. Something interesting was happening, or simply finding it funny. It was that simple. In a way that they would not find with someone screaming and yelling at them, better than being yelled at . . . There were lovely moments. A friend of mine said, for example, that he talked with people watching in the park who'd not really been political who said, "we saw the clown army and we understood for the first time what it was all about." There were moments when we saw people in cafés who'd smile and would wave through the windows and just all of that in a way that they wouldn't if it was the spectacle. But in their imagination, they have a reference point which was about pleasure, the circus, and clowns. And their reference point with the black bloc would

be terror and violence. Suddenly you are opening a reference of plea-sure, where people can smile and wave out their window. And there were funny moments. There were funny, funny moments.

Still, Jordan left the G8 protests with an acute awareness that while clown-ing diffused police pressure and helped push a critique into newspapers around the world, the model was filled with holes. Without being con-nected to an ongoing organizing campaign that connected aspirations with concrete action, the limitations became glaring. Clowning was not able to provide "life rafts" for those with little else.

Yet, it had proven profoundly effective at garnering attention to a given issue. Over the next five years, the Time's Up! Bike Lane Liberation Clowns kept experimenting with bike lane street theatrics. "Come Ride with the Clown Bicycle Brigade as they Ticket Motor Vehicles & Liberate the Bike Lanes," declared a flyer announcing three more rides at the end of 2005. "The Bicycle Clowns will ride through the bike lanes of Manhattan search-ing out cars illegally parked in their lane," the flyer explained. "If any cars are caught in their lane, the clowns will issue the driver a parking ticket for $115, the official fine for parking in the bike lane," it instructed, describ-ing the action's mode of operation. "Knowing how dangerous, sometimes deadly, cars in the bike lane are for cyclists, the Clowns will search out policeman harassing cyclists without bells and bring them over to take care of the real traffic violators." The call ended with an eye on the big picture. "Once the bike lanes are liberated from all nasty petroleum suck-ing machines, the clowns will head back to Washington Square Park to rejoice and take a victory lap." For the rest of the decade, the group honed the use of clowning, street theater, and direct action to draw attention to enforcement of traffic laws and nonpolluting transportation and the city started paying attention. (For a full extended case study, see Shepard and Smithsimon, 2011.)

David Solnit left the 2005 G8 protests and continued with his work on a campaign which used play as well as provided life rafts. The success-ful campaign by the Coalition of Immokalee Workers (CIW) for better pay from Taco Bell offers striking examples of the use of creative direct action and community organizing, yet in a strikingly different context than CIRCA or the Time's Up! Clowns.

For years, Taco Bell had neglected the CIW's simple request: an increase of one penny per pound of tomatoes picked for their tacos, with a guarantee that the increase go to the farmworkers. And it's no wonder: such slim mar-gins translate into large profits. The demands of migrant and immigrant workers, such as the mostly Haitian, Latino, and Mayan Indians subsisting on subpoverty wages throughout Florida who constitute the coalition, are a low priority for companies such as Taco Bell which stand to profit from their labor. Poverty among migrant farmworkers saves consumers some fifty dollars per year (Schlosser, 2003). At first, Taco Bell refused to even acknowledge the CIW's requests. But the company reached out after the CIW staged a guerilla performance of a mock wedding between a ten-foot-tall Queen Cheap Tomato and King Taco Bell in the street facing their corporate headquarters in Irvine, California.

"I think it's essential to think below the surface, from the gut; if we don't learn to articulate the core roots of the problems we face, we'll always be on the defensive," noted Solnit. And the CIW was anything but defensive. The group was able to explain what it wanted from the very beginning. Using this demand, it helped up the ante. Facing a mounting boycott and pressures from workers, students, and activists around the world, Taco Bell agreed to the core demands advanced by the CIW on March 8, 2005. The CIW could celebrate what amounted to a complete victory against one of the largest fast-food corporations in the world (D. Solnit, 2005).

The campaign gained vitality by mixing a number of organizing ingredients. A few of these elements included: a well-articulated claim, art, research, well-targeted theatrics, nonhierarchical organizing, expansive social networking, and a jigger of play. Through its use of guerilla theater, the campaign successfully bridged the movement's broad critique with an effective organizing and messaging. "We were able to show through their use what the reality of our lives is really like," Solnit elaborated. Along the way, the campaign helped highlight the social and economic issues involved in engaging ways. This in turn helped bring new workers into the campaign. After all, "People join campaigns that are fun and hopeful," explained Solnit. "It's always been there—in the civil rights movement, for example, art helped shut down the WTO."

Much like the Lower East Side Community Labor Coalition, which achieved victory for greengrocery workers in New York City in 2001 (see Ness, 2002), the organizing done by the CIW brought together many of the same boisterous coalitions—including neighborhood, public space, labor, student, and immigrant groups—that fueled the Global Justice Movement's ascendance. Yet, those most affected—in this case, immigrant community groups—led the campaign. "We Are All Leaders," was the campaign slogan.

A vital part of this consciousness-raising included an engagement between art, play, and creative community building. The CIW worked from local bases to transform the isolated struggle of one of the least visible communities in the world into one of the most well-publicized struggles in North America. In the same way that the Zapatista movement built an ethos that allowed anyone to connect with their community, the CIW invited citizens from around the world to participate in their struggle. In this way, leadership and community building intersected in bountiful ways. As the CIW explain: "Our network spread and grew like wildfire. And suddenly, wherever we would go and mention that we were from Immokalee, it would elicit the reaction, 'Oh, the tomato pickers'" (quoted in D. Solnit, 2005). And win by win, the group made inroads.

Finally, the campaign benefited from an appreciation of the possibilities of creative play. "We were able to catch people's attention by making our marches and protests colorful and fun," suggested Solnit. Combined with a willingness to make use of the tools of popular education, storytelling, and art, this spirit supported a winning organizing strategy. "We have to be creative about communicating our story. Art, images, and theater played a very important role," Solnit explained. "And through the images and signs, we were able to more effectively communicate our message to anyone who might have driven by or seen us on the news or in the newspapers" (quoted in D. Solnit, 2005).

Along the way, the campaign offered an alternative, a "yes" to community and the rights of workers. By connecting creativity and a coherent organizing strategy, play informed the campaign, providing it with energy and theatrics. For Solnit, CIW victory was an inspiration and a best-practice model for those involved in campaigns for global justice.

Notes toward a Conclusion
Reflections on the Study of Play in Social Movements

Throughout the final months of work on this manuscript the dynamics of social movement activity shifted and shifted again. The stage seemed to widen with debate about the merit of organizing practices during the US electoral cycle in 2008. Throughout the period, regular people organized any number of events—from stoop sales to bike rides. The second weekend in August 2008, two groups in New York organized street parties. The first party began on the West Side of the City, where it ebbed and flowed, zigged and zagged from Battery Park City, through a peace labyrinth near Ground Zero, off to the Staten Island Ferry, and eventually into Brooklyn. Later that night, a second street party began at Union Square. There activists, borrowing a tactic from early RTS, descended into the subway, jumped on the L train traveling east out to Brooklyn, where they ascended from the underground in Williamsburg and transformed Bedford Avenue into a makeshift street party. An RTS veteran of its first actions passed out free beer from a grocery cart, carrying drinks and a sound system. And music filled the air. Not long after, the police arrived, arrested the DJ, and tried to clear the streets as the two groups played chase all night long.

All this took place just hours after Summer Streets in which the city of New York heeded the call of public space activists and opened up seven miles of streets for biking and play, with all cars blocked up and down Broadway and Fifth Avenue. Members of Time's Up! met at the Astor Place cube where they danced, hula hooped, and boogied away to Queen's "I Want to Ride My Bicycle" as the city was transformed into a space for play and imagination, a celebration of nonpolluting transportation and possibility.

For two decades, members of the group had been arguing that bikes are part of the solution to the city's environmental woes. August 16, 2008, the group was able to really show the city what car-free streets could look like. The Summer Streets was really about finding a space to play in a global city. And people from all walks of life—joggers, parents with kids in strollers, bikers, clowns—everyone seemed to revel in their right to the city.

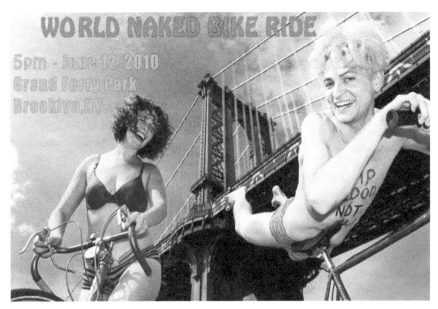

Figure C.1   In Summer 2010, Time's Up! helped organize the raucous and fun World Naked Bike Ride attended by hundreds of semi-clad bikers. Activists rode across the Williamsburg Bridge, dancing to a sound system attached to a bike, through the East Village, where they chanted "less gas, more ass" at a BP station, before dipping into a few fountains, visiting the UN, and taking it back to Brooklyn for an after party.

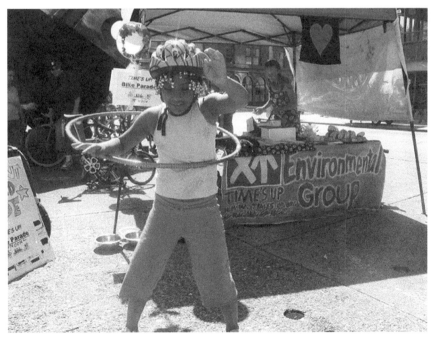

Figure C.2   Photo of Time's Up! at Summer Streets. Courtesy http://times-up.org/

A week later, the city finally agreed to pay off activists swept off the streets by the New York Police Department in front of the Carlyle Group on April 7, 2003 (Dwyer, 2008). "Antiwar Activists Win $2 Million Settlement from New York City in Major Victory for Free Speech Rights," declared the Center for Constitutional Rights, who represented the arrestees, including myself, in the lawsuit. "My question is, why did the NYPD send over one hundred police in riot gear, along with vehicles to block the street and disrupt the flow of morning rush hour traffic, all to stop a legal, peaceful protest?" asked Ahmad Shirazi, a film editor, grandfather, and one of the plaintiffs in the case. "Aren't there more important matters they could be pursuing?" he wondered. "And why did they fight us in court so doggedly when they knew the evidence proved that we were arrested without any police orders to leave?" An NYPD videotape of the demonstration depicts a group of demonstrators lined along the sidewalk of West Fifty-Sixth Street between Fifth and Sixth Avenues— with ample space for pedestrians—ninety-four of whom were arrested without any police warning or opportunity to leave. The arrests took place outside the offices of the Carlyle Group, an investment firm with ties to the Bush family and an extensive portfolio of holdings in the military-defense sector. The police tactics used that day became the model used by the NYPD during the 2004 Republican National Convention held in New York in which some eighteen hundred people were arrested and jailed (Dwyer, 2008).

Two weeks after the settlement, a similar crackdown took place in St. Paul, Minnesota, with activists and videographers swept from the streets and rounded up (Moynihan, 2008). Most vexing were the preemptive arrests of members of Eyewitness Video and Glass Bead Video collective, who compile the sort of video used to win the case against the Carlyle Group (see Dwyer, 2005). "This is the America . . . where dissent is no longer tolerated," explained Starhawk (2008), who witnessed the police raid on the St. Paul Convention center firsthand. "[P]re-emptive strikes have become the strategy of choice for those who hold power, where any group can be accused of 'bombmaking' or 'terrorism' on no evidence whatsoever in order to deter dissent" (ibid.).

The lesson continues to be that activists have to pick and choose their battles, while striving to reinvent movement repertoires. No one tactic or approach can be fetishized after its utility has run its course. As the final chapter of this work suggests, convergence actions feel decreasingly like spaces for social transformation. Certainly, they sometimes offer spaces for theatrical presentation, yet they feel less open to the possibility for social change than do long-term campaigns. It is hard to imagine changes in everyday life at convergence actions. Instead other spaces for organizing are always opening up. From Naked Bike Rides to Drag Rides, new forms of spontaneous direct action take shape all the time in the streets of New York and around the globe. And elements of play remain a part of many such moments. Yet, instead of taking place at convergence actions, fighting for a space to play, rather than perform, has increasingly become a contest of the everyday (Stout, 2011). And in so doing, it functions as a means to challenge social hierarchies.

A news report from Thailand highlights the ubiquity of the model. "On 5th Day of Thai protests, a Carnival Atmosphere," the Associated Press (2008) reported. The dispatch noted that the activists looked amazingly loose, even festive for a group of people who had faced tear gas from riot police just hours before. "The thousands of Thai demonstrators who ran Prime Minister Samak Sundaravej out of his compound looked like a crowd at a folk concert Saturday, singing, clapping and smiling on the grounds of the Government House, the seat of Thailand's government." Another witness would observe, "It's like a carnival," as activists passed out apples, oranges, sticky rice, eggs, and other assorted snacks (Associated Press, 2008).

Protest and play, democracy and tear gas—they are themes which run throughout the cases presented throughout this volume. At its core, a festive spirit often sustains and nourishes movement activity. Not to mention, it feels good. I'm certainly not alone in making such an observation. "[T]here is another aspect to it that I think we should talk and act on more," noted movement scholar Frances Fox Piven, unprompted, in an interview with me.

> And that is the recognition that collective action is really a lot of fun
> . . . And all these political veterans who portray themselves and their
> lives as bitter struggles, as virtually martyrdom, even though the strug-
> gle part might have been only a year or two. They are not telling the
> truth. They did it because they wanted to and because it was so joyful
> and so satisfying. . . . It's a lot of fun to act with your comrades. And
> we should also use our imaginations to make the interior of the move-
> ment even more fun. (Shepard, 2008, p. 14)

IN SUM

"Children know a simple truth that many administrators seem to have forgotten: play is a necessary part of growing up," writes Sheila Flaxman (2000, p. 39). Yet it is more than children who benefit from such behavior. "Free play is a critically important factor" (ibid.), but not just for children—for everyone. The cases presented herein build on this sentiment. Today space for such behavior is being squeezed out of schools, public space, and everyday lives. If we are "homo ludens," as Johan Huizinga suggested, today we must ask what happens if we lose a space for play. Do we become less human? Faced with such a dilemma, many are fighting back (Stout, 2011).

For Johan Huizinga (1950, p. 3), "[t]he *fun* of playing resists all analysis, all logical interpretation." Despite the elusiveness of the concept, this study has tried to offer a history and analysis of the play element in social movement action over five decades of community organizing for social change.

At the beginning of his film *Caravan Prague: Bicycling to Utopia/ Protesting Globalization*, RTS New York member Zack Weinstein describes a picture of activists playing soccer on the field of an airport occupied by activists, followed by a caption with the words: The most important thing is participation. The point, of course, was that everyone should be able to play a part in the game of social change. Play invites people to participate in an expanding public conversation, in which movements and community groups interact. Throughout the cases traced in *Play, Creativity and Social Movements*, we see how these different movements are connected within a story of social action. "Reclaim the Streets stuff helped build Seattle and created support for efforts in the Global South," concluded John Jordan as his interview for the project came to an end. Echoing this sentiment, George Katsiaficas (2002) has argued that the lineage of actions from 1968 to the Battle of Seattle is connected by a cumulative, ever-expanding eros effect. "Through the power of exemplary people's actions leading to involvement by others, small groups are able to detonate social explosions in which millions of ordinary people unexpectedly take the direction of society into their hands to make long overdue changes," writes Katsiaficas (2002). This process can be understood as "the eros effect." Here, eros expands with social action, each gesture building on the preceeding one. It expands from a lusty connection between minds and possibilities, actions and movements—and their yearning to create something better of this world. It is a sensibility which transcends self interest or rational action, toward a desire for something better for everyone. Play contributes to social eros by bringing people together, creating means for people to connect, build communities, engage power, resist social controls, and feel pleasure (Turner, 1982).

In doing so, such practices help us imagine new ways of thinking and being. As the case examples here suggest, play is an intricate part of a bountiful DIY community-building activity. Through it, audience and spectator, leader and follower blur as people are invited to participate in the story themselves (Bakhtin, 1981, 1984). Here stories and songs, music and food, winks and banter lull and seduce rather than hammer. Along the way, once-passive spectators join the action. Many do.

Yet, as the chapters suggest, the fun of social change works best as part of a holistic approach to organizing which includes a clear goal or question, a great deal of research on an issue, accompanied by a coherent approach to communicating a goal, mobilization around it, a legal strategy, direct action to achieve it, and sustainability strategies to keep the campaign going. Here, play is but one ingredient of a larger mix of strategies which help create power. "We're talking about it as one tool within a repertoire of tools that a social movement has," explained Andrew Boyd. "On its own I don't think that it can do that much." Without a connection to a full organizing schema, play is little more than a way to blow off steam (Marcuse, 1955). This text names this phenomenon, attempting to examine a long-standing element of movement strategy and practice.

FINDINGS

For the Situationists and Yippies, play involved the creative prank or gesture; for Gay Liberationists, play was a code word for pleasure and sexual exchange; for AIDS activists, safe play became the order of the day, while subversive humor, street theatrics, pranks, and zaps were used to disarm opposition and move an agenda; for DIY activists, play was part of a prank tradition, now known as culture jamming, that originated with the Situationists. The contrast between the Yippies and the Young Lords considered in the second chapter suggests that play takes on any number of different social and cultural contexts, with different meanings attached. For Gay Liberationists, punks, and ACT UP, play fostered innovation; creating spaces for play was respected as a legitimate movement aim. Here. defending civic space overlapped with struggles to create a different public sphere. For public space activists, the imperative to act involved an effort to create and defend places to play with a burlesque of DIY protest. For global justice activists, play was part of an effort to counter the privatization of public space, a way to help people build their own commons; it was also a way to counter social controls. For antiwar activists, play was part of an effort to offer a counternarrative to war. Here, play offered a life-affirming response to death and violence, as well as a counterbalance to disengagement; it was a way to stay engaged rather than slip into depression or alienation.

After all, in difficult times, many activists have borrowed from and sustained themselves by incorporating ludic elements into their efforts. Here, play serves as an embodiment of an alternative way of being in the world, and a way of creating space and energy, thereby helping activists to stay engaged. It offers a generally—but not always—nonviolent way of engaging and playing with power while creating communities.

In this way, play contributes to a culture of resistance which supports social change. Chapter 3 highlights the stories of queer activists who used every tool in their activist tool chest, from play to research, to pleasure to direct action, sophisticated use of media and so on, to shift the terms of a racist, sexist, and homophobic cultural discourse which allowed the AIDS catastrophe to run rampant (Gould, 2009; Shepard, 2009). If activists were to be successful in their struggle, they would need to shift hearts and minds as well as policies. By 2003 when the Supreme Court overturned its homophobic 1986 *Bowers v. Hardwick* decision with *Lawrence v. Texas*, repealing federal sodomy laws, one could argue queer activists had made some headway. For Mary Bernstein (2005), the Lawrence decision was a discursive victory. Through nearly two decades of challenging public beliefs, the views of society were radically changed in profound and unexpected ways. She argues that those who study movements must consider more than the political implications of a mobilization, they should also consider cultural impacts, the shifts in social discourse, the organization of communities, and the networks they create (Bernstein, 2005).

After all, social change is more akin to a labyrinth than a straight shot from conception to execution. Instead, it takes shape in a wide variety of sometimes obscure ways. Radical historian Howard Zinn (2002) suggests the historical record offers any number of examples of just these kinds of changes. Consider the campaign in Albany, Georgia, during the civil rights movement. Unable to point to any one specific policy change which it produced, observers have described the campaign as a failure. Yet, Zinn (2002) suggests this positivist interpretation misses the mark. After waves of civil disobedience, no one in Albany ever looked at the city or its laws in the same way. Nothing would be the same. The same could be said for the worldwide protests of the Global Justice Movement. "We've had victories if one looks at it in not a linear way, but in a very networked kind of way," explained John Jordan. "It's hard to see direct physical changes that have happened when you've prevented something . . . Things get better and they get worse at the same time."

Chapter 7 of this study highlights a similar dynamic with the contemporary antiwar movement. While the movement did not stop the war, the movement helped to create February 15, 2003, a day of protests in cities worldwide that is considered the largest day of protest in world history (Cortright, 2005; Kauffman, 2004; Solnit, 2004). And the world would know there were a lot of people who took enormous risks to stand up and say no.

"I can honestly say the real motivating factor. It was heartbreak when the bombs started," explained Joan Wile, organizer of the Grandmothers Against the War in New York, a group which has held a weekly antiwar vigil since the war started. "I can't measure our effect." History is far more porous and slippery. Like many of the activists in this study, she was particularly down after Bush's reelection in 2004. "But the day after he was elected, we had a vigil and we felt so much better." Sometimes this is just it—just taking part in the actions helps everyone feel better. In this way, the active process of staying engaged and finding a sense of agency makes for happier lives (see Chakrabortty, 2010). This pleasure keeps movements churning forward.

While it is not generally clear what effects a movement is having, a recognition of the gamelike dynamics of politics helps. "The core truth of basketball is there's always another game," said Todd Muller. "There is another opportunity. If we lose, there is another game. We'll start over," Muller continued. "As Chuck D said in *He Got Game*: don't let a win get to your head, or a loss to your heart. There is always a game. We won now, but there is another tomorrow." An appreciation of the connection between play and politics informs this Zen-like disposition. "If we invade Baghdad and tear down a statue, don't jump around, 'cause we still got another game. We gotta lace 'em up tomorrow. If the Sunnis beat us up, we got another game tomorrow."

Playing games teaches participants to cope with the ebb and flow of life and politics. "Losing and coming back—that takes character. Anybody can win; look at W [President Bush]" explained Muller. The impacts of our actions are often elusive, especially if their primary influence is on the creation of communities. Countless interviewees suggested that these communities are the most important things they have. Sometimes the community impact leads to cultural changes that in turn change hearts and minds as Bernstein suggests (2005). In other cases, they lead to further democratic participation or simply keep people engaged in the game and the struggle. Throughout the study, interviewees were asked to discuss how creative play contributes to or undermines social change activism. The final pages highlight a few of the themes which came out of these interviews.

THE STRENGTHS OF PLAY

As the case exemplars suggest, savvy activists have utilized elements of play and political performance to comment on and influence the tragicomic dimensions of a modern life of constant flux. In so doing, they have altered the way people understand the work and play of social change.

As far as strengths, interviewees suggested that play is useful for social movements because, among other things:

- It helps activism feel invigorating.
- It animates culture.
- It helps keep things light—even during dark times.
- It fosters creativity, which can help achieve movement aims.
- It recognizes pleasure.
- It creates and supports stories.
- It expands the public commons and makes democracy more colorful.
- It helps garner media attention to new narratives of action, helping actors propel their culture tales into the larger public discourse.
- It reduces alienation.
- It cultivates humor.
- It creates hope.
- It gets people to think.
- It supports individual and community strengths.
- It fosters nonhierarchical leadership networks.
- As a low-threshold activity, it brings people into organizing.
- It helps combat mechanisms that control the body and inhibit political activity.
- It makes social change work feel compelling and inviting.

When social actors organize in engaging, thoughtful ways, their work usually attracts followers. And others are seduced to join in the action. From the

264 Play, Creativity, and Social Movements

Yippies to ACT UP to RTS, when groups offered a low-threshold entry point that seemed accessible and fun, many people got involved. Sometimes people join groups to dance. And then the change bug grabs them. It's the hook. In other cases, play involves a high-octane cat and mouse game of chase between activists and police. Here, participating has more to do with the contact high. From the Young Lords to today's black bloc types, there are those activists who find the fantasy of battling police much more compelling than dancing in the street. Such high-risk actions can be understood as a form of dark play (Schechner, 2002).

Yet, as the Esperanza coqui sleepovers and stories of the cruising at ACT UP meetings suggest, social eros constitutes another dimension of movement culture. Sometimes attraction to a specific person can be an important part of the passion to build a better world for everyone. This was often the case with members of LESC, who made socializing a primary part of their organizing work. Many have worked from this ethos. "Sarah Schulman once said in the Lesbian Avengers, if you are not helping someone find a girlfriend, then you are not doing your job," recalled writer and activist Kirk Read, after seeing her give a talk on the Lesbian Avengers in San Francisco. For Read, it was a moment he would never forget. In the years to come, it would become an abiding principle for him. When I asked Sarah Schulman about the quote, she explained, "[I]t came from my mother's experience of The Communist Party (which she never joined) as the place that provided free beer." The point is that organizing has to actually make people's lives better. After all, "people are fighting for themselves—not like solidarity movements. So that organizations organizing lesbians had to be a place where lesbians could have a better life—which included meeting friends and lovers." This is why Schulman suggested ACT UP's parade of boyfriends was the group's greatest recruitment strategy. "You can't expect people to be in movements because it's 'right,' there has to be something in it for them," Schulman concluded.

Yet, there is always more to play than fun or pleasure. Play has been viewed as a useful approach to diffuse power. It was thought of as a way to effectively present a point without engaging in violent conflict. Wavy Gravy, the Yippie clown, helped everyone put on red noses as they eluded the police in 1976. Referring to just this kind of situation, Andrew Boyd mused:

> It's like what Saul Alinsky says, "Ridiculousness is the most potent weapon we have. There is no defense against it." But this was against the unsophisticated targets he was dealing with in the 1960s. Now everyone is a lot more sophisticated. Everyone is operating in this whole other rarified hipster symbolic media game. But in the 1960s, the targets were not that used to this and they would sort of respond in this kind of unimaginative organization man law-and-order kind of way. And if you were using humor against them, basically a cop beating up a clown looks really bad for the cop.

Decades later, CIRCA included the police in their theater of the absurd during the 2005 G8 meetings in Scotland. Both gestures helped diffuse power. "It does this thing where it can ramp down the violence and bring down the tension in the situation," explained Andrew Boyd. "It can make cops laugh." Yet this is hard to predict. The New York chapter of CIRCA did not receive similar treatment during the Republican National Convention in 2004: the police had no interest in playing or being played. Yet when the Critical Mass bike ride in New York was attacked by police in 2004, the subsequent addition of a clown ride provided bike activists with a needed lift. While play is often misunderstood, supporters tend to appreciate the energy created through combinations of its sheer silliness, camp, and ethos of freedom.

For others, the struggle involves an embodied approach to breaking through a grand mystification, a one-dimensional element flattening process that reduces social actors to passive spectators (Marcuse, 1978). Here, play helps break down systems of discipline which drain power from the body and the social imagination (Foucault, 1980).

"Capital," John Jordan speculated. "[I]t needs sadness, the social and individual sadness. The tyrant needs sadness. Break sadness. Make people laugh and give pleasure, enable them to disobey the fundamental docile body." Here, play overlaps with a set of embodied experiences. "It's fundamental to breaking the famine," Jordan explained. "And it's also giving people the potential to see another way of being. And then to take that into other parts of their lives." In this way, the affective logic of play opens up a space for different kinds of social knowledge.

A spirit of play allows a place for many to participate, including "the crazies," who Bob Kohler always suggested activists would be well advised to pay attention to. "[H]uman salvation lies in the hands of the creatively maladjusted," argued Martin Luther King (quoted in Freedman and Combs, 1996, p. 42). His point was that social change takes place through recognition of nonexpert paradigms of social knowledge. In contrast to professionalized models of social change practice, play inspires low-threshold models of organizing which help create spaces where people with a wide range of experiences can participate and feel included. Here, individual strengths are appreciated and celebrated. AIDS activist Andy Vélez recalled different "talents" people brought to ACT UP. Early in ACT UP, the group held a talent show. Rather than sing or perform, many brought distinct skills not recognized outside the movement. Michelangelo, for example, put a whole banana into his mouth and showed he could remove it without leaving teeth marks to roars of approval. "Use who you are," Vélez noted, smiling. "This is where it becomes fun."

Kate Crane offers another example. "In these great fun actions that we do I'm like, oh my God, this person who I thought was a little nutty, they just brought all the colorful hats," Crane explained. "Or they just showed up with food for all of us or they're singing loudest of all, or look at that crazy costume that everybody's taking pictures of and laughing at." Here, less serious approaches to organizing create a context that allows social actors to be truly valued for what they have to contribute. It can be life changing when one is supported and loved for those distinct qualities of oneself. If a movement does this, then the tie between the individual and the group takes on powerful dimensions. Social eros takes shape in any number of forms.

At its best, play keeps social activism vital. As Saul Alinsky counseled (1989), a good approach to activism is to use tactics people enjoy. "It can't drag on. If you keep doing the same thing over and over again, nobody cares," Andrew Boyd, the founder of Billionaires for Bush (or Gore), explained. "[Y]our enemy, your target, figures out how to deal with it. You can't reinvent Seattle, you have to be doing something new." Some play and some performances are better at communicating messages than others. "I always try to turn this stuff around," explained Boyd.

> Like you are some legislator who is pro-choice. And there are some wacko protestors outside. And they have a better puppet than last time. Are you going to feel more pressure? No. Only if it's getting more at-tention, people to laugh, or getting people into the street or fall in the message. But then you might worry.

It is useful for organizers to be clear about what play can and cannot do.

Perhaps the most fundamental role of play is to foster gratification (Lan-tos, 1943). And this is valuable in and of itself, especially for organizing. As Cindra Feuer of ACT UP explained: "If you are not enjoying what you are doing . . . people won't come back. They can't sustain it. You can only go so far in your anger and then you really need to be getting enjoyment and fulfillment." Without some element of pleasure, people drop out. "People get their needs met or they book," explained queer activist Eric Rofes.

Questions about the viability of play-based practices to achieve any kind of lasting or radical social change permeate this work. Yet, as the cases—from ACT UP to the gardens—indicate, there are many programs and poli-cies which took shape from campaigns which made use of play. The work of ACT UP to create effective AIDS policies, the Garden activists to create green space, the LESC Community Labor Coalition to win back wages for vulnerable workers—these were all campaigns which linked play within a broader organizing framework. "The metaphor I always use is it's one tool in the toolbox," Andrew Boyd elaborated.

> Then the next question becomes how does that tool articulate what other tools can't do? When do you think that tool works? It's a Swiss Army knife with a hundred tools in it. Which blade do you use when? So you have the straight tool and the humor tool, how do you build the house? The answer is, it's one tool . . .

In terms of all the things it provides, it's a huge dimension. Every social movement should be a microcosm of the human community, of all the things that we are, all the things that we aspire to. It should have gravitas. It should have play in it. It should have mythology. It should have narrative. It should have love. It probably should have hate. It should have id and it should have superego. You know, it should have authority. And I think it should have leadership and recognized leadership. It also has to have openness and democracy. I mean these are all dialectics and how they work together.

There's certain things play has to offer. It's humanizing . . . It can kind of empathize with a common humanity on either side of the picket line. In the same way that in CD nonviolence training that you are supposed to look the guy in the eyes, it makes it harder to dehumanize. It's an obvious media attractor. It's something that nurtures, that makes everyone have a better time. It's a whole mode of communication unto itself.

All the world's a stage, says Shakespeare. "I think it's actually essential to think in those frames," David Solnit concurred. "It dramatically shifts the quality." From this vantage point, most activism—from direct action to radical street performance—can be recognized as a form of performance. The play's the thing, after all. Subcomandante Marcos (2001) of the Zapatistas has written about their struggle as a performance in which the spectators join the actors on stage then refuse to leave. "The play is a problem," Marcos (2001, p. 154) contends. Here, play is intricately connected with a highly participatory conversation about democracy.

Andrew Boyd cited the example of the Yes Men as a group which connected play and performance with a larger struggle for social change.

They are incredible at using play and humor and trickery to expose the underlying ideology of neoliberalism. And also do a reduction ad absurdum [reductive and absurd] to extrapolate what it really means into the true human costs of it. Like in their last action when they disbanded the WTO and everyone was kind of happy with that. They bring out the sort of invincible operations of even that capitalist class. Like this conservative guy in Australia says, "It's about time we gave back to the people we've been taking from." So it has a way to bring all of that stuff out. They are not going to bring down the WTO on their own. They are part of this large social movement. If it was not for a mass global movement and ten thousand little NGOs clawing away at the beast, it would just be art. It would be a noble heroic, tragic, esoteric thing in costumes.

Play is part of a tradition of organizing which links art with performance and social struggle. Many view it as an important alternative. As

Starhawk suggested, "Traditional models of organizing and politics really haven't gotten us very far. So we have to be willing to try other things."

Sometimes the most important step is thinking of an alternative plotline (Freedman and Combs, 1996; Polletta, 2006; Somers, 1994). Far too many live in dead-end stories. Capitalism is inevitable, etc. Yet, there has to be something else to living than a struggle for simple means of necessity (Marcuse, 1955). By its very connection to inductive thinking, play helps open up any number of less linear approaches to considering social reality. If the stories highlighted here suggest anything, they indicate there are any number of ways of reconsidering social life and the practice of organizing.

Not only does play make activism more fun, but it also transforms the way social actors think about efficacy and power. As Subcomandante Marcos (2001, 2004) and Doug Crimp (Takemoto, 2003) have suggested, play helps direct action groups transform politics and power, moving from the conventional tropes into more abundant, less reactive models of social movement practice.

Writing about contemporary ludic performance groups such as the Billionaires for Bush and Ya Basta, philosopher Simon Critchley (2007, p. 124) described some of the distinct logic of such activism:

> These comical tactics hide a serious political intent: they exemplify the effective forging of chains of equivalence or collective will formation across diverse and otherwise conflicting protest groups. Deploying a politics of subversion, contemporary anarchist practice exercises a satirical pressure on the state in order to show that other forms of life are possible. Picking up on my thoughts about humor, it is the exposed, self-ridiculing and self-undermining character of these forms of protest that I find most compelling as opposed to the pious humorlessness of most forms of vanguardist active nihilism and some forms of contemporary protest (I name no names). Groups like the Pink Bloc or Billionaires for Bush are performing their powerlessness in the face of power in a profoundly powerful way. Politically, humor is a powerless power that uses its position of weakness to expose those in power through forms of self-aware ridicule.

Here, Critchley suggests play and ridicule are rightful ingredients within a social battle against often insurmountable targets. The anti-heroic aesthetics of ludic activist practices are indeed appealing for those who have grown weary of the overused rhetoric of the Left (Isserman, 1993). Douglas Crimp found this aspect of ACT UP's organizational culture tremendously refreshing. It allowed him to stay engaged with the group for over five years, as the AIDS carnage ran rampant without a cure in sight (Takemoto, 2003). It is just this recognition of the need for emotional sustenance which eludes the analyses of critics of ludic protest (Weissberg, 2005).

Here, not only does play fashion a different relationship to power and social knowledge, it helps create an outlet for direct action groups to take themselves less seriously. A post on an anarchist listserv highlights some of the complications of the interplay between playful responses and movement engagement. "[P]ersonally [I] think the question of taking ourselves seriously is the wrong question and I don't think it's semantics," Jameson (2006) explained. As the accounts of radical clowns and pranksters, guerilla gardeners and philosophers imply there is a counterintuitive, yet powerful logic to ludic engagement (Critchley, 2007). Here, the aim is to create a different kind of a game of social change. "[W]hat I think is important to mention," Jameson (2006) argued:

> is that social protest is often routinized and when it's routinized sometimes it often not only becomes boring to the participants (not the worst of it) but fails in its mission to capture the imagination of wider groups of people. I see playful protest as a tactic and strategy. It's a way of illuminating a problem effectively that sometimes militant protest or boring protest cannot. It's a way of creating social knowledge, an effective way of bridging divides among organizers. It's a communicative act like all others, just a nontraditional way of communicating.

Given the limitations of convergence actions, the realm of activism must contend with questions about the capacity of movements to both "communicate effectively" and "illuminate new social knowledge." In other words Jameson (2006) mused: "Can we play? Can we kick it?" To a degree, this book offers a long response to Jameson's post. The point has been to tease out the instructive and expressive elements in which play supported, influenced, or undermined the distinct character of social movements.

LIMITATIONS OF PLAY

"Camp which knows itself to be camp is usually less satisfying," cautioned Susan Sontag (1964/2001, p. 58). Some of the limitations of play mentioned by interviewees include the following:

- It does not consistently function as an effective response to political repression.
- It can be easily misunderstood.
- It can become stale quickly.
- Lack of resources limits its efficacy.
- It does not work in a vacuum.
- It can be seen as just entertainment.
- It can become fetishized.

- It is not a substitute for a clear policy proposal.
- It is not a substitute for a holistic organizing strategy.

While interviewees were happy to talk about what worked about play, they were also eager to talk about what did not. Many of the best uses of play involve affective uses, including humor, jokes, and group process. When reaching out to larger publics, ludic play works well when its expression is well matched with a clearly articulated goal—such as the defense of a community space or a bike ride. Yet, the style of the protest does not always match the end goal. Michael Shenker explained:

> There was a style of things that came out after the gardens where you can't really go to a demonstration unless you give out the party toys. You know, I can't get with that. The mode of the expression and the tenor of the expression needs to be proportional to the injury being inflicted. So if a quarter million people have died, it's a little difficult to say we are going to go have a good time without paying some type of tribute through the collective expression which could actually create a deeper level of human experience. Some type of tribute needs to be made to the people who are suffering. There comes a time when we need to transcend ourselves.

Ludic play is not as well tailored for many heavy issues such as police brutality, to name just one example. It is hard to laugh when people are dying. But sometimes people still do. As George Bernard Shaw famously observed: "Life does not cease to be funny when people die, any more than it ceases to be serious when people laugh," (quoted in Shepard, 2005, p. 50). While certainly, there is gallows humor which is powerful, it can sometimes be off-putting if not carefully explained and contextualized. Such humor has to be culturally specific, clear, and savvy. While David Feinberg's (1994) AIDS comedies are profoundly moving, sometimes there is too much pain to laugh. In such cases, the use of ludic tactics can backfire, be misunderstood, or be seen as belittling.

It is useful to be aware of what play can and cannot do in relation to social movements. Andrew Boyd addressed this issue in terms of the Billionaires:

> We didn't try to overreach. We did at times. But we tried to check ourselves for what we are not good for. There's all these zillions of groups and there are all these coalitions of closely networked movements now. And so it's an ecology. Every group has what they are good at and what they are not. We're good at getting a lot of media attention.

Yet, play does not consistently speak across lines of class or race. "We weren't good at organizing base communities in working-class and underclass populations, who were not diggin' on [it], who have a very different kind of irony," Boyd confessed. Understandings of pleasure and play and community building are culturally bound. Such performance is highly subject to misinterpretation, and prone to becoming insular.

Within this context, John Sellers noted:

> Mainly my biggest critique of it is that too often we do it for ourselves. Why are we singing for the choir all the time? Why are we creating theater for our own fucking troop? I love some of that. I think it's incredibly creative, but I question why aren't we asking ourselves basic questions about who we are trying to reach with that piece? What are their values? How do we meet them at their value set and then take them a little bit further? And so often creative people are doing stuff that is so inside. Don't get me wrong, it can be really great when it's time to laugh at ourselves or recharge. [But] I don't think that we can turn our backs on Babylon.

Sellers aspires to bring a creative politics to organizing which does not alienate, but rather speaks in culturally specific and intelligent ways.

To do so, activists have come to think very tactically about the uses of irony. For example, after 9/11 Andrew Boyd recognized that he sometimes had to go out of character when doing Billionaire performances (Hitt, 2004). Irony and satire are effective to the extent that their uses and limitations are clearly identified and acknowledged.

The lesson remains that if activists do not keep reinventing their approaches, then opponents get the upper hand. When play or any other tactic is overused, it becomes stale and loses its capacity to actually produce effective action or reaction. No longer "fresh," such pranks stop being "newsworthy." And the media gravitates to other stories (Bogad, 2005B). For the Yippies, this limitation started to become clear even after the 1968 Democratic National Convention. While the frantic, ludic pranks of the Yippies were not expected in 1968, they quickly became routine. Elites adapt and create counter-responses. And repression becomes all that much easier. After the first two RTS New York street parties, police caught on to the group's methods and started conducting massive arrests during the actions. The group grew weary of the same tactics and moved closer to guerilla theater, updating its repertoire over the next four years (Duncombe, 2002A). Much of this work is about this process of adaptation.

Obviously, part of the process is recognizing the limits of what one can and cannot do with a given tactic. The politics of play tend to hit a wall when faced with the question of political economy. "I look at people and I think 'fuck, maybe it's time to build real external differences,'" John Jordan bemoaned. A tension between community building and policy change ran throughout the interviews. "The ideal is to build both," Jordan explained.

> I'm always trying to do both. If you just create alternatives, you forget why you were creating the alternatives in the first place. You create

alternatives to the system and then you get sucked into the system. You have to resist and create at the same time. It's really hard, but they are both as important. Before I pop off this planet, I would love to be part of something that does both at the same time.

Jordan helped create the RTS story line that expanded around the globe: "It was part of a transnational community. It's lined up with the poetic and the pragmatic and the symbolic." But, its limitations became glaring. "It can become just symbolic, with no real policy or external changes." After a while, symbolic actions that fail to create visible changes in the external environment wear thin.

Yet, success and social change is not always easy to assess or measure. As Rebecca Solnit (2005) notes:

> The glum traditional left often seems intent upon finding the cloud around every silver lining. And joy is one of our weapons and one of our victories. Non-activists sometimes chide us for being joyous at demonstrations, for having fun while taking on the serious business of the world, but in a time when alienation, isolation, and powerlessness are among our principal afflictions, just being out in the streets *en masse* is not a demand for victory: it is a victory.

One of the complicating features of studying collective action is that because groups are always innovating, predicting "success" is trickier than it might be in settings where people are using established strategies and tactics. Figuring out what is effective is more akin to figuring out what kind of aesthetic tools to use in a given moment (e.g., plays, paintings, dance, etc.). Arts and songs, chants and stories speak to people in multiple ways. They create different illusions (Nardi, 2006). If reality is made of countless stories and illusions, the challenge for social activism is to advance different kinds of stories and games of social change. It is useful to steer away from a positivist-style prediction by thinking about innovation and the mix of the aesthetic/political activism. "Play has a tendency to be beautiful," Huizinga (1950, p. 10) reminds us. While this study considers ends, much of its focus is on means. By asserting there are different ways of studying social change, we acknowledge there are different forms of social knowledge, which find expression in any number of creative expressions described throughout this book. Given the alternatives—war, violence, mind-numbing monoculture—these gestures offer a hopeful alternative trajectory for human experience and interaction.

IN THE END

Summer 2009, my family and I traveled around Germany, returning to Berlin for the first time in two decades. One finds bits and pieces of the Wall throughout the city. In some locations, it is a location for memory. In others, such as Mauerpark, an open field cum DIY public commons in Prenzlauer Berg which had been enclosed by the Berlin Wall from 1961 to 1989, it is a space for expression. On a bright Saturday afternoon, a diverse group of people hung out and spray-painted murals; DJs played music as people BBQed, napped, threw Frisbees, or danced. Kids climbed through a Dali-esque wooden tree house cum jungle gym. And my daughters and I swung on the swings—adjacent to a space which only two decades prior was an epicenter of a decades-long Cold War. Play finds itself in the strangest places and bits of history.

In the midst of a bloody civil war in El Salvador, a group of women organized three committees per refugee camp: one for education, another for construction/sanitation, and a third for joy—the comité de alegría (Hollyday, 1995). School teachers set up a space for children to play in Tahrir Square during the recent uprising in Egypt (Goldmark, 2011). We are homo ludens after all. This study has documented a number of cases in which play contributed to campaigns that utilized holistic approaches to organizing for social change, in their own given context. These include groups that worked for economic justice, education, health care, green space, and basic needs, as well as pleasure—not one or the other. Just as in the civil war in El Salvador, the committee for joy was not formed outside of the work of the committees for education and construction/sanitation. Yet, without the committee for joy, or LESC's Ministry of Love, the other work of change becomes more than many can bear. The limitations of play in politics are easy to understand. McKay (1998) has noted that DIY politics can easily fall into repeating anarchism's limitations: poor organization, a partial narrative, micropolitics, naive utopianism, and preference for spectacle over long-term organizing strategy. Yet, with these limitations in mind, play can complement a larger organizing campaign; here, play can offer profound energy and resources to such an effort. It can also be end unto itself.

In sum, play is useful to movements in any number of ways.

- It helps create community as well as bring new political actors into the arena.
- It is profoundly useful for group development.
- It helps sustain organizing efforts.
- It bridges the gap between hearts and minds.
- It helps validate different ways of knowing and working within the world.
- It supports a holistic organizing strategy that includes: a clear request, research, mobilization, legal tactics, direct action, and a clear workable policy alternative.

In this way, the politics of play offers more than a "no." Rather it helps advocates demonstrate what they want the world to look like. As Aresh of More Gardens! explained, it is part of being a "yes" group. "I think we very much have to be able to articulate and embody what we're for, not just what we're against," explained organizer David Solnit. Here, it can also be a profoundly effective part of a plan of social action.

To build on this resource, organizers must realize that there are different forms of expertise. In an era of a dwindling welfare state, play can be a useful way to expand social and mutual aid networks. Here, social actors animate culture, organize, socialize, and build connections with those creating coalitions aimed at creating a better world today. This is part of the eros effect George Katsiaficas (2002) describes. Through such an interplay between minds and bodies, new social relations take shape.

"If fear and destructiveness are the major emotional sources of fascism, eros belongs mainly to democracy," argued Theodor Adorno and the other authors of the *Authoritarian Personality* in 1950 (quoted in Martin, 1973, p. 86). Here, play opens up space for conviviality (Illich, 1973). When the eros effect gains momentum and people enter the streets, crack through a wall, or even share a beer as they did in Berlin in 1989, then the world is rarely the same.

Yet, there is no point in trying to recreate these moments. There is no point in trying to fashion another Tompkins Square Park Riot, Seth Tobocman ruminated as we stood outside the same park, some two decades later. There is no point in trying to create another Seattle or another 1968. History is far more fluid. Rather than fixate on one event at the expense of others, I hope we can move beyond narratives which imply the movement of movements rose from the late 1990s to 9/11 and then declined. As the immigrant rights rallies attended by well over a million people in 2006, the bike rides in support of non-polluting transportation, or the waves of direct action from Egypt to Tunisia suggest, stories of social change move in any number of directions.

Groups form and tribes expand their own communities of resistance, while others wane. When Joe Tuba and the Hungry March Band traveled to Rome, they found a vast new network of radical marching bands:

> It's not restricted to wires or being in a club, it's not restricted to anything; it's kind of like this democratic thing where you can play for everybody for free as soon as you walk out the door. And you can have this whole other network of other bands. It's amazing. People go crazy.

People get to know each other, dance, and build communities which stretch across the globe. Networks take shape. Many live for the sort of space created at the shows, the streets, the gardens, the public commons form through this connection of bodies, politics, and an ever-evolving ludic carnival. Tuba continued:

> It's the same thing RTS was doing. That the gardens were really doing. You are creating a space. And it's like the commons that people are

always talking about. It just doesn't exist in the mind-set in the United States at all. In England there is a history of it. Here there is no recollection of that kind of thing. That's what this whole scenario is trying to remind people about and make people create.

Tuba broke out into laughing as we finished our conversation. The show and the interview were over. Today, the Hungry March Band are less politicized, but the Rude Mechanical Orchestra spawned from the group supports a wide range of movements with their dancing beats. All the while picnics are happening; kids are romping through public space and their parents are talking about ways to organize daycare collectives and getting together for additional playdates. Gardens are expanding and contracting as movement gains remain in constant flux (as agreements end and others take shape). All that is solid melts into air, Marx and later Berman (1982) remind us. But we can still dance amidst the wreckage (Ollman, 2003).

Is play everything to a social movement? Certainly not. Yet it is better for people to form tribes to expand alienation-reducing social networks (Maffesoli, 1993, 1996) than to leave public life or watch TV. Without this dance, many fall into despair and isolation (Ehrenreich, 2007a). While serious politics often mirrors the very power structures activists oppose, playful responses open up questions, stories, and spaces. And the eros effect, it goes on and on. And struggles for a place to play continue to extend from the classroom to the streets and the social imagination (Stout, 2011; Vaneigem, 1967/2003).

"Play begins and then at a certain point it is over. It plays itself to the end," counsels Johan Huizinga (1950, pp. 9–10). Through this process it changes and alters itself. "[I]t at once assumes a fixed form as a cultural phenomena." And its story, like this story and the groups it considers, comes to an end. There is no use replaying or trying to recreate what was. New stories, plays, and actions take shape. Yet, Huizinga reminds us there is a final feature of play worth bearing in mind. "Once played, it endures as a newfound creation of the mind, a treasure to be retained by memory."

Interviews

The primary data source for this study is interviews.
The following individuals participated in interviews for the study.

Vicente "Panama" Alba
Mark Anderson
Walter Armstrong
Dana Beal
Tim Becker
Johnathan Berger
Jeanne Bergman
Barton Benes
Jay Blotcher
L.M. Bogad
Andrew Boyd
Ariane Burgess
Allan Clear
Kate Crane
Julie Davids
Bill DiPaola
Tim Dooty
Todd Eaton
Beka Economopoulis
Abby Ehmann
William Etundi
Cindra Feuer
Donald Gallagher
Greg Gonsalvez
Jason Grote
Mark Harrington
Ron Hayduk
Amanda Hickman

Wayne Hoffman
Melissa Hope
Lidell Jackson
Aresh Javadi
JKtheCat aka Judith Candela
JoeTuba aka Joe Keady
Louis Jones
John Jordan
Aron Kay
Charles King
Bob Kohler
Jamie Leo
Jarrett Lovell
Bonfire Madigan
Ben Mauers
Mike McGuire
Elizabeth Meixell
Todd Muller
Urania Mylonas
Ann Northrop
Steve Questor
Karen Ramspacher
Kirk Read
Chuck Reinhart
Eric Rofes
Matthew Roth
Eric Sawyer
John Sellers
Michael Shenker
Marina Sitrin
David Solnit
Starhawk aka Miriam Simos
Marla Stevens
Seth Tobocman
James Tracey
Andy Vélez
James Wagner
Joan Wile
Lesley Julia Wood
Susan Wright

A Brief Glossary of Groups

The following is a brief overview of groups covered throughout this book. It is by no extent an exhaustive source on ludic protest.

Absurd Response to an Absurd War 2002–2003. RTS/LESC project anti-war group designed to fulfill the Masquerade Project's goals to bring color into the movement as well as to highlight the absurdity of the rush to war in Iraq. Featured in Chapter 7.

ACT UP AIDS Coalition to Unleash Power—1987 to the present. The seminal AIDS activist group of the movement, ACT UP brought civil rights era direct action combined with queer aesthetics and a sophisticated understanding of media and graphics to the AIDS struggle. Featured in Chapter 3.

Art & Revolution 1995 to the present. A contemporary activist practice featuring David Solnit. It combines art, theater, puppetry, and direct action, born in the tradition of the Diggers, Yippies, and Situationists. Referred to in Chapter 6.

Billionaires for Bush (or Gore) 2000–2008, reformed as Billionaires for Wealthcare in 2009. Started by Andrew Boyd, the group was organized to critique the role of money in US elections. Used irony to make its point. Featured in Chapters 2, 6, 7, and Conclusion.

Biotic Biking Brigade Late 1990s loosely affiliated group of activists organized around the practice of humiliating political opponents by throwing pies in their faces. The practice of pieing dates back to the early 1970s, although the Brigade is most famous for its 1998 pieing of San Francisco Mayor Willie Brown. Featured in Chapter 2.

CIRCA Clandestine Insurgent Rebel Clown Army—2003–2005. A radical clowning group created by some of the organizers from RTS London to protest President George Bush's visit to London in 2003. Also protested 2004 Republican Convention in New York and the Group of 8 meetings in

Scotland in 2005. More of a meme than a group, the concept continues to find expression. Featured in Chapters 7 and 8.

CIW Coalition of Immokalee Workers—1993 to the present. A community-based group of farmworkers in Florida, the majority of whom are Latino, Mayan Indians, and Haitian immigrants, organizing for fair wages for vulnerable workers. Featured in Chapter 8.

Cockettes 1970–1972. Anarchist queer theatrical San Francisco performance group. Briefly featured in Chapter 2.

Dada 1915–1923. Post-WWI New York and European absurdist, antiwar arts group. Hugo Ball and Tristan Tzara were its founders. Tzara (1918) described its aims with the Dada Manifesto. Featured in Introduction and Chapter 2.

Diggers 1966–1968. San Francisco anarchist, performance group famous for passing out free food.

Direct Action Network New York 1999–2002. A post-Seattle network of anarchist groups organized to put support campaigns and convergence actions in New York and the East Coast. Featured in Chapters 5 and 6.

Earth First! 1979–present. A radical environmental movement which favors the use of direct action, civil disobedience, and grassroots organizing to defend wilderness. Featured in Chapters 4 and 5.

Fed Up Queers (FUQ) 1998–2000. New York City queer direct action group, in the tradition of ACT UP, which helped organize the 1998 Matthew Shepard Political Funeral (although not as FUQ) and later initiated a wave of civil disobedience after the NYPD shot unarmed African immigrant Amadou Diallo. Referred to in Chapter 3.

Global Justice Movement 1994 to the present. Also described as antiglobalization or alterglobalization movement, flashpoints the Zapatista rebellion, 1999 Seattle World Trade protests, and many other convergence actions. Featured in Chapters 3 to 7.

Grandmothers Against the War. 2004 to the Present. Led by Joan Wile, this group has held a weekly vigil against the Iraq War for since 2004. On October 17th, 2005, some eighteen grannies, including Wile, went to the military recruiting station in Times Square to volunteer to fight so their grand children would not have to. And were later arrested.

Housing Works 1990–present. Started as the ACT UP Housing Committee, Housing Works is the nation's largest, most militant, minority-controlled AIDS service organization. Featured in Chapter 3.

Lower East Side Collective (LESC) 1997–2000. LESC is a pro-fun Lower East Side organizing collective of project groups. These include a public space group working on issues including the community gardens, a labor group—the Community Labor Coalition, a culture-jamming group—the Strike Team, a support entity—the Ministry of Love, and Reclaim the Streets, another public space group. Profiled in Chapters 3 and 4. Its offshoot groups are featured throughout the rest of the text.

Masquerade Project 2001. LESC global justice project group organized to inject some color and queer flamboyance into global justice convergence actions. Plans halted by September 11, 2001, attacks. Featured in Chapter 5.

OutRage 1990–2006. Formed by Peter Tatchell, the London-based queer direct action group with a similar disposition to ACT UP used camp, performance, and confrontation to fight homophobia. Featured in Chapter 2.

Provos 1965–1967. Dutch countercultural group of anarchists who performed pranks and provocations while advocating for bike safety and cannabis awareness. Later a few members formed the Kabouters, some of whom were elected to political office. Referred to in Introduction and Chapter 1.

Quakers 1965 to the present. A religious movement, the Society of Friends, their emphasis on nonviolence influenced US social movements, including antinuke and civil rights. Referred to in Chapter 6.

Radical Faeries 1979–present. Founded by Harry Hay, the loosely knit worldwide affiliation of queer people which reject commercial models of gay life in favor of gay and pagan models of sustainability, environmentalism, and spirituality. Referred to in Introduction and Chapter 5.

Reclaim the Streets New York (RTS) 1998–2004. Inspired by the London group, the New York group was formed as a Lower East Side Collective project group which put on street parties. The group spawned project groups including the Students for an Undemocratic Society, the Absurd Response to an Absurd War, and others. Referred to throughout the entire text.

Red Army Faction Late 1960s–1998. German antiwar group which, like the Weather Underground, rejected nonviolence in favor of urban guerilla armed resistance. Referred to in Introduction and Chapter 2.

Reverend Billy and the Church of Stop Shopping 1998 to the present. Global justice, anticonsumer movement group organized to challenge consumerism in silly tongue-in-cheek manner. Referred to in Chapters 5, 6, and 7.

Situationists 1957–1972. Guy Debord (1967) and Raoul Vaneigem (1967/2003) were intellectual leaders of this highly influential avant-garde group, which viewed much of modern life as a 'Spectacle.' Terms *detournment* and *derive* come from them. Featured in Chapter 1 and throughout.

Stand Up Harlem Early 1990s. A Harlem-based AIDS housing direct action program, rooted in squatting and AIDS activism. Featured in Chapter 3.

Students for a Democratic Society (SDS) 1960–1969. New Left student group, which advocated nonviolent civil disobedience to challenge US militarism and racism in its 1962 Port Huron Statement. A new SDS was formed in 2006. Referred to in Chapters 1, 2, and 5.

Students for Undemocratic Society (SUDS) 2001. RTS spin-off group organized as a spoof of the Students for a Democratic Society. Organized for the Bush inauguration protests. Featured in Chapters 6 and 7.

Surrealists 1924 to 1930s. An arts and cultural movement which looked to fantasy to challenge social mores. Andre Breton (1924/1972) described its aims with *Manifestos of Surrealism*. While it peaked in the 1930s, it continued well into the postwar period, with an active chapter in Chicago. Featured in Chapter 1.

Time's Up! 1987 to present. Time's Up! is a long-standing Lower East Side environmental group which calls for nonpolluting transportation. Spawned project groups including the Bike Lane Liberation Clowns. Featured in Chapter 3 and Introduction.

Up Against the Wall Motherfucker (UAW/MF) 1966–1971. Anarchist-inspired Lower East Side direct action counterculture group formed in 1966. In 1968, changed their name to UAW/MF. Inspired the Yippies and the Weather Underground. Referred to in Chapters 1 and 3.

Weather Underground (or The Weathermen) 1969–1973. A spin-off of the SDS, in 1969 The Weathermen, named after a Bob Dylan song, rejected nonviolence in their efforts to halt the US involvement in the Vietnam War. Over the next few years it set off bombs. Referred to in the Introduction and Chapter 1.

Yippies 1968 to end of Vietnam War, active period. Highly influential youth counterculture group in Lower East Side of New York founded by Abbie Hoffman. Famous for use of theater as a political intervention. Its living leader, Dana Beal, still advocates for free, legal use of pot and ibogaine. Beal and the remaining Yippies remain active. Profiled in Chapter 2.

Young Lords 1969–1973. National Puerto Rican direct action group, which grew out of a mid-1960s Chicago gang. It became a militant organization in New York, igniting direct action campaigns and a form of militant activism similar to the Black Panthers. Its members continued with projects related to the group in future years. Profiled in Chapter 2.

Zapatista Army of National Liberation 1983 to the present. Based in Chiapas, this highly influential Mexican movement group sees itself as the heirs to Eliliano Zapata, the hero of the Mexican Revolution. The group ignited anticapitalist movements around the world with their 1994 uprising challenging NAFTA. The poetry of their spokesman Subcomandante Marcos helped the Global Justice Movement reimagine movement activity and struggles against corporate and state targets. Referred to in Introduction, Chapter 6, and Conclusion.

References

Abramson, Michael, et al. 1971. *Palante: Young Lords Party*. New York: McGraw-Hill Book Company.

Abu-Lughod, Janet, ed. 1994. *From Urban Village to East Village: The Battle for New York's Lower East Side*. Oxford, UK: Blackwell.

Addams, Jane. 1910/1998. *Twenty Years at Hull House*. New York: Penguin.

Addams, Jane. 1914. *The Spirit of Youth in the City Streets*. New York: The Macmillan Company.

Adlam, Carol, ed. 1997. *Face to Face: Bakhtin in Russia and the West*. Sheffield Academic Press.

Aeschylus. 1984. *The Oresteia: Agamemnon; The Libation Bearers; The Eumenides*. Trans. Robert Fagles. New York: Penguin Classics.

Alba, Vicente "Panama." 2004. *The Journey: Memories of Former Member of the Young Lords Party*.

Alex in Pictures. 2007. "Clowns Kicked KKK Asses." http://www.neatorama.com/2007/09/03/clowns-kicked-kkk-asses/ (accessed June 8, 2010).

Algarin, Miguel and Pinero, Migue, eds. 1975. Nuyorican Poetry: An Anthology of Puerto Rican Words and Feelings. New York: William Morrow and Company.

Alinsky, Saul. 1989. *Rules for Radicals*. New York: Vintage Books.

Anderson, L. 1998. "Auction Disrupted, but Charas Is Sold." *The Villager*, July 22.

Anderson, L. 2001. "Activists Confront Anti-Union at Fifth Ave Groceries." *The Villager*, May 2.

Anderson, L. 2004. "Gotta Have Park, Say G.O.P. Convention Protesters." *The Villager*. June 9–15, 73 (6). http://www.thevillager.com/villager_58/gottahave-parksaygop.html (accessed January 29, 2005).

Apple, R.W. 2001. "The Inauguration, News Analysis, Tradition, and Legitimacy." *New York Times*, January 21, 1.

Aronowitz, Stanley. 1972/1992. *False Promises: The Shaping of American Working Class Consciousness*. Durham, NC: Duke University Press.

Archives of Global Protests. 2001. http://nadir.org/nadir/initiativ/agp/free/genova/leaflet.htm (accessed August 9, 2001.)

Associated Press. 1998. "Activists Unleash Crickets at Auction." *New York NEWSDAY*, July 21.

Associated Press. 2008. "On 5th Day of Thai Protests, a Carnival Atmosphere." *International Herald Tribune*, August 30.

Aufheben. n.d. "What Ever Happened to the Situationists?" http://www.geocities.com/aufheben2/auf_6_situ.html (accessed January 27, 2006).

Ayers, B. 2001. *Fugitive Days*. Boston, MA: Beacon Press.

Bakhtin, Mikhail. 1981. *The Dialogic Imagination: Four Essays*. Ed. Michael Holquist and Trans. Caryl Emerson and Michael Holquist. Austin: University of Texas Press.

Bakhtin, Mikhail. 1984. *Rabelais and His World*. Bloomington: Indiana University Press.

Barash, Mauer. 1961/1979. "Translator's Introduction." *May, Play and Games*, by Roger Caillois. New York: The Free Press.

Barry, D. 1999a. "Giuliani Seeks Deal to Sell 63 Community Gardens to Land Groups to End Suits." *New York Times*, May 12, B1.

Barry, D. 1999b. "Sudden Deal Saves Gardens Set for Auction. Bette Midler Clears Way for Purchase of 112 Lots." *New York Times*, May 13, B1.

Barto, S. 1983. "'Nuclear Saints' Take over Senior's Lab." *Michigan Daily*, November 15, 1.

Bateson, Gregory 1972. *Steps to an Ecology of Mind*. New York: Ballantine Books.

Beauregard, Robert A. 2002. *Voices of Decline: The Postwar Fate of U.S. Cities*. New York: Routledge.

Benjamin, Walter. 1978. "Surrealism." In *Reflections: Essays, Aphorisms, and Autobiographical Writings*. Translated by Edmond Jephcott (p. 177–92). Schocken Books: New York.

Benjamin, Walter. 1999. "Paris: Capital of the 19ᵗʰ Century." In *The Arcades Project*. Translated by Howard Eiland & Kevin McLaughlin. Edited by Rolf Tiedemann (pp. 1–26). Cambridge: Belkap Press.

Berman, Marshall. 1982. *All That is Solid Melts into Air*. New York: Simon and Schuster.

Berman, Marshall. 1999. *Adventures in Marxism*. New York: Verso.

Berman, Marshall. 2007. "Introduction." In *New York Calling: From Blackout to Bloomberg*. Ed. Marshall Berman and Brian Berger (pp. 9–38). London: Reaktion Books.

Bernstein, Mary. 2005. Liberalism and Social Movement Success: The Case of Sodomy Statutes." In *Regulating Sex: The Politics of Intimacy and Identity*. Ed. Elizabeth Bernstein and Laurie Schaffner (pp. 3–18). New York: Routledge.

Bérubé, Allan. 1990. *Coming Out Under Fire*. New York: The Free Press.

Bevington, David. 1962. *From Mankind to Marlowe*. Cambridge, MA: Harvard University Press.

Bey, Hakim. 1991. *T.A.Z. The Temporary Autonomous Zone*. Brooklyn, NY: Autonomedia.

Bey, Hakim. 2003. *Immediatism*. Oakland, CA: AK Press. http://www.sterneck.net/musik/bey-immediatism/index.php (accessed October 18, 2010).

Bial, Henry. 2004. Part IV Play, Section introduction. In *The Performance Studies Reader*. Ed. H. Bial (pp. 115–16). New York: Routledge.

Blank, Rebecca. 2000. "Fighting Poverty: Lessons from Recent U.S. History." *Journal of Economic Perspectives* 14 (2): 3–19.

Blumenfeld, Larry. 2007. "Band on the Run in New Orleans: Police Have Cracked Down on Funeral Processions … But Musicians Vow to Play On." www.salon.com/news/feature/2007/10/29/treme (accessed October 29, 2007).

Boal, Augusto. 1990. *Theater of the Oppressed*. Trans. C.A. McBride and M.-O. Leal McBride. Theatre Communications Group.

Bogad, L.M. 2003. "Facial Insufficiency: Political Street Performance in New York City." *TDR: The Drama Review* 47:4.

Bogad, L.M. 2005a. *Electoral Guerrilla Theatre: Radical Ridicule and Social Movements*. New York: Routledge.

Bogad, L.M. 2005b. "Tactical Carnival: Social Movements, Demonstrations, and Dialogical Performance." In *A Boal Companion*. Ed. J. Cohen-Cruz and M. Schutzman (pp. 46–58). New York: Routledge.

Boyd, Andrew. 1999. *The Activist Cookbook: Creative Actions for a New Economy*. Boston: United for a Fair Economy.

Boyd, Andrew. 2000. "The Birth of a Movement, Extreme Costume Ball: A New Protest Movement Hits the Streets in Style." *Village Voice*, July 19–25.

Boyd, Andrew. 2002. "Irony, Meme Warfare and the Extreme Costume Ball." In *From ACT UP to the WTO*. Ed. B. Shepard and R. Hayduk (pp. 245–53). New York: Verso.

Boyd, Andrew and Duncombe, Stephen. 2004. "The Manufacture of Dissent: What the Left Can Learn From Las Vegas." *Journal of Aesthetics and Protest* 1 (3): 34–47.

Breton, Andre. 1924/1972. *Manifestos of Surrealism*. Trans. R. Seaver and H.R. Lane. Ann Arbor: University of Michigan Press.

Briody, Dan. 2003. *The Iron Triangle: Inside the Secret World of the Carlyle Group*. John Wiley and Sons.

Brown, Stuart. 2009. *Play: How it Shapes the Brain, Opens the Imagination, and Invigorates the Soul*. New York: Penguin Group.

Buhle, Paul and Schulman, Nicole. 2005. *Wobblies! A Graphic History of the Industrial*. New York: Verso.

Burdell, Linda. 2003. "Play and Performance in Sabina Berman's Entre Pancho Villa y una mujer desnuda." Presented at The Red River Conference on World Literature. North Dakota State University.

Bureau of Public Secrets. n.d. "The Joy of Revolution, Foreplay. Chapter 2." http://www.bopsecrets.org/PS/joyrev2.htm#Oppression%20versus%20playfulness (accessed October 9, 2005).

Burghardt, Steve. 1982. *The Other Side or Organizing*. Cambridge, MA: Schenkman Publishing Company, Inc.

Butters, S. 1983. "The Logic of Inquiry of Participant Observation." In *Resistance through Rituals. Youth Subcultures in Post-War Britain*. Ed. S. Hall and T. Jefferson (pp. 253–73). London: Hutchinson University Library.

Caillois, Roger. 1961/1979. *Man, Play, and Games*. New York: Shocken Books

Caillois, Roger. 2003. *The Edge of Surrealism: A Roger Caillois Reader*. Ed. Claudine Frank. Trans. Claudine Frank and Camille Naish. Durham, NC: Duke University Press.

Carr, C. 1993. *On Edge: Performance at the End of the Twentieth Century*. Middletown, CT: Wesleyan University Press.

Carter, David. 2004. *Stonewall: The Riots that Sparked the Gay Revolution*. New York: St. Martin's Press.

Cauvin, H. 1998. "Activists Bugged by City Land Auction." *Daily News*, July 21.

Chakrabortty, A. 2010. "Activism Makes You Happy—New Research Shows There Is a Link between Being Politically Active and Wellbeing." *The Guardian*, March 2. http://www.guardian.co.uk/science/2010/mar/02/brain-food-activism-makes-you-happy (accessed March 10, 2010).

Chang, Jeff. 2005. *Can't Stop Won't Stop: A History of the Hip-Hop Generation*. New York: St. Martin's Press.

Chivers, C.J. 2000. "After Uprooting Gardeners, City Razes a Garden." *New York Times*, April 16, A1.

Chrysler, Robert. 2003. "The REAL Revolutionary Party: Reclaim the Streets!" http://www.getunderground.com/underground/features/article.cfm?Article_ID=11 39 (accessed June 8, 2003).

Cho, M. 2004. "Presidential Cockfight." *In These Times Magazine*. http://www.inthesetimes.com/site/main/article/1387/ (accessed November 1, 2005).

Chvasta, Marcyrose. 2006. "Anger, Irony, and Protest: Confronting the Issue of Efficacy Again," in *Text and Performance Quarterly* 26(1): 5–16.

Clarke, Richard. 2004. *Against All Enemies: Inside America's War on Terror*. New York: The Free Press.

Clover, J. 2005. "The Mirror Sage." *Village Voice*, November 16–22, 36.

Cockettes, The. 2009. *Elevator Girls In Bondage starring Rumi Missabu*. http://www.youtube.com/watch?v=bhV3sbhvW9A (accessed October 18, 2010).

Complacent. 2000. "Money Falls." http://www.complacentnation.org/money/ (accessed April 10, 2006).

Cortright, David. 2005. "The Peaceful Superpower: The Movement against the War in Iraq." In *Charting Transnational Democracy: Beyond Global Arrogance*. Ed Janie Leatherman and Julie Webber (pp. 75–100). New York: Palgrave MacMillan.

Crane, K. 2004. "Review of *PIE ANY MEANS NECESSARY*." *NY Press*. www.nypress.com (accessed January 11, 2005).

Crenson, Matthew A. and Ginsberg, Benjamin. 2002. *Downsizing Democracy*. Baltimore, MD: The Johns Hopkins University Press.

Crimp, Douglas. 2002. *Melancholia and Moralism. Essays on AIDS and Queer Politics*. Cambridge, MA: MIT Press.

Crimp, Douglas. 2007. "ACT UP Oral History Interview with Sarah Schulman. 16 May." www.actuporalhistory.org/ (accessed August 15, 2008).

Crimp, Douglas and Rolston, Adam. 1990. *AIDS DEMOGRAPHICS*. Seattle: Bay Press.

Critchley, Simon. 2007. *Infinitely Demanding: Ethics of Commitment, Politics of Resistance*. New York: Verso.

Csikszentmihalyi, Mihaly. 1975. *Beyond Boredom and Anxiety: The Experience of Play in Work and Games*. London: Jossey-Bass Publishers.

Debord, Guy. 1967. *The Society of the Spectacle*. Trans. Ken Knabb. Bureau of Public Secrets. http://www.bopsecrets.org/SI/debord/6.htm (accessed January 16, 2010).

Deconstructive Institute for Surreal Topology. 2001. "We Made the Catapult, Judy Rebick Got the $$$." *Rabble. CA*, April 25. http://www.rabble.ca/news/we-made-catapult-judy-rebick-got (accessed June 8, 2010).

Delany, Samuel. 1998/2005. "Notes on the Star-Pit." http://www.pseudopodium.org/repress/TheStarPit/SamuelRDelany-NotesOnTheStarPit.html (accessed December 26, 2007).

Denning, Michael. 1997. *The Cultural Front*. New York: Verso.

Deparle, Jason. 1990. "Rude, Rash, Effective, ACT UP Shifts AIDS Policy." *New York Times*, January 3, B1 and B4.

Diva TV. 1990. *Like a Prayer: Stop the Church*. Diva TV Productions.

Dobbs, Bill. 2006. "ACT UP Oral History Interview with Sarah Schulman. 21 November." www.actuporalhistory.org/ (accessed August 15, 2008).

Doepfner, Thomas P. and Sweet, Kerry R. 2004. New York City Police Department Legal Guide for the Republican National Convention. Raymond W. Kelly, Police Commissioner. Georgia Grasso, First Deputy Commissioner, Stephen L. Hammerman, Deputy Commissioner, Legal Matters. March 10.

Dominguez, Ricardo. 2001. "Re: And Introducing." E-mail to RTS Listserv. April 18.

Dominguez, Ricardo. 2002. "Electronic Disturbance." In *From ACT UP to the WTO*. Ed. B. Shepard and R. Hayduk (pp. 274–89). New York: Verso.

Dowd, Maureen. 2006. W's Mixed Messages. *New York Times* (11 March). Accessed 18 October, 2010 from http://query.nytimes.com/gst/fullpage.html?res=9C0DEFDA1331F932A25750C0A9609C8B63&sec=&spon=

Duncombe, Stephen. 2000. "Reclaim the Land! An Action Report. May 2." http://www.infoshop.org/octo/m1_nyc1.html (accessed June 5, 2005).

Duncombe, Stephen. 2001. "Big Meeting! Traveling Carnival! DC Protest! Sept 5!" E-mail to RTS Listserv. August 30.

Duncombe, Stephen. 2002a. "Introduction." In *Cultural Resistance: A Reader* (pp. 1–15). Ed. Stephen Duncombe. New York: Verso.

Duncombe, Stephen. 2002b. "Stepping off the Sidewalk: Reclaim the Streets/ NYC." In *From ACT UP to the WTO*. Ed. B. Shepard and R. Hayduk (pp. 215–29). New York: Verso.

Duncombe, Stephen. 2003. "The Poverty of Theory: Anti Intellectualism and the Value of Action." *Radical Society* 30 (1): 11–17

Duncombe, Stephen. 2004. *Carnival against Capitalism: Culture and Politics in Contemporary Activism. Pugwash Magazine.* http://216.122.222.203/pugwash/duncombe_2004_1.asp (accessed October 21, 2005).

Duncombe, Stephen. 2007. *Dream: Re-Imagining Progressive Politics in an Age of Fantasy.* New York: The New Press.

Dunlap, David. 2000. "In City Canyons, Slivers of Public Space Erode." *New York Times,* September 28.

Dunn, C., et al. 2004. "Arresting Protest—A Special Report of the NYCLU on New York City's Protest Policies at the February 15, 2003 Antiwar Demonstration in New York City." http://www.rncprotestrights.org/pdf/arrestingprotest. pdf (accessed August 26, 2006).

Dunn, Christopher, Eisenberg, Arthur, Lieberman, Donna, Silver, Alan, Vitale, Alex. 2003. Arresting Protest—A special report of the NYCLU on New York City's protest policies at the February 15, 2003 antiwar demonstration in New York City. http://www.nyclu.org/files/publications/nyclu_pub_arresting_pro-test.pdf (Accessed MONTH? 18, 2010).

Dwyer, Jim. 2005. "Videos Challenge Hundreds of Convention Arrests." *New York Times,* April 12, A1.

Dwyer, Jim. 2006a. "Aggressiveness of Bike Chasers Stirs Questions for the Police." *New York Times,* February 24, B1.

Dwyer, Jim. 2006b. "City Rebuffed in Trying to Bar Mass Bike Rides." *New York Times,* February 16.

Dwyer, Jim. 2006c. "Police Memos Say Arrest Tactics Calmed Protest." *New York Times,* March 17, B1.

Dwyer, Jim. 2008. "One Protest, 52 Arrests And a $2 Million Payout." *New York Times,* August 20, B1.

Earth Celebrations. 2004. "14th Annual Rites of Spring Procession." Flyer. May 22.

Ebert, Theresa. 1996. *Ludic Feminism and After.* Ann Arbor: University of Michigan Press.

Economopolis, Beka. 2003. "Class Post Miami." In possession of the author.

Ehrenreich, Barbara. 2007a. "Dance, Dance Revolution." *New York Times,* June 3, WK 14.

Ehrenreich, Barbara. 2007b. *Dancing in the Streets: A History or Collective Joy.* New York: Metropolitan Books.

Eliade, Mercea. 1958. *Rites and Symbols of Initiation.* Woodstock, CN: Spring.

El Diario. 1998a. "Community Group: 0, Real Estate Interests: 1." Editorial. July 23.

El Diario. 1998b. "SOLD—Amid Crickets and Police, CHARAS/El Bohio Cultural Center Is Auctioned Off to an Anonymous Buyer." July 21.

Ellis, Michael. 1998. "Republican Tax Photo Opportunity Backfires." *Reuters,* April 15.

Epstein, B. 1991. *Political Protest & Cultural Revolution.* Berkeley: University of California Press.

Epstein, Steven. 1998. *Impure Science.* Berkeley: University of California Press.

Eyerman, Ron and Jamison, Andrew. 1998. *Music and Social Movements.* Cambridge: Cambridge University Press.

Eyerman, Ron and Jamison, Andrew. 2003. "Movements and Cultural Change." In *The Social Movements Reader: Cases and Concepts.* Ed. Jeff Goodwin and James Jasper (pp. 367–69). Malden, MA: Blackwell Publishers.

FAIR. 2003. "NYC Newspapers Smear Activists Ahead of WEF Protests." Press Release. January 28.

FBI. 2001. "Statement for the Record, Louis J. Freeh, Director, Federal Bureau of Investigation, on the Threat of Terrorism to the United States before the United

States Senate Committees on Appropriations, Armed Services, and Select Committee on Intelligence." May 10. http://www.fbi.gov/congress/congress01/freeh051001.htm (accessed June 23, 2002).

Feinberg, David. 1994. *Queer and Loathing: Rants and Raves of a Raging AIDS Activist*. New York: Viking Press.

Ferguson, Sara. 1999. "Garden Wars—Mayor's Threat to Sell Off Community Plots Has Created Angry Revolt in Unlikely Places." http://www.pacificnews.org/jinn/stories/5.10/990511–gardens.html (accessed July 18, 2009).

Ferrell, Jeff. 2001. *Tearing Down the Streets: Adventures in Urban Anarchy*. New York: Palgrave/St. Martin's Press.

Fine, Gary Allen. 1995. "Public Narration and Group Culture: Discerning Discourse in Social Movements." In *Social Movements and Culture*. Ed. Hank Johnson and Bert Klandermans (pp. 127–43). Minneapolis: University of Minnesota Press.

Flaubert, Gustave. 1869/2008. *A Sentimental Education*. http://books.google.com/books?id=x4fX_9zMJ24C&printsec=frontcover&dq=flaubert+on+the+students+in+the+french+revolution&source=bl&ots=Ug8fUhSKgE&sig=WpiDe GakVQsFllEFoRGrBpGyKc0&hl=en&ei=HlHoS5GQE4K0lQfw6eSRAw&sa =X&oi=book_result&ct=result&resnum=7&ved=0CDAQ6AEwBg#v=onepage& q&f=false (accessed May 10, 2010).

Flaxman, Sheila G. (2000, September). Play an Endangered Species. *Instructor*, 110 (2), 39–41.

Flynn, Jennifer and Smith, Eustacia. 2004. Fed Up Queers. In *Thats Revolting: Queer Strategies for Resisting Assimilation*. Ed. Mattilda, AKA Matt Bernstein Sycamore. (p. 219–35). Brooklyn: Soft Skull Press.

Foote, N. N. 1954. "Sex as Play." *Social Problems* (April) 1 (4): 159–63.

Foucault, Michel. 1980. *Power/Knowledge. Selected Interviews and Writings 1972–77*. Ed. Colin Gordan. New York: Pantheon.

Foucault, Michel and Deleuze, Gilles. 1977. "Intellectuals in Power: A Conversation between Michel Foucault and Gilles Deleuze." In *Language, Counter-Memory, Practice, Selected Essays and Interviews*, by Michel Foucault. Ed. Donald Bouchard (pp. 205–18). Ithaca, NY: Cornell University Press.

Freedman, Gene and Combs, Jill. 1996. *Narrative Therapy: The Social Construction of Preferred Realities*. New York: WW Norton.

Freeman, Joshua. 1990. *Working Class New York*. New York: The Free Press.

Freud, Sigmund. 1914. "Remembering, Repeating, and Working Through." In *The Standard Edition of Freud's Psychological Works*, Vol. XII. Ed. Strachey, J. (pp. 147–56). London: Hogarth.

Freud, Sigmund. 1961. *Civilization and Its Discontents*. Standard Edition. Trans. and ed. James Stachey. New York: WW Norton.

Fuchs, Cynthia. 2004. "Freedom Dues: A Review of THE SPOOK WHO SAT BY THE DOOR." *PopMatters*, March 29. www.popmatters.com/film/reviews/s/spook-who-sat-by-the-door.shtml (accessed September 23, 2005).

Fuoss, Kirk. 1997. *Striking Performances/Performing Strikes*. Jackson: University of Mississippi Press.

Gaffney, Dennis. 2008. "Familiar Voice of Protest Keeps a Roadside Vigil." *New York Times*, June 22, 26.

Gallagher, Bob and Wilson, Alexander. 1987/2005. "Sex and the Politics of Identity: An Interview with Michel Foucault." In *Gay Spirit: Myth and Meaning*. Ed. Mark Thompson (pp. 25–35). Maple, NJ: Lethe Press.

Gamson, Joshua. 1991. "Silence, Death, and the Invisible Enemy: AIDS Activism and Social Movement "Newness." in *Ethnography Unbound: Power, Resistance in the Modern Metropolis* by Buraway et al. Berkeley: University of California Press. P. 43–9.

Gardiner, Michael. 1997. "Review of *Time of the Tribes*." Canadian Journal of Sociology 22 (4): 535–40.

Geertz, Clifford. 1973. *The Interpretation of Cultures*. New York: Basic Books.

Ghazvinian, John. 2000. "Dancing in the Streets: A Dash of Britain's Rave Culture Has Brought a New Style to Global Protests." *The Nation*, April 24, 23.

Ginsberg, Allen. 1965/2000. "Demonstration or Spectacle as Example, as Communication or How to Make a March Spectacle." In *Deliberate Prose: Selected Essays 1952–95*, Ed. Edward Sanders (pp. 9–13). New York: Perennial/HarperCollins.

Ginsberg, Allen. 1969/2001. "Interview with Paul Carroll." In *Spontaneous Mind. Selected Interviews 1958–1996*. Ed. David Carter (pp. 159–96). New York: Perennial/HarperCollins.

Goffman, Erving. 1959. *The Presentation of Self in Everyday Life*. New York: Anchor Books.

Goldberg, Ron. 2003. "Interview with Sara Schulman. ACT UP Oral History Project." October 25. http://www.actuporalhistory.org/ (accessed September 1, 2005).

Goldberg, RoseLee. 1988. *Performance Art*. New York: Harry N. Abrams., Inc.

Goldmark, Alex. 2011. Did You Know There Was a Pop-Up Kindergarten in Tahrir Square? *Good Culture*. Accessed 15 Feb 2011 from http://www.good.is/post/a-moving-letter-from-egypt-about-the-role-of-children-in-tahrir-square/

Gordan, Mel. 2000. *Voluptuous Panic: The Erotic World of the Weimar Cabaret*. Los Angeles, CA: Ferel House.

Goodwin, Jeff, Jasper, James M., and Polleta, Francesca. 2001. "Introduction: Why Emotions Matter." In *Passionate Politics: Emotions and Social Movements*. Ed. Jeff Goodwin, James Jasper, and Francesca Polleta (pp. 1–26). Chicago: University of Chicago Press.

Gould, Deborah, 2009. *Moving Politics: Emotion and ACT UP's Fight against AIDS*. Chicago: University of Chicago Press.

Graeber, David. 2002. "The New Anarchists." In *Movement of Movements: Is Another World Really Possible?* Ed. Tom Mertes (pp. 202–15). New York: Verso.

Graeber, David. 2004. "Lying in Wait." *The Nation*, April 1.

Graeber, David. 2009. *Direct Action: An Ethnography*. Oakland, CA: AK Press.

Gramsci, Antonio. 1971/1992. *Selections from the Prison Notebooks*. New York: International Publishers.

Grantham, Barry. 2001. *Playing Commedia: A Training Guide to Commedia Techniques*. Portsmouth, NH: Heinemann Drama.

Grele, Ronald. 1996. "Oral History: Method and Theory." *Radical History Review* 65 (Spring): 131–35.

Grote, Jason. 2001. "Bariojason." E-mail to RTS Listserv. April 14.

Grote, Jason. 2002. "KNEEL BEFORE BUSH!: The Origin of Students for an Undemocratic Society." In *From ACT UP to the WTO*. Ed. B. Shepard and R. Hayduk (pp. 254–59). New York: Verso.

Guttman, Cheryl. 2007. "A Brief History of the Yippies and An Interview with Dana Beal." In *Resistance: A Radical Social and Political History of the Lower East Side*. Ed. Clayton Patterson (pp. 507–20). New York: Seven Stories Press.

Haden-Guest, Anthony. 1997. *The Last Party*. New York: William Morrow.

Harvey, David. 1991. Afterward to Henri Lefebvre. In *The Production of Space*. Trans. by David Nicholson-Smith (pp. 425–34). Malden, MA: Blackwell.

Harvey, David. 2005. *A Brief History of Neoliberalism*. New York: Oxford University Press.

Henricks, Thomas. 2006. *Play Reconsidered: Sociological Perspectives on Human Expression*. Chicago: University of Illinois Press.

Herbst, M. 2002. "The Masquerade Project." *Journal of Aesthetics and Protest* 1 (1). http://www.journalofaestheticsandprotest.org/1/masquerade/index.html (accessed March 11, 2006).

Herodotus. 1942. *The Persian Wars*. New York: Random House.

Highleyman, Liz. 2004. "Emma Goldman." In *The Encyclopedia of Social Movements*. Ed. Immanuel Ness (Vol. 2, p. 501). New York: ME Sharpe.

Hitt, Jack. 2004. *"The Birth of the Meta-Protest Rally?"* New York Times Magazine, *March 28*.

Hoffman, Abbie. 1989. *The Best of Abbie Hoffman, Selections from Revolution for the Hell of It, Woodstock Nation, Steal This Book, and New Writings*. New York: Four Walls and Eight Windows.

Holland, Dorothy, Skinner, Debra, Lachicotte Jr., William, and Cain, Carole. 1998. *Identity and Agency in Cultural Worlds*. Cambridge, MA: Harvard University Press.

Hollyday, J. 1995. "Living the Word." *Sojourners Magazine*, September–October.

Holtzman, B., Hughes, C., and Van Meter, K. 2004. "Do It Yourself . . . and the Movement Beyond Capitalism." *Radical Society* 31 (1): 7–20.

Hopkins, David. 2004. *Dada and Surrealism: A Very Short Introduction*. New York: Oxford University Press.

Hudema, Mike. 2004. *An Action a Day Keeps Global Capitalism Away*. Toronto: Between the Lines.

Huizinga, Johan. 1950. *Homo Ludens: A Study of the Play Element in Culture*. Boston: Beacon.

Huizinga, Johan. 1950/2004. "The Nature and Significance of Play as a Cultural Phenomena." In *The Performance Studies Reader*. Ed. H. Bial (pp. 117–20). New York: Routledge.

Hume, Lynne and Mulcock, Jane. 2004. "Introduction: Awkward Spaces, Productive Places." In *Anthropologists in the Field: Cases in Participant Observation*. Ed. Lynne Hume and Jane Mulcock (pp. xiv–xxvii). New York: Columbia University Press.

Humm, Andy. 2008. "NYPD Buffers Pope from Protest." *Gay City News*, April 24. http://www.gaycitynews.com/site/news.cfm?newsid=19515872&BRD=2729&PAG=461&dept_id=569341&rfi=6 (accessed April 25, 2008).

Hungry March Band. n.d. "Urania Mylonas, HMB Twirl Like You Mean It." http://www.dvdojo.com/hmb/members/hmbplayas.php?member_id=126 (accessed November 1, 2005).

Hyde, Lewis. 1998. *Trickster Makes This World: Mischief, Myth, and Art*. New York: Farrar, Straus, and Giroux.

Illich, Ivan. 1973. *Tools for Conviviality*. London: Marion Boyers.

Isserman, Maurice. 1993. *If I Had a Hammer: The Death of the Old Left and the Birth of the New Left*. Chicago: University of Chicago Press.

Jameson, Jamie McCallum. 2006. "Re: [anarchisms] Can We Play?" E-mail to RTS Listserv. April 18.

Jasper, James. 1997. *The Art of Moral Protest: Culture, Biography, and Creativity in Social Movements*. Chicago: University of Chicago Press.

Jordan, John. 1998. "The Art of Necessity: The Subversive Imagination of Anti-Road Protest and Reclaim the Streets." In *DiY Culture: Party and Protest in Nineties Britain*. Ed. G. McKay (pp. 129–51). London: Verso.

Jordan, John. 2003. "Deserting the Art Bunker." http://amsterdam.nettime.org/Lists-Archives/nettime-l-0304/msg00016.html (accessed October 1, 2005).

Jung, Carl. 1923. *Psychological Types*. Trans. H. Godwyn Baynes. Princeton, NJ: Princeton University Press.

Juris, Jeffrey. 2007. "Practicing Militant Ethnography." In *Constituent Imagination: Militant Investigations//Collective Theorization in the Global Justice Movement*. Ed. S. Shukaitis and D. Graeber (pp. 164–78). Oakland, CA: AK Press.

Juris, Jeffrey. 2008. *Networking Futures: The Movements Against Corporate Globalization*. Durham, NC: Duke University Press.

Kaes, Anton, Jay, Martin, and Deiendberg, Edward. 1994. *The Weimar Sourcebook*. Berkeley: University of California Press.

Kantrowitz, Arnie. 1977/1996. *Under the Rainbow: Growing Up Gay*. New York: St. Martin's Press.

Karmazin, Eugene. 2005. "Riding for Critical Mass." *Guernica: A Magazine of Art and Politics*. May. http://www.guernicamag.com/features/riding_with_critical_mass/index.php (accessed May 25, 2005).

Katsiaficas, George. 2002. "Eros and the Battle of Seattle." www.eroseffect.com (accessed January 1, 2009).

Kaufman, David. 2002. *Ridiculous: The Theatrical Life and Times of Charles Ludlam*. Applause. New York: New York.

Kauffman, L.A. 2000. "The New Unrest." *The Free Radical* 1 (February). http://www.free-radical.org/issue1.shtml (accessed September 23, 2003).

Kauffman, L.A. 2001. "Text of FBI Report Calling RTS Terrorist." E-mail to RTS Listserv. June 28.

Kauffman, L.A. 2004. "A Short, Personal History of the Global Justice Movement." In *Confronting Capitalism: Dispatches from a Global Movement*. Ed. Eddie Yuen, Daniel Burton-Rose, and George Katsiaficas (pp. 375–88). New York: Soft Skull Press.

Kifner, John. 1999. "Giuliani's Hunt for Red Menaces, From Transit Union to Gardeners, May Sees Marx's Shadow." *New York Times*, December 20, B3.

Klein, Naomi. 2000. Remarks during the Panel: "Can Movement and Party Challengers Work Together?" at "Independent Politics in a Global World Conference," at the CUNY Graduate Center, NY, October 7.

Klein, Naomi. 2004. "Reclaiming the Commons." In *Movement of Movements*. Ed. Tom Mertes (pp. 219–29). New York: Verso.

Kohut, Heinz. 1959/1978. "Introspection, Empathy and Psychoanalysis: An Examination between Mode of Observation and Theory." In *The Search for the Self: Selected Writings of Heinz Kohut, 1950–1978*. Ed. P. Ornstein (pp. 205–32). New York: International Universities Press.

Lantos, Barbara. 1943. "Work and the Instincts." *International Journal of Psychoanalysis* 24: 114–19.

Lasn, k. 1999. *Culture Jam*. New York: Harper Paperbacks.

Laursen, Eric. 2006. "Re: [dan] NYT: Police Memos Say Arrest Tactics Calmed Protest(re:World Economic Forum)." E-mail to RTS Listserv. March 17.

Le Bon, Gustave. 1896. *The Crowd: A Study of the Popular Mind*. New York: Macmillan.

Lear, J. 1998. *Open Minded: Working Out the Logic of the Soul*. Cambridge: Harvard University Press.

Lederman, R. 2001. "Giuliani's 'Jerks, Idiots, Morons.'" *Newsday*, June 29.

Lee, Jennifer. 2009. "For a Latino Group, A Legacy Continues." *New York Times*, August 25, A16.

Lefebvre, Henri. 1947/1991. *Critique of Everyday Life*. Vol. 1. Trans. John Moore. New York: Verso.

Lefebvre, Henri. 1974/1991. *The Production of Space*. Trans. Donald Nicholson-Smith. Malden, MA: Blackwell.

Lichterman, Paul. 2002. "Seeing Structure Happen: Theory Driven Participant Observation." In *Methods of Social Movement Research*. Ed. B.K. Andermand and S. Staggerborg. Minneapolis: University of Minnesota Press.

Linn, Susan. 2008. *The Case for Make Believe: Saving Play in a Commercialized World*. New York: The New Press.

Loew, Karen. 2005. "What's the Point of Protest? After Two Years of Massive Public Demonstrations, the War's Still On and Bush Will Be Inaugurated Again."

http://www.commondreams.org/views05/0118–30.htm (accessed January 18, 2001).

Logan, John R. and Molotch, Harvey L. 1987. *Urban Fortunes: The Political Economy of Place*. Berkeley: University of California Press.

Longman, Jore. 2010. "Youth Soccer League Fights AIDS with Soccer." *New York Times*, June 10. http://www.nytimes.com/2010/06/11/sports/soccer/11aids.html?emc=eta1 (accessed June 10, 2010).

Lukas, Ian. 1998. *Outrage!: An Oral History*. London: Cassell.

M26. n.d. "NYC Attempts to Jail Non-Violent Protesters." http://www.m26.org/index.php?name=homepage (accessed April 24, 2006).

Maffesoli, Michael. 1993. *The Shadow of Dionysus: A Contribution to the Sociology of Orgy*. Trans. C. Linse and M.K. Palmquist. Albany: State University of New York Press.

Maffesoli, Michel. 1996. *Time of the Tribes: The Decline of Individualism in Mass Society*. Thousand Oaks, CA: Sage Press.

Mailer, Norman. 1986. *Miami and the Siege of Chicago: An Informal History of the Republican and Democratic Conventions of 1968*. New York: Plume.

Mains, Geoff. 1984/2002. *Urban Aboriginals: A Celebration of Leathersexuality*. 20th Anniversary Issue. Los Angeles, CA: Deadalous Publishing Company.

Marcos, Subcomandante Insurgente. 2001. *Our Word is Our Weapon. Selected Writings*. New York: Seven Stories Press.

Marcos, Subcomandante Insurgente. 2004. "The Hourglass of the Zapatista. Interviewed by Gabriel Garcia Marquez and Roberto Pombo." In *Movement of Movements. Is Another World Really Possible?* Ed. Tom Mertes (pp. 3–15). New York: Verso.

Marcus, Greil. 1989. *Lipstick Traces: A Secret History of the Twentieth Century*. Cambridge, MA: Harvard University Press.

Marcuse, Herbert. 1955. *Eros and Civilization: A Philosophical Inquiry into Freud*. New York: A Vintage Book.

Marcuse, Herbert. 1964. *One Dimensional Man: Studies in the Ideology of Advanced Industrial Society*. Boston: Beacon Press.

Marcuse, Herbert. 1969. *An Essay on Liberation*. Boston: Beacon Press.

Marcuse, Herbert. 1972. *Counterrevolution and Revolt*. Boston: Beacon Press.

Marcuse, Herbert. 1978. *The Aesthetic Dimension: Toward a Critique of Marxist Aesthetics*. Boston: Beacon Press.

Martin, Douglas. 2006. "tew Albert, 66, Dies; Used Laughter to Protest a War." *New York Times*, February 1, A23.

Martin, Jay. 1973. *The Dialectical Imagination*. New York: Little Brown.

Martinez, Miranda. 2009. "Attack of the Butterfly Spirits." *Social Movement Studies* 8 (4): 323–40.

Mattson, Kevin and Duncombe, Stephen. 1992. "Public Space, Private Place: The Contested Terrain of Thompkins Square Park." *Berkeley Journal of Sociology* 37:129–61.

McAdam, Doug. 1988. *Freedom Summer*. New York: Oxford University Press.

McAdam, Doug. 1996. "The Framing Function of Movement Tactics." In *Comparative Perspectives on Social Movements*. Ed. Doug McAdam, John McCarthy, and Mayer Zald (pp. 338–56). Cambridge: Cambridge University Press.

McAdam, Doug, McCarthy, John D., and Zald, Mayer N. 1988. "Social Movements." In *Handbook of Sociology*. Ed. N.J. Smelser (pp. 695–730). Newbury Park, CA: Sage Press.

McAdams, Dan. 1985. *Power, Intimacy, and the Life Story*. Homewood, IL: Dorsey Press.

McCarthy, J. and Zald, M.N. 1973. *The Trend of Social Movements in America*. Morristown, NJ: General Learning.

McClish, Carmen. 2009. "Activism Based in Embarrassment: The Anti-Consumption Spirituality of the Reverend Billy." *Liminalities: A Journal of Performance Studies* 5(2): 1–20. http://liminalities.net/5-2/mcclish.pdf (accessed October 20, 2010).

McCracken, Grant. 1988. *The Long Interview*. Newbury Park, CA: Sage Press.

McKay, George. 1998. "Notes Toward an Intro." In *DiY Culture: Party and Protest in Nineties Britain*. Ed. George McKay (pp. 1–53). London: Verso.

McWilliams, Nancy. 2004. *Psychoanalytic Psychotherapy: A Practitioner's Guide*. New York: The Guilford Press.

Media Matters. 2005. "*NY Times* Downplayed Powell's Responsibility for False Weapons Claims in U.N. Address." October 5. http://mediamatters.org/items/200510270014 (accessed April 24, 2006).

Mele, Christopher. 2000. *Selling the Lower East Side*. Minneapolis: Minnesota University Press.

Melendez, M., Torres, J., and Newfeild, J. 2003. *We Took the Streets: Fighting For Latino Rights with the Young Lords*. New York: St. Martin's Press.

Merrifield, Andy. 2002. *Metromarxism: A Marxist Tale of the City*. New York: Routledge.

Mertes, Tom, ed. 2003. *The Movement of Movements: Is Another World Really Possible?* London and New York: Verso.

Mink, Janis. 2006. *Duchamp*. Hong Kong: Taschen.

Mitchell, Tony. 1999. *Dario Fo: People's Court Jester*. London: Methuen.

Molesworth, Helen. 1998. "Work Avoidance: The Everyday Life of Marcel Duchamp's Readymades." *Art Journal* 57 (Winter): 50–61. http://www.accessmylibrary.com/article-1G1-53747210/work-avoidance-everyday-life.html (accessed October 16, 2010)

Moore, Patrick. 2004. *Beyond Shame: Reclaiming the Abandoned History of Radical Gay Sexuality*. Boston: Beacon.

Moshenberg, Simon. 2001. "Subject: March 23: JOIN THE ANTI-DISPLACEMENT CIRKUS OF THE STREETS!" E-mail.

Moynihan, Colin. 1999. "Still Mourning, Latino Group Loses 2 Treasured Murals." *New York Times*, November 21, 8.

Moynihan, Colin. 2001. "Yippie Central." *New York Times*, April 29, C1.

Moynihan, Colin. 2008. "Dozens Detained ahead of Convention." *New York Times*, August 30.

Myerhoff, Barbera and Ruby, Jay. 1982/1992. "A Crack in the Mirror: Reflective Perspectives Anthropology." In *Remembered Lives: The Work of Ritual, Storytelling, and Growing Older*. Ed. Mark Kaminsky (pp. 307–40). Ann Arbor: University of Michigan Press.

Mylonas, Urania. n.d. "NOLA Memories. A Gathering of the Tribes." http://www.tribes.org/cgi-bin/form.pl?karticle=657 (accessed October 1, 2005).

Nardi, Peter. 2006. "Sociology at Play, Or Truth in the Pleasant Disguise of Illusion." *Sociological Perspectives* 49 (3): 285–95.

Nelson, J.A. 2001. "Feminism, Nationalism, and the Politics of Reproduction among New York City's Young Lords." *Journal of Women's History* 13 (1):157–80.

Nepstad, Sharon Erickson. 2002. "Creating Transnational Solidarity: The Use of Narrative in the US-Central America Peace Movement." In *Globalization and Resistance: Transnational Dimensions of Social Movements*. Ed. J. Smith and H. Johnston (pp. 133–52). Lanham, MD: Roman and Littlefield Publishers.

Ness, Immanuel. 2002. "Community Labor Alliances." In *From ACT UP to the WTO*. Ed. B. Shepard and R. Hayduk (pp. 256–73). New York Verso.

Neumann, Osha. 2008. *Up Against the Wall Motherf**r: A Memoir of the 1960's with Notes for the Next Time*. New York: Seven Stories Press.

Neumann, Rachel. 2000. "A Place for Rage." *Dissent* (Spring): 89–92.

Newman, Saul. 2004. *I Am Not a Man, I am Dynamite! Frederich Nietzche and the Anarchist Tradition.* Edited by John Moore with Spencer Sunshine. Brooklyn, NY: Autonomedia.

Newton, E. 1972. *Mother Camp: Female Impersonators in America.* Chicago: University of Chicago Press.

Nietzsche, Friedrich. 1967. *The Birth of Tragedy and The Case of Wagner.* Translated with Commentary by Walter Kauffman. New York: Vintage.

notbored. 1999. "Reclaim The Streets NYC." http://www.notbored.org/rts.html (accessed November 1, 2005).

Notes from Nowhere. 2003. *We Are Everywhere: The Irresistible Rise of Global Anti-Capitalism.* London and New York: Verso.

Ollman, Bertell. 2003. *Dance of the Dialectic.* Chicago: University of Chicago Press.

Ollman. Bertell. 2005. "The Philosophy of Basketball and its Relation to Capitalism, Democracy, and Socialism." *Logos* 4 (1). www.logosjournal.com (accessed March 17, 2006).

Ornstein, Claudia. 1998. *Festive Revolutions.* Jackson: University of Mississippi Press.

Parascandola, Rocco. 2010. "NYPD Intel Division Not Going Soft on Public Events like Pillow Fights." *New York Daily News,* April 20. http://www.nydailynews.com/news/2010/04/20/2010–04–20_nypd_intel_division_not_going_soft_on_public_events_like_pillow_fights.html#ixzz0leaabRoe (accessed April 20, 2010).

Patterson, Clayton, ed. 2007. *Resistance: A Radical Social and Political History of the Lower East Side.* New York: Seven Stories Press.

Patterson, Clayton and Rensaa, Elsa. 2009. "Worst Court Transcript: 'Crickett Justice.'" In *The Worst Book I Ever Read.* Ed. the Unbearables (pp. 267–77). New York. Unbearables Books/Autonomedia.

Patton, Michael. 2002. *Qualitative Research & Evaluation Methods.* 3rd edition. Thousand Oaks, CA: Sage Publications.

Payne, C. 1995. *I've Got the Light of Freedom: The Organizing Tradition and the Mississippi Freedom Struggle.* Berkelely, CA: University of California Press.

Perez, Richie. 2000. "A Young Lord Remembers. Boricua Tributes." http://www.virtualboricua.org/Docs/perez_00.htm (accessed January 29, 2006).

Piaget, Jean. 1962. *Play, Dreams and Imitation in Childhood.* New York: WW Norton.

Pietri, Pedro. 1974. *Puerto Rican Obituary.* New York: Monthly Review Press.

Piven, Frances Fox. 2008. "Commentary." Presented at the New Spatial Scales of Democracy and Resistance, CUNY Graduate Center, May 4.

Plant, Sadie. 1992. *The Most Radical Gesture: The Situationist International in a Postmodern Age.* New York: Routledge.

Polletta, Francesca. 2002. *Freedom Is an Endless Meeting: Democracy and American Social Movements.* Chicago: University of Chicago Press.

Polletta, Francesca. 2006. *It Was like a Fever: Storytelling in Protest and Politics.* Chicago: University of Chicago Press.

Powell, Michael. 2002. "Domestic Spying Pressed Big-City Police Seek to Ease Limits Imposed After Abuses Decades Ago." *Washington Post,* November 29.

Pranksters. 1987. *Pranks! Research #11.* San Francisco: Last Gasp of San Francisco.

Rabble Staff. 2001. "Free Jaggi Singh." May 4. http://www.rabble.ca/news/free-jaggi-singh (accessed June 8, 2010).

Rashbaum, William K. 2003a. "Police Stop Collecting Data on Protestor's Politics." *New York Times,* April 11, D1.

Rashbaum, William K. 2003b. "Police Try to Defend Practice of Debriefing Demonstrators." *New York Times,* April 11, D2.

Reed, T.V. 2005. *The Art of Protest.* Minneapolis: University of Minnesota Press.

Reel, Monte and Fernandez, Manny. 2002. "100,000 Rally, March against War in Iraq." *Washington Post*, October 17, A01.

Reich, Robert. 2006. "The Poor Get Poorer." *New York Times Book Review*, April 2, 21.

Reich, Wilhelm. 1970. *The Mass Psychology of Fascism*. New York: Farrar, Straus, and Giroux.

Rein, L. 1999. "Gardeners Plant Selves in Street." *New York Daily News*, May 6, 77.

Renfrew, Alastair. 1997. The Carnival without Laughter. In *Face to Face: Bakhtin in Russia and the West*. Eds. Adlam, Carol, Pinfield, Leslie, Makhlin, Vitalii, and Falconer, Rachel (p. 185–95). Sheffield England: Sheffield Academic Press.

Reverend Billy. 2009. "The Yes Men and Reverend Billy Levitate an Immigrant Detention Center." http://www.youtube.com/watch?v=UsnehHqLMik (accessed October 18, 2009).

Rosemont, Franklin and Radcliffe, Charles, eds. 2005. *Dancin' in the Streets!* Chicago: Charles H. Kerr Publishing Company.

Rosemont, Penelope. 2002. "Toward a Politics of the Pleasure Principle." In *Surrealist Subversions*. Ed. Ron Sakolsky (pp. 395–96). Brooklyn, NY: Autonomedia.

Rosenbaum, David. 2001. "Thousands Speak Out on Election and Other Issues." *New York Times*, January 21, 17.

Russo, Vito. 1988. "Why We Fight." www.actupny.org/documents/whfight.html (accessed January 18, 2010).

Sakolsky, Ron, ed. 2002. Surrealist Subversions. Oakland, CA: AK Press.

Sanders, Ed. 2004. *Tales of Beatnik Glory*. New York: Da Capo Press.

Schalk, David. 2000. "A Historian's Engagement." *Peace and Change: A Journal of Peace Studies* 25 (4): 297–515.

Schechner, Richard. 2002. *Performance Studies: An Introduction*. New York: Routledge.

Schechter, Joel. 2001. *The Pickle Clowns*. Edwardsville: Southern Illinois University Press.

Schlosser, Eric. 2003. *Reefer Madness: Sex, Drugs, and Cheap Labor in the American Black Market*. New York: [PUBLISHER NAME?]

Sedgwick, Eve Kosofsky. 1997. "Paranoid Reading and Reparative Reading." In *Novel Gazing: Queer Reading in Fiction*. Ed. E.K. Sedgwick (pp. 1–40). Durham, NC: Duke University Press.

Seeger, Pete. 1963. *We Shall Overcome: The Complete Carnegie Hall Concert, June 8, 1963*. Sony.

Shepard, Benjamin. 1997. *White Nights and Ascending Shadows: An Oral History of the San Francisco AIDS Epidemic*. London: Cassell Press.

Shepard, Benjamin. 2003. "Absurd Responses Versus Earnest Politics." *Journal of Aesthetics and Protest* 1 (2): 95–115.

Shepard, Benjamin. 2004. "Playin' It Straight: Fighting to Turn NYC into a Patriot Act Free Zone." *Journal of Aesthetics and Protest* 1 (3): 62–73.

Shepard, Benjamin. 2005. "Creative Direct Action in the Era of the Patriot Act: Arrested for Stickerring, Biking and Other Misadventures." *Counterpunch*, June 18–19. http://www.counterpunch.org/shepard06182005.html (accessed September 1, 2008).

Shepard, Benjamin. 2005. Play, Creativity, and the New Community Organizing. *Journal of Progressive Human Services* 16 (2): 47–69.

Shepard, B. 2007. "From Connection to Separation (and Back): Social Movements and Mayday." *Working USA: The Journal of Labor and Society* 10:357–66.

Shepard, B. 2008. "On Challenging Authority: An Oral History Interview with Frances Fox Piven." *Reflections: Narratives of Professional Helping* 14 (2): 3–15.

Shepard, B. 2009. *Queer Political Performance and Protest: Play, Pleasure, and Social Movement*. New York: Routledge.

Shepard, B. 2010. "Play and World Making: From Gay Liberation to DIY Community Building." In *The Hidden Seventies Confidential: Histories of Radicalism.* Ed. Dan Berger (pp. 177–94). New Brunswick, NJ: Rutgers University Press.

Shepard, Benjamin and Hayduk, Ron. Eds. 2002. *From ACT UP to the WTO: Urban Protest and Community Building in the Era of Globalization.* New York: Verso.

Shepard, Benjamin and Moore, Kelly. 2002. "Reclaim the Streets for a World without Cars." In *Critical Mass: Bicyclings's Defiant Celebration.* Ed. Chris Carlsson (Full draft page #'s p. 195–203). Oakland, CA: AK Press

Shepard, Benjamin and Smithsimon, Greg. 2011. *The Beach beneath the Streets: Contesting New York City's Public Spaces.* New York: SUNY Press.

Simon, Daniel. 1989. "Preface." In *The Best of Abbie Hoffman*, by Abbie Hoffman. New York: Four Walls and Eight Windows.

Simon, Herbert. 1957. *Administrative Behavior: A Study of Decision-Making Processes in Administrative Organization.* 2nd Edition. New York: Macmillan Co.

Simmonds, Alecia. 2007. The Humorless State: Power hates the laughter of the carnival. *Arena Magazine* (August–September):12–14.

Sites, William. 2003. *Remaking New York: Primitive Globalization and the Politics of Urban Community.* Minneapolis: University of Minnesota Press.

Situationist International. 1958. "Contribution to a Situationist Definition of Play." *Situationist International* 1 (June). Trans. Reuben Keehan. http://www.cddc.vt.edu/sionline/si/play.html (accessed October 5, 2005).

Slackman, Michael and Cardwell, Diane. 2004. "Anger of Demonstrations Gets Little Media Attention." *New York Times*, September 2.

Smith, Neil. 1996. *The New Urban Frontier: Gentrification and the Revanchist City.* New York: Routledge.

Snow, David and Trom, Danny. 2002. "The Case Study of Social Movements." In *Methods of Social Movement Research.* Ed. Bert Lkandermans and Suzanne Staggenborg (pp. 146–72). Minneapolis: University of Minnesota Press.

Solnit, David, ed. 2004. *Globalize Liberation: How to Uproot the System and Build a Better World.* San Francisco: City Lights Press.

Solnit, David. 2005. *The New Face of the Global Justice Movement: Taco Bell Boycott Victory—A Model of Strategic Organizing. An interview with the Coalition of Immokalee Workers. t r u t h o u t | Perspective*, Wednesday 24 August 2005. http://www.truth-out.org/article/david-solnit-taco-bell-boycott-victory (accessed October 21, 2010).

Solnit, Rebecca. 2005a. "Acts of Hope: Challenging Empire on the World Stage." *Women's World.* http://www.wworld.org/crisis/crisis.asp?ID=444 (accessed January 12, 2009).

Solnit, Rebecca. 2005b. *Hope in the Dark: Untold Histories, Wild Possibilities.* New York: Nation Books.

Somers, Margaret. 1994. "The Narrative Construction of Identity: A Relational and Network Approach." *Theory and Society* 23:605–49.

Sontag, Susan. 1964/2001. "Notes on Camp." In *Come Out Fighting: A Century of Essential Writing on Gay & Lesbian Liberation.* Ed. Chris Bull (pp. 52–66). New York: thunder's mouth press/nation books.

Spitzer, Elliot. 2002. "Memorandum of Agreement between Attorney General and Community Gardeners." http://www.oag.state.ny.us/environment/community_gardens_agreement.pdf Summary of Community Gardens Agreement. http://www.oag.state.ny.us/environment/community_gardens_sum.html (accessed July 1, 2010).

Stallman, Honorable Michael D. 2006. "Supreme Court of the State of New York. The City of New York against Times Up, Inc. Index # 400891/05 Decision and Order." http://times-up.org/uploads/pdf/2006–02–14–decision.pdf (accessed January 12, 2009).

Starhawk. 2008. "RNC2Raid on the Convergence Center. 31 August." http://www.opednews.com/articles/RNC2-Raid-on-the-Convergen-by-Starhawk-080831-765.html (accessed September 1, 2008).

Stiglitz, Joseph. 2002. *Globalization and Its Discontents*. New York: WW Norton.

Stout, Hillary. 2011. The Movement to Restore Children's Play Gains Momentum. *New York Times*, 5 January. Accessed 13 January 2011 from http://www.nytimes.com/2011/01/06/garden/06play.html?_r=1

Strauss, Anselm and Corbin, Juliet. 1990. *Basics of Qualitative Research: Grounded Theory Procedures and Techniques*. Newbury Park, CA: Sage Press.

Sunshine, Spencer. 2003. "On the Disenchantment Thesis." Unpublished manuscript.

Sutton-Smith, Brian. 1997/2004. "The Ambiguity of Play." in *The Performance Studies Reader*. Ed. H. Bial (pp. 132–38). New York: Routledge.

Taibbi, Matt. 2004. "Because the protests of the last week in New York were more than a silly, off-key exercise in irrelevant chest-puffing. It was a colossal waste of political energy," *New York Press*, September 13. Accessed November 1, 2007 from http://www.nypress.com/17/36/news&columns/Taibbi2.cfm?CFID=6575263&CFTOKEN=90763892.

Takemoto, Tina. 2003. "The Melancholia of AIDS: Interview with Douglas Crimp." *Art Journal* (Winter). http://findarticles.com/p/articles/mi_m0425/is_4_62/ai_1116558. . . (accessed October 21, 2010).

Tarrow, 1998. *Power in the Movement: Social Movements and Contentious Politics*. 2nd Edition. Cambridge, UK: Cambridge University Press.

Tatchell, Peter. 2000. "Protest as Performance." http://www.petertatchell.net/OutRage/protestasperformance.htm (accessed August 15, 2008).

Tawney, R.H. 1937. *Religion and the Rise of Capitalism*. New York: The New American Library.

Tedlock, Barbara. 1991. "From Participant Observation to Observation of Participation: the Emergence of Narrative Ethnography." *Journal of Anthropological Research* 47:69–94.

Tent, Pam. 2004. *Midnight at the Palace: My Life as a Fabulous Cockette*. Los Angeles: Alyson Books.

Thompson, Nato and Sholette, Gregory, eds. 2004. *The Interventionists: User's Guide to Creative Disruption of Everyday Life*. Boston: Mass MOCA.

Tobocman, Seth. 1999. *War in the Neighborhood*. Brooklyn, NY: Autonomedia.

Turner, Victor. 1969. *The Ritual Process: Structure and Anti-Structure*. Chicago: Aldine Publishing Company.

Turner, Victor. 1982. *From Ritual to Theatre: The Human Seriousness of Play*. New York: Performing Arts Publications.

Tzara, Tristan. 1918. "DADA, the DADA Manifesto." http://www.ralphmag.org/AR/dada.html (accessed October 9, 2005).

Vaneigem, Raoul. 1967/2003. *The Revolution of Everyday Life*. London: Rebel Press.

Varon, Jeremy. 2004. *Bringing the War Home*. Berkeley: University of California Press.

Vega, M. 1998. "City Sells 'Charas/El Bohio' Cultural Center." *El Diario*, July 21.

Waldman, A. 1998. "Cricket Invaders Turn an Auction into 'Madness.'" *New York Times*, July 21.

Weber, Max. 1930/1992. *The Protestant Ethic and the Spirit of Capitalism*. New York: Routledge.

Weber, Max. 1946/1968. *Economy and Society, Volumes 1 and 2*. Ed. G. Roth and C. Wittich. Berkeley and Los Angeles: University of California Press.

Weissberg, Robert. 2005. *The Limits of Civic Activism: Cautionary Tales on the Use of Politics*. New Brunswick, NJ: Transaction Publishers.

Weissman, Harold. 1990. *Serious Play: Creativity and Innovation in Social Work.* Silver Spring, MD: NASW Press.

Wenner, Melinda. 2009. "The Serious Need for Play." *Scientific American*, January 28. http://www.sciam.com/article.cfm?id=the-serious-need-for-play (accessed February 20, 2009).

Wheeler, Jacob. 2004. "United for Peace and Justice, Today's Protestors are Mature, Artful, and Productive." *Utne.com* (August). http://www.utne.com/web_special/web_specials_2004–08/articles/11368–1.html (accessed August 29, 2004).

william, e. 2000. "A16 SUCCESS!" E-mail to RTS Listserv. April 17.

Williams, Timothy. 2008. "Long-Tenured Drummers, Guardians of a Park, Draw New Neighbor's Ire." *New York Times*, July 6, 23.

Wilson, R. Rawdon. 1990. *In Palamedes' Shadow: Explorations in Play, Game and Narrative Theory.* Boston: Northeastern University Press.

Winnicott, D.W. 1971. *Playing and Reality.* Philadelphia: Routledge.

Wood, L.J. and Moore, K. 2002. "Target Practice." In *From ACT UP to the WTO.* Ed. B. Shepard and R. Hayduk (pp. 21–34). New York: Verso.

Yin, Robert K. 1994. *Case Study Research: Design and Methods.* Thousand Oaks, CA: Sage Press.

Yuen, Eddie. 2004. "Introduction." In *Confronting Capitalism: Dispatches from a Global Movement.* Ed. Eddie Yuen, Daniel Burton-Rose, and George Katsiaficas (pp. vii–xxix). New York: Soft Skull Press.

Young Lords Party and Abramson, Michael. (1971). *Palante: Young Lords Party.* New York: McGraw-Hill Book Company.

Zernike, Kate. 2002. "Rally in Washington Is Said to Invigorate the Antiwar Movement." *New York Times*, October 30, A1.

Zinn, Howard. 2002. *You Can't Be Neutral on a Fast Moving Train: A Personal History of Our Times.* Boston: Beacon Press.

About the Author

Benjamin Shepard, PhD, is an Assistant Professor of Human Service at New York School of Technology/City University of New York. He is the author/editor of six books including *Queer Politics and Political Performance: Play, Pleasure, and Social Movement, White Nights and Ascending Shadows: An Oral History of the San Francisco AIDS Epidemic*, and *From ACT UP to the WTO: Urban Protest and Community Building in the Era of Globalization* (coedited with Ron Hayduk). His upcoming works include: *Community Projects as Social Activism: From Direct Action to Direct Services*, and *The Beach Beneath the Streets: Contesting New York's Public Space* (coauthored with Greg Smithsimon). Further, his writing has appeared in anthologies including: *Nobody Passes, That's Revolting: Queer Strategies for Resisting Assimilation, Democracy's Moment: Renewing Democracy for the 21st Century*, and *Teamsters and Turtles: Leftist Movements Today and Tomorrow*, and journals including: *Working USA, Radical Society, Lambda Book Review, Monthly Review, Sexualities, Journal of Progressive Human Services, Antioch Review, Monthly Review*, and *Drain*. He has done organizing work with ACT UP, SexPanic!, Reclaim the Streets New York, Time's Up!, CIRCA, CitiWide Harm Reduction, Housing Works, and the More Gardens! coalition. To reach him contact: http://www.benjaminheimshepard.com/.

Index